Current Medicine 3

Royal College of Physicians of Edinburgh

Current Medicine 3
Royal College of Physicians of
Edinburgh

Edited by

David H. Lawson MD FRCP (Ed) FRCP (Glas)
Consultant Physician at Glasgow Royal Infirmary;
Visiting Professor at School of Pharmacy,
Strathclyde University, Glasgow, UK

Foreword by
John Richmond MD PRCP (Ed) FRCP
President, Royal College of Physicians. Edinburgh, UK

CHURCHILL LIVINGSTONE
EDINBURGH LONDON MELBOURNE NEW YORK AND TOKYO 1991

CHURCHILL LIVINGSTONE
Medical Division of Longman Group UK Limited

Distributed in the United States of America by Churchill
Livingstone Inc., 1560 Broadway, New York, NY
10036, and by associated companies, branches and
representatives throughout the world.

First published 1991

ISBN 0-443-04598-4

British Library Cataloguing in Publication Data
Current medicine: 3. – (Current medicine)
  I. Lawson, David H. II. Series
  615

  ISBN 0-443-04598-4

Library of Congress Cataloging in Publication Data
Current medicine 3: Royal College of Physicians of
  Edinburgh/edited by David H. Lawson; foreword by
  John Richmond.
      p.   cm.
  Includes index.
  ISBN 0-443-04598-4
  1. Internal medicine. I. Lawson, David H. II. Royal
College of Physicians of Edinburgh. III. Title: Current
medicine three.
  [DNLM: 1. Clinical Medicine.   WB 100 C9768]
RC46.C96 1991
616—dc20
DNLM/DLC
for Library of Congress   91–15711
                              CIP

Printed and bound in Great Britain by
Butler & Tanner Ltd, Frome and London

Foreword

It gives me great pleasure to introduce Current Medicine 3 which presents a further series of present day topics. These publications were started primarily for the College's own Fellows and Members, but they have appealed to a wider readership, not only to physicians in training, but also to established physicians who know that the good doctor has to be committed to continuing medical education.

The 'Best management' articles have proved very popular in the two previous editions and have been continued. They give a common sense approach to common problems and perhaps with current emphasis on clinical audit there will be increasing scope for consensus papers of this kind.

Again there is tribute to senior Scottish physicians who taught and influenced the present generation and stamped us by their teaching, with the foundations of todays 'current medicine'.

The College is extremely grateful, once more, to Dr David Lawson for gathering together a group of excellent contributors, undertaking the burden of editorship and bringing this endeavour to successful fruition.

Edinburgh, 1991   J.R.

Preface

The task facing the physician in the latter part of the 20th century is a daunting one. Not only has he to keep abreast of developments in his own field, but he has also to be aware of the constant march of science and the effect this is likely to have on his chosen speciality in the future. Physicians must resist the temptation to over-specialize—patients rarely present neat problems which are confined to highly-specialist areas. The complete physician must therefore be aware of advances in other fields and sensitive to his patients' needs in areas other than his own.

The increase in resources directed towards prevention is one of the characteristic features of medicine in the last decade. This is most marked in the cardiovascular field and presents a major challenge to clinicians—to select carefully both those individuals who should be screened for 'risk factors' and the proportion of such individuals who should be exposed to long-term treatment to correct the abnormal risk factor. There is a danger of creating more dis-ease than benefit in the general population if this approach is adopted uncritically.

This third volume of Current Medicine aims to address some aspects of these problems. Topics from programmes to reduce the burden of cardiovascular disease, through the difficult area of prevention, diagnosis and management of thromboembolic disease to the advancing fronts of bone marrow transplantation are addressed in detail. With the increase in international travel, the spectre of resistant malaria should always be kept in mind to explain obscure pyrexias. We therefore present an up to date review of this topic. Newer diseases in other species such as bovine spongiform encephalopathy (BSE) are reviewed, as are advances in membrane technology insofar as this affects the physician.

A regular feature of this series is the section dealing with an individual physician's personal approach to a common clinical problem. This popular section is likely to be of particular value to aspiring and newly qualified members of the College as they begin to build up their own personal clinical experience of common conditions.

The dramatic advances in the management of gallbladder disease are discussed by Professors Bouchier and Cuschieri, who outline the major changes which have occurred in this field over the last generation.

Finally, I make no apology for including a historical section in this book on Current Medicine. On this occasion I have asked two eminent cardiologists to look at the life and times of their distinguished predecessors, Dr A. Rae Gilchrist—former President of the Royal College of Physicians of Edinburgh, and Dr J. H. Wright—former President of the Royal College of Physicians and Surgeons of Glasgow. The younger generation has much to learn from the careers and exploits of its predecessors. The depth and breadth of knowledge shown by these great Scottish physicians are a challenge to their successors.

No book can be written without the enthusiastic collaboration of a number of people. My thanks are due to our contributors, who have adhered to tight schedules, my secretary Mrs Ann Rodden, who has orchestrated the entire exercise from beginning to end, and our publishers whose assistance and expertise have been of the highest calibre.

Glasgow, 1991   D.H.L.

Acknowledgement

These papers are published by the Royal College of Physicians of Edinburgh with the aid of an educational grant from Norwich Eaton Ltd, a division of Procter and Gamble.

D.H.L.

Contributors

I. A. D. Bouchier CBE MD FRCP (Ed) FRCP FRS (Ed)
Professor of Medicine, University of Edinburgh

A. K. Burnett MD FRCP (Glas) FRCPath
Consultant Haematologist, Royal Infirmary, Glasgow

J. A. Burton MB BDS FRCP (Glas)
Consultant Physician, Raigmore Hospital, Inverness

A. Calin MD FRCP
Consultant Rheumatologist, Royal National Hospital for Rheumatic
Diseases, Bath

A. Cuschieri MD FRCS (Ed) FRCS (Eng)
Professor of Surgery, Ninewells Hospital & Medical School, Dundee

J. W. Dobbie MD FRCP (Glas) FRCPath
Vice-President Advanced Scientific Development, Baxter R & D Europe,
Nivelles, Belgium

N. J. Douglas MD FRCP (Ed)
Senior Lecturer, Respiratory Medicine Unit, City Hospital, Edinburgh

R. Fife MB FRCP FRCP (Glas)
Retired Consultant Physician, Glasgow

A. Forbes BSc, MD MRCP (UK)
Senior Registrar, Gastrointestinal Unit, Charing Cross Hospital, London

C. D. Forbes MD DSc FRCP (Ed) FRCP FRCP (Glas) FRSA
Professor of Medicine, Ninewells Hospital & Medical School, Dundee

H. M. Gilles MD DSc FRCP FFPHM
School of Tropical Medicine, University of Liverpool

M. J. Godman MB FRCP (Ed)
Consultant Paediatric Cardiologist, Royal Hospital for Sick Children,
Edinburgh

S. A. Greene MB MRCP (UK)
Consultant Endocrinologist, Department of Child Health, Ninewells Hospital & Medical School, Dundee

D. A. Henry MB FRCP (Ed)
Senior Lecturer, University of Newcastle, Australia

A. C. MacCuish MD FRCP (Ed) FRCP (Glas)
Consultant Physician, Royal Infirmary, Glasgow

I. Murray-Lyon MD FRCP (Ed) FRCP
Consultant Gastroenterologist, Charing Cross Hospital, London

M. F. Oliver CBE MD PPRCP (Ed) FRCP FACC FFPHM FRSE
Emeritus Professor of Cardiology, University of Edinburgh, Director, Wynn Institute for Metabolic Research, London

A. C. Parker MB PhD FRCP (Ed) MRCPath
Senior Lecturer, Department of Haematology, Royal Infirmary, Edinburgh

B. M. Rifkind MD FRCP (Ed) FRCP (Glas)
Chief, Lipid Metabolism-Atherogenesis Branch, National Institutes of Health, Bethesda, Maryland, USA

J. Thomson MD FRCP (Glas) DObstRCOG
Consultant Dermatologist, Royal Infirmary, Glasgow

R. G. Will BA MB FRCP (Ed)
Consultant Neurologist, Western General Hospital, Edinburgh

Contents

SECTION 2
Best management

SECTION 3
History of medicine

SECTION 4
20th century Scottish physicians

Topical reviews

1. Artificial membranes and the physician

J. W. Dobbie

INTRODUCTION

Membranes are the stuff of life. In the unicellular organism the cell membrane is the condensation of organic material which separates the living world from the non-living medium it inhabits. Biological membranes are composed of molecules arranged such that they constitute both a barrier and a selective filter for the maintenance of different chemical and physical conditions on either side of the divide. An electron micrograph of any cell in the human body displays a plethora of internal membranes arranged to form vesicles, cisternae, endoplasmic reticulum, and mitochondria stuffed with interdigitating double-membraned cristae. Thus in any one cell in any organ, there is an extensive area of membrane material which provides innumerable compartments where separate processes of biosynthesis or degradation may continue unhindered by the activity which is occurring all around. Slowly over the past century there was a steadily growing appreciation of the paramount importance of membranes in providing a vast surface area for chemical reaction. In the 1950s the dawning realization of the essential role of biological membranes was an important catalyst to the conceptual revolution which overtook therapeutics. In a short space of time artificial membranes were eagerly sought for replacement or repair of deficient or impaired bodily functions. Until then we had been restricted to the use of membranes of animal or vegetable origin. In the last decade, advances accruing from 50 years of research in organic and polymer chemistry have provided us with the ability to synthesize more membranes than there are biologists, time or money to evaluate. Thus, unfortunately, we can expect a considerable lag-period before the physician may have an opportunity to fully test the therapeutic potential of this embarrassment of riches.

The process by which artificial membranes came to play a significant role in modern therapeutics began in 1854 when Thomas Graham in his paper 'On Osmotic Force' first described the phenomenon of dialysis. Using a membrane fashioned from an ox bladder, he observed the movement from one compartment to the other of different types of solutes of varying concentration. The following year, the German physiologist Adolph Fick demonstrated the selective permeability of an artificial membrane made of collodion. In 1889 Richardson, also working with collodion membranes, was able to differentiate the properties of crystalline and colloidal solutions and apply this concept to the nature of solutions separated by natural membranes in the human body. He probably made the first reference to the use of collodion membranes in the dialysis of blood. At Johns Hopkins University in the early 1900s, Abel, Rowntree & Turner (1914) began research on a device using collodion membranes which allowed them to perform in the experimental animal a technique they called 'vividiffusion'. This was the progenitor of the process which we now know as haemo-dialysis. This first artificial kidney consisted of numerous delicate tubes of collodion contained within a glass cylinder. Blood entered the device at one end, being distributed by manifolds to the collodion tubes through which it passed to the venous end, where a similar set of manifolds conducted the blood into one channel for delivery to the vein (Fig. 1.1). The space in the glass cylinder surrounding the collodion tubes was filled with a dialysis solution which was delivered and removed at one end of the cylinder. The dialysing tubes were simply and easily made in their own laboratory by mixing collodion with ether and ethyl alcohol to make a paste which was used to coat the inside of glass cylinders. Following drying, the collodion tubes could be carefully removed from the cylinders and attached to the manifolds.

In 1923 Necheles constructed a dialyser using lamb's peritoneum as the membrane and a sandwich technique which minimized the internal volume of the membrane envelope, and so increased the surface area of blood in contact with dialysate. In 1938 Thalheimer found that the membrane (cellophane) used in the sausage industry, could be used for removal of solutes from blood. Cellophane (cellulose acetate), in contrast to any of the

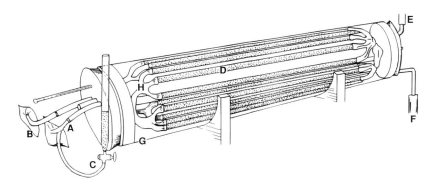

Fig. 1.1 Diagrammatic representation of the Abel, Rowntree, Turner 'vividiffusion' apparatus which uses the progenitor of the haemodialysers of today. A, Blood inflow, B, Blood outflow, C, Anticoagulant (Hirudin), D, Colloidin tubes, E, F, Dialysate inflow and outflow, G, Jacket, H, Manifolds.

previous membranes used, was strong, of uniform thickness, and could be manufactured in large quantities. Indeed, it was this membrane which was used in the rotating drum kidney machine of Kolff which ushered in the era of effective treatment of acute and chronic renal failure. The use of artificial membranes in therapeutics was firmly established from that day forth (Kolff 1950).

Material science and the creation of artificial membranes

The rapid advances in the material sciences of the past 30 years have given rise to new terms, new concepts and new disciplines. Thus, therapeutics have come to rely heavily on biomaterials of continually improving biocompatibility, devised and evaluated by biophysicists and bioengineers. It increasingly behoves the physician to attain some familiarity with the applicability, limitations and toxicology of these materials, for there is still considerable ignorance in the medical world of what can and what cannot be done with plastics and polymers, and considerable confusion in the minds of 'green' activists over the necessity for a variety of additives in many of the biomaterials now widely used in artificial membranes and devices.

Polymers and plastics

Polymers have revolutionized modern medical and surgical practice. They are light, usually strong but highly flexible and often have low bioreactivity. Indeed, in comparison to more traditional material, polymers provide a far better balance between weight and mechanical, chemical and physical properties. Several polymers which have been used in artificial membranes are described briefly:

Collodion. This form of cellulose nitrate used in the first artificial kidney experiments, has in recent years been used to coat activated carbon granules for use in haemoperfusion systems, employed in the treatment of acute liver failure and poisoning. The affinity of collodion for albumin confers on the membrane a reasonable degree of compatibility with blood.

Cellulose. Membranes prepared by the regeneration of cellulose and usually plasticized with glycerol are widely employed in haemodialysis, where they are available in flat sheets, tubular and hollow fibre forms.

Cellulose acetate. This membrane is increasingly used in haemodialysis where it provides for greater ultrafiltration than cellulose (cuprophane) membrane, with some advantages in additional biocompatibility.

Polyacrylonitrile. A polymer which gives a membrane possessing advantages in blood biocompatibility, it is used in hollow fibre dialysers.

Polycarbonate. Co-polymerized with silicones, these membranes have been used in blood oxygenators.

Polypropylene, polytetrafluoroethylene. The microporous varieties of these polymers can function as effective membranes for blood oxygenation and plasma separators.

Polymethylmethacrylate. Membrane preparations of the polymer generally referred to as acrylic have been used for plasma membrane filtration.

Polyvinylalcohol. Used in membrane plasma filtration.

Polyurethane. This polymer has good mechanical and biocompatibility properties.

Polyvinylchloride. This polymer, extensively used for tubing in delivery sets and medical devices, tops the green list for proscription. Its loss to medical devices and blood storage containers would be a major problem.

Other ingredients in polymers

It is unlikely that one could ever obtain a completely pure material. A large number of chemicals are required for the manufacture of any polymer and the final product may therefore contain variable amounts of substances whose toxicology must be carefully scrutinized. These substances are required as inhibitors, catalysts, initiators, emulsifiers, chain transfer agents, plasticizers, curing agents, accelerators, anti-oxidants and fillers. Any may be leached from the polymer matrix during contact with biological systems and give rise to local or systemic reaction. This is a large, complex and rapidly expanding field of industrial development, and unfortunately tends to become a battleground where politics rule and science suffers. Diethylhexylphthalate (DEHP), a plasticizer which has been used extensively for the past several decades in innumerable devices in medical practice, has been a bone of contention as regards its human toxicity. Despite the fact that its use in plastics in haemodialysis alone probably constitutes one of the largest and longest clinical trials of all time in which no associated syndrome of attributable toxicology has been unequivocally identified, this agent is now being actively replaced by materials whose properties can only be judged from simple animal trials. As we move forward into an age where material science becomes more and more important, the physician should be aware that many ill-founded arguments advanced for the elimination of certain substances and the introduction of others could have disastrous consequences.

In addition to the problems of fabrication, polymers in medical devices pose yet further difficulties in their sterilization. In recent years this has developed into a branch of material science of daunting complexity. The physician should be aware that although scientists invent materials with considerable potential for use in biological systems, many of these are abandoned because no effective method of sterilization can be found which does not alter or degrade the substance. Most polymers cannot be sterilized by dry heat (160–190°C). Steam autoclaving is limited to polymers with softening points above the normal autoclaving of 134°C. Sterilization by ionizing radiation has many advantages, but again its application is limited since it tends to promote cross-linking and polymer degradation. Gaseous sterilization is extensively employed and is particularly suited for heat-sensitive polymers. Ethylene oxide (ETO) is the commonest agent used in this form of sterilization, but it is well-recognized that its use is associated with allergic-type reactions in patients using ETO-sterilized haemo-dialysers. Thus, patients on haemodialysis may show high serum IgE concentration and a positive IgE-RAST for antibodies to ETO. Formaldehyde, an effective sterilant, has also been widely used for artificial membranes. However, its removal through extensive washing with expensive sterile saline before the device can be used, detracts from its use. Despite exponentially increasing knowledge on the properties of plastics and polymers, their safe application in medical devices is not an easy undertaking.

BIOMATERIALS AND BIOCOMPATIBILITY

The term biomaterial is applied to natural or synthetic materials which are used in contact with living tissue and/or biological fluids. In 1974 a study group of the US-National Institutes of Health first proposed a definition for biocompatibility, whose revised version (Klinkman et al 1984), the so-called 'No-definition', is now widely accepted by the medical community. A biomaterial is defined as having clinically acceptable biocompatibility if there is no thrombogenic, toxic, allergic or inflammatory reaction to its use; no destruction of formed elements or changes in plasma proteins or enzymes; no immunological reactions, carcinogenic effect or deterioration of adjacent tissues.

Thrombogenicity of foreign surfaces

Most of the early studies on the biocompatibility of biomaterials were restricted to an examination of the thrombogenic and haemolytic properties of artificial membranes in contact with blood during haemodialysis. A biocompatible membrane should not trigger surface sensitive plasma proteins such as the Hageman factor or perturb platelet function and so activate the coagulation cascade (Basile & Drueke 1989). Some of the membranes first used extensively in haemodialysis, e.g. cuprophane, were recognized as having tolerably low thrombogenicity in a heparinized patient, but it was nevertheless appreciated that their use gave rise to a transient though significant thrombocytopenia and platelet activation during dialysis. That membranes possessed different thrombogenic potential became apparent when in vitro and in vivo testing of dialysers made of polyacrylonitrile, polycarbonate and polymethylmethacrylate were shown to be measurably less thrombogenic than cuprophane. Nowadays most membranes used in extracorporeal devices possess functionally acceptable low propensity to activate coagulation, while research and development efforts continue, by whatever means, to improve their biocompatibility and so progressively lessen the need for anticoagulation.

Complement activation by artificial membranes

In the early decades of haemodialysis, little interest was shown in the phenomenon of dialysis-induced leucopenia. When in 1977 Craddock et al presented evidence that the leucopenia resulting from pulmonary sequestration of leucocytes was causally associated with the activation of complement through the alternative pathway, there was a sudden upsurge in interest which has continued to date (Basile & Drueke 1989).

The complement system consists of a series of proteins which form two interrelated enzyme cascades, termed the classical and alternate pathways, providing two routes to the cleavage of a key component, C3. This is a central event in an amplifying system of enzyme activation which in turn leads to the formation of membrane attack complexes. These are biologically potent substances capable of producing lytic lesions in cell membranes.

In the alternative pathway activation of complement it was subsequently demonstrated that the cascade could be triggered by a large number of substances, including polysaccharides, lipopolysaccharides, endotoxin and a variety of synthetic materials, without the involvement of antigen–antibody complexes. It was soon realized that regenerated cellulose membranes constructed of repetitive polysaccharide units mimicked the lipopolysaccharide structure of the bacterial cell wall, a powerful initiator of the alternative pathway of complement. With further enquiry into the surface chemistry of regenerated cellulose, the distribution and density of hydroxyl radicles were correlated with the membrane's potential to interact with leucocyte cell surfaces and initiate complement activation. Thus, membranes were modified to replace some of the hydroxyl with less reactive acetate or amino groups. These have resulted in the construction of newer membranes (e.g. haemophane) whose improved biocompatibility with respect to complement activation is believed to be substantiated by demonstrably lower serum concentrations of C3a and lesser degrees of leucopenia during haemodialysis.

Complement activation is now firmly tied to intradialytic morbidity with respect to the occurrence of anaphylaxis-type of reactions, smooth muscle contraction, microcirculatory disturbances, hypotension and pyrogenic reactions (Klinkmann 1987). More chronic effects ascribed to complement activation and interleukin release are those of hypercatabolism and depression of host defence mechanisms. One lasting effect of the work carried out on complement activation in haemodialysis is the realization that contact of an artificial membrane and a biological system involves highly complex interactions between the energetics and kinetics of all physical, chemical and biochemical processes which occur at the interface, both during and after the time of contact.

Foreign body reaction to tissue-implanted membranes

The histopathological reaction of human and animal tissue to the implantation of foreign structures has been recognized and studied extensively over the last century. Virtually all foreign substances introduced into body tissues will evoke a response which consists of formation of multinucleated giant cells, chronic inflammatory cells and usually significant local fibroneogenesis. Nevertheless, it could be argued that our understanding of the mechanics of this reaction has advanced but little since its first description.

The field of artificial organ development is littered by abandoned devices, the work of material scientists and others who, forging ahead with their inventions, disregard the inevitable consequence of the appearance of foreign body giant cells around their implant.

ARTIFICIAL MEMBRANES

Artificial membranes in modern therapeutics can be categorized according to the basic nature of their composition and their mode of employment:

Membranes used for the extracorporeal manipulation of blood and body fluids

1. Haemodialysis
2. Haemofiltration
3. Haemodiafiltration
4. Haemoperfusion
5. Membrane plasma filtration
6. Immune adsorption
7. Blood oxygenation

Artificial cells

1. Internalized artificial organs
2. Liposomes

Implanted non-biodegradable membranes

1. Bioprostheses
2. Membranes as biosensors

Artificial membranes in the extracorporeal manipulation of blood

When artificial membranes first became available, they were put to use in a manner which did not deviate from medieval European concepts of the causation of disease. They were thus applied to the purification of blood, as a modern magic filter to rid the body of the toxins. To date the greatest application of membranes in therapeutics has been in the alteration of the constituents of blood in order to achieve a temporary or curative effect on an illness, to maintain life or reduce morbidity of a chronic life-threatening disorder. Extracorporeal processing of blood depends on the mass transport mechanism of molecular diffusion which is the movement of a chemical species from a region of high to one of lower concentration (Colton 1987).

Haemodialysers and their descendents

The early membranes were used in acute renal failure to remove low molecular weight 'toxins' (potassium, urea and creatinine) from the blood. The search for the ultimate uraemic poison continued, as did the quest for a suitable membrane to filter out larger molecules, the so-called middle molecules arraigned as the prime suspects. Thus, the development of membranes with very high hydraulic permeabilities led to the birth of a new species of haemodialysers. These provided high clearance rates of solutes up to moderate molecular weights, predominantly through convective transport, a process which more closely mimicked the natural filtering capabilities of the normal human glomerulus. The acquisition of more porous membranes in a pressure driven system thus gave rise to the technique now known as haemofiltration (Colton 1987).

Currently there a dozen or so membranes available for treatment of acute or chronic renal failure. These can be conveniently placed in three categories according to the nature of the material used in their construction— cellulose, derivatized cellulose and synthetics. The latter may be further subdivided into hydrophilic or hydrophobic classes (Lysaght 1988). Some 80% of contemporary dialysers are made from cellulose. Of the derivatized cellulose membranes, cellulose acetate and haemophane hollow fibres are being increasingly utilized, while the high flux, hydrophobic, synthetic membrane, polysulphone, is gaining in popularity.

Haemodialysis, representing predominantly diffusive, and haemofiltration, representing predominantly convective transport, lie at opposite ends of the spectrum of solute removal in renal replacement therapy. In the 1970s, new treatment modalities were developed combining controlled rates of ultrafiltration higher than those employed in haemodialysis but lower than those used in haemofiltration (Colton 1987). This technique retains the high clearance capabilities of haemodialysis for low molecular weight solutes while adding enhanced clearance rates for high molecular weight solutes characteristic of haemofiltration. Increasing numbers of patients are now being maintained on regimes which incorporate these advances.

As regular haemodialysis now sustains hundreds of thousands of patients worldwide, most current research and development in artificial membranes has concentrated on the problems attributed to regular, long-term extra-corporeal circulation of blood. Although complications associated with chronic haemodialysis such as arthropathies and tissue deposition of amyloid have engaged the attention of many researchers, there is still considerable dispute as to what associated pathologies can reasonably be ascribed to long-term exposure of blood to membranes of low biocompatibility. As time passes and more experience with newer membranes of vaunted biocompatibility accrues, then comparison of mortality of sizeable cohorts of patients stratified by exposure to different membranes may provide a clear answer.

Driven by the need to cut cost and maintain profit, large numbers of dialysis centres in the USA have devised techniques to sterilize hollow fibre dialysers for multiple re-use. Surprisingly, and to their pecuniary delight, it was found that some procedures conferred enhanced biocompatibility on the re-used dialysers. Either through coating of the lumenal surfaces by plasma proteins or modification of surface chemistry by the sterilizing procedures, the re-used dialysers exhibited improved biocompatibility as evidenced by decreased complement activation. Currently these practices have raised the ire of renal patients' associations who are naturally concerned over the multiple re-use of disposable dialysers.

The brave new world of the 1970s and early 1980s has passed, an epoch when the plethora of new membranes and new devices promised untold control over human disease. At present we are in a less glamorous phase of stepwise, slow improvement of the biocompatibility of artificial membranes.

Membrane plasma filtration

In a companion paper to their publication on vividiffusion, Abel, Rowntree and Turner in 1914 described another form of blood purification which they called 'plasmapheresis'. Following collection of blood from an animal, they allowed the red cells to sediment and, removing the plasma, replaced it with an isotonic salt solution. The reconstituted blood was then reinfused back into the animals. There ensued a delay of over half a century before the development of a rotating seal and adequate anticoagulation permitted separation of blood and plasma in a spinning centrifuge bowl.

Diseases believed to be caused by macromolecules such as antibodies, circulating immune complexes or protein-bound toxins have now been successfully treated, particularly in the acute life-threatening phase of an illness, by plasma exchange (Horiuchi, Malchesky & Nosé 1987). Initially, centrifugation of blood was exclusively used to achieve separation of the cellular from the fluid element. However, recently the development of the technique of plasma membrane filtration has allowed greater operational flexibility and discrimination in removing plasma solutes. Although centrifugal plasma separation is a relatively simple technique, the equipment is bulky and separation of plasma from blood cells is incomplete. In contrast, in membrane plasma separation, equipment is minimal and exclusion of cells or cellular debris from the plasma filtrate is complete. Despite the fact that membranes suitable for membrane plasmapheresis have been available since the 1950s, progress in development was retarded by difficulties caused by haemolysis, plugging and flux decay. However, by 1972 it had been established that these problems could be circumvented through modifications of channel geometry and blood flow. In 1978, with the advent of hollow fibres made from microporous polypropylene, the stage was set for the rapid advancements in development and application of plasma filters which occurred in the 1980s.

Membrane plasmapheresis occurs when blood passes in shear flow over a porous surface. Flux increases with the strength of the shear flow. Ideally the pore diameter should lie between 0.1–1.0 μm. Haemolysis may occur if the pores are too large or the shear rate exceeds a critical value. Although plasma separators are closely related to dialysers and haemofilters, there are significant differences which account for their ability to satisfy specific clinical and operational demands. Haemodialysers require higher trans-membrane pressures for operation and have lower filtrate fluxes than membrane plasma separators. Haemofilters yield filtrate fluxes similar to membrane plasma separators but do not allow passage of plasma proteins. Functional plasma separators have been constructed from a wide variety of polymers which are hydrophilic or can be rendered hydrophilic; these include cellulose acetate, polyvinyl chloride, polyethylene, polypropylene and polymethylmethacrylate.

Driven largely by the high cost of albumin replacement, there has been a determined effort to develop more selective techniques for elimination of pathogenic macromolecules. No one denies the fact that simple plasma exchange throws several precious babies out with the bath water! Thus, a variety of manipulations of technique and operating conditions have evolved, including cascade or double step filtration, thermal filtration and cryofiltration. In cascade filtration the procedure, which is performed at ambient temperature, relies on the membrane properties with respect to pore size and distribution. With thermal filtration the technique takes advantage of the effect on sieving of varying operational temperature. In this procedure the solution is warmed above physiological temperature. Conversely, cryofiltration exploits the fact that a decrease in temperature promotes aggregation of plasma solutes and therefore the plasma is cooled to between 4–10°C to obtain an increase in selectivity.

An important consideration which is often overlooked in the debate on the benefits attributable to the use of plasmapheresis, is the fact that additional to the elimination of incriminated macromolecules, the removal of the mediators of an over-zealous inflammatory response, tissue destruction and persistent coagulopathy possibly contribute more to patient survival in fulminant illness than is appreciated. In this regard it may not be inappropriate to remind the would-be practitioner that peritoneal dialysis expertly performed may make a significant contribution to the continual removal of mediators in the intervals between courses of plasmapheresis. This is particularly applicable in patients with incipient or established renal failure where the generation by haemodialysis of yet more mediators is obviously undesirable. Foregoing the convenience of haemodialysis for high flow hypertonic tidal peritoneal dialysis, one can achieve more than adequate dialysis and in 5–10 litres of ultrafiltrate, remove accumulating mediators between courses of plasmapheresis. Continuing in the same vein, the success of plasmapheresis in acute illness may not solely depend on the sophistication of the devices or the aggressiveness of the procedure. A regime which stabilizes the patient and buffers him from the rigours of extracorporeal assault is to be commended. Thus, although albumin is both scarce and expensive, miserly replacement of this vital substance may exact a cost. One must not forget that the normal level of albumin in plasma is 45 g/l not 25 g/l. Through its capacious adsorptive properties, albumin acts as a vascular dustbin for most of the debris of the complement and coagulation cascades. Moreover, its importance to normal rheology in the face of endothelial failure should not be underestimated. Thus, for those few practitioners who have had access to adequate supplies of high quality albumin and enjoyed the luxury of titrating their patients back to normal plasma levels between courses of plasmapheresis, any arguments to the contrary are singularly unconvincing.

The therapeutic potential of plasmapheresis has been avidly tested on a wide variety of conditions. The following list details those in which most benefit has been obtained in modifying or arresting progression. In most conditions so treated, the patients receive plasma filtration as an adjunct to contemporaneous treatment with traditional medication which, in many instances, is immunosuppression.

Neurological conditions

1. Myasthenia gravis.
The detection of the pathogenic role of antibodies against acetylcholine receptors gave a rational basis for the establishment of immunosuppression and plasmapheresis. The efficacy of plasmapheresis has been proven in many open trials.
2. Chronic demyelinating inflammatory polyradiculoneuropathy.
These disorders, which encompass the Guillain–Barré syndrome, are now regularly treated by plasmapheresis.
3. Lambert–Eaton syndrome.
A chronic disease due to circulating antibodies against components of the motor nerve terminal.

4. Refsum's disease.
Due to a rare inborn error of lipid metabolism (phytanic acid).

Haematological conditions

1. Thrombotic thrombocytopenic purpura.
2. Haemolytic uraemic syndrome.
3. Paraproteinaemias and hyperviscosity syndromes.
4. Rhesus incompatibility.

Rheumatology

1. Rheumatoid vasculitis.

Glomerulonephritides

1. Rapidly progressive glomerulonephritis.
This is due to either antiglomerular basement membrane antibody or antineutrophil cytoplasmic antibody.

Hyperlipoproteinaemias

Further evaluation of therapeutic role

As with all new concepts it could be argued that indiscriminate deployment of this attractive new membrane technology by enthusiastic amateurs has not contributed significantly to a sober evaluation of its true merit in checking the progression of disease. Nevertheless, it must be recognized that its careful application to conditions otherwise refractory to medical treatment should in no way be discouraged. As time passes and the noise in the system is itself subject to filtering through a cognitive membrane of suitable porosity, a better appreciation of the most appropriate applications will surely emerge!

Therapeutic immunoadsorption

The development of this modality represents the next logical step in the drive for ever more selective removal of pathogenic macromolecules from blood and circumvention of the difficulties of using replacement solutions. The majority of systems utilize an extracorporeal arrangement involving a cell centrifuge or hollow fibre device to separate plasma which is then passed over an immunoadsorption column. The treated plasma is recombined with cells for return to the patient. Adsorption columns have used a variety of ligands of specificity ranging from monoclonal and polyclonal antibodies, specific antigenic determinants, through to non-specific adsorbants such as charcoal. Ligands have been immobilized on silica particles, beads, collodion, and hollow fibre polymers. Considerable use has been made of protein A, a cell wall component of *Staphylococcus aureus*, which specifically binds the Fc portion of all IgG subclasses except 3. The development of parallel columns with continual regeneration of spent columns by elution with buffer solutions has greatly increased the system's capacity for removal of target molecules. A major concern, however, is sensitization of the patient through leaching of ligands from the column. Biocompatibility varies with the ligand and support matrix used. Protein A activates complement and its use is associated with fever, hypotension, hypertension and respiratory distress.

Therapeutic immunoadsorption has been successfully used in the treatment of ABO and Rhesus incompatibility, in addition to familial hypercholesterolaemia through removal of low density lipoprotein. Although much of the endeavour in this field has been highly creative, it is still largely experimental and at this stage not all clinical goals have been achieved.

ARTIFICIAL CELLS

There are many bioreactive materials, particularly adsorbents, which are highly efficacious in removing unwanted substances from the blood of acutely ill patients. Unfortunately most of these materials are not only incompatible with blood, but also release fine particles which give rise to microembolism. Thus, the high hopes for haemoperfusion of activated charcoal columns in conditions such as fulminant hepatic failure and acute poisoning were never realized. However, the coating of each granule of activated charcoal with an ultrathin polymer conferred more acceptable biocompatibility, while still retaining most of the charcoal's adsorptive potential through leaving the surface pores uncovered. These coated granules have been termed artificial cells (Chang 1987) (Fig. 1.2). This manoeuvre also prevented release of particulates into the circulation and allowed blood compatible granules to be used in haemoperfusion devices. Many bioreactive materials such as enzymes, ion exchange resins and immunoadsorbents have been microencapsulated in systems which provide a large surface to volume relationship where the ultrathin membrane permits rapid equilibration of molecules across these artificial cells. The membrane most commonly used for coating granules is collodion (cellulose nitrate), while other polymers such as cellulose and cellulose acetate have been occasionally employed.

Artificial cells of this nature have been used in the routine treatment of acute poisoning for removal of aluminium and iron overload and in the treatment of FHF. However, their use in chronic renal failure as an adjunct treatment for removal of 'middle molecules' has not met expectations. Experimental work on the formation of artificial erythrocytes through microencapsulation of cross-linked haemoglobin is underway.

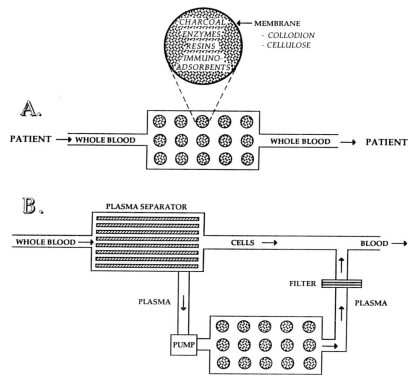

Fig. 1.2   Diagrammatic representation of the use of artificial cells in two different types of extracorporeal circuits. In A, whole blood is passed directly through a container loaded with membrane-coated granules. In B, plasma alone is subjected to 'purification' by passage over the artificial cells which, in practice, have been filled with a wide variety of bioreactive materials. Such complex systems have been used in the treatment of poisoning, liver failure and immune disorders.

Internalized artificial organs

This field of endeavour which is still largely experimental, seeks to employ permeability-selective membranes to encapsulate living cells from the same or different species. A membrane is chosen whose porosity does not permit host antibodies to penetrate to the donor cells but allows secretory molecules of lower molecular weight to diffuse into the host tissue to replace deficient, vital agents. Many centres throughout the world are now feverishly engaged in seeking this Holy Grail. However, until we can dissuade tissues of their ingrained distaste for foreign bodies and prevent induction of giant cells and their lymphocytic camp followers, we will be continually frustrated in achieving an important further contribution from artificial membranes. Employing such basic design, the construction of an artificial pancreas for implantation in a tissue of suitable vascularity is high on the priority list of many engaged in the development of artificial organs.

Liposomes

Discovery of the relative ease with which manipulation of phospholipids in solution produced micelles whose walls mimicked the basic structure of the cell membrane, has given to modern therapeutics the liposome. Currently these artificial membranes are being used to package drugs and biologics for highly focused delivery to specific regions of the body. Much of this effort has concerned the targeting of tumour tissue with cytotoxic agents where the logic of delivering systemic-sparing biodegradable capsules is a commendable pursuit. Nevertheless, the frustrating complexities of intra-tumour hypertension, washout and fickle microcirculation have to date frustrated the establishment of this form of therapy in widespread clinical practice.

Permanent (non-biodegradable) membranes

Bioprosthesis

Here material, which may either be synthetic or denatured animal protein, is used as a membranous scaffolding for the internal reconstitution of a vital anatomical structure, e.g. heart valves, major arteries, vascular shunts, etc. Cardiovascular surgeons have accumulated several decades of experience in employing such techniques.

Membranes as biosensors

In this development artificial membranes are used at an interface between body compartments to sense changes in chemistry to provide the physician, the patient or an automatic device, the opportunity to respond in a negative feedback loop.

CONCLUSIONS

Future medical historians may well chronicle the introduction of artificial membranes as a landmark in the treatment of human disease when, for the first time, material science and advanced technology were successfully harnessed to the old chariot of therapeutics. Perhaps other more cynical commentators may regard this epoch of 'high tech' blood letting as but the culmination of an ancient and persistent European fetish for purging the body of noxious substances. Whatever the verdict, it seems likely that the use of artificial membranes in the treatment of life-threatening illnesses will continue to develop and grow in the next few decades. On the other hand, their current dominant role in long-term life support systems in irreversible organ failure, will in due course be supplanted by more effective biological measures.

REFERENCES

Abel J J, Rowntree L G, Turner B B 1914 The removal of diffusible substances from the circulating blood of living animals by dialysis. Journal of Pharmacology and Experimental Therapeutics 5: 275–316

Basile C, Drueke T 1989 Dialysis membrane biocompatibility. Nephron 52: 113–118

Chang T M S 1987 Applications of artificial cells in medicine and biotechnology. Biomaterials, Artificial Cells, and Artificial Organs 15: 1–20

Colton C K 1987 Analysis of membrane processes for blood purification. Blood Purification 5: 202–251

Craddock P R, Fehr J, Dalmasso A P et al 1977 Hemodialysis leukopenia: Pulmonary vascular leukostasis resulting from complement activation by dialyzer cellophane membranes. Journal of Clinical Investigation 59: 879–888

Graham T 1854 The Bakerian lecture—On osmotic force. Philosophical Transactions of the Royal Society of London 144: 177–228

Horiuchi T, Malchesky P S, Nosé Y 1987 Overview: Selective macromolecules removal by secondary filtration. In: Bambauer R, Malchesky P S, Falkenhagen D (eds) Therapeutic plasma exchange and selective plasma separation. Schattauer, Stuttgart, 5–15

Klinkmann H 1987 Biocompatibility problems in membrane separation processes. In: Bambauer R, Malchesky P S, Falkenhagen D (eds) Therapeutic plasma exchange and selective plasma separation. Schattauer, Stuttgart, 17–32

Klinkmann H, Wolf H, Schmitt E 1984 Definition of biocompatibility. Contributions to Nephrology 37: 70–77

Kolff W J 1950 Artificial kidney—Treatment of acute and chronic uremia. Cleveland Clinic Quarterly 17: 216–228

Lysaght M J 1988 Hemodialysis membranes in transition. Contributions to Nephrology 61: 1–17

Thalheimer W 1938 Experimental exchange transfusions for reducing azotemia: use of artificial kidney for this purpose. Proceedings of the Society for Experimental Biology and Medicine 37: 641–643

2. Current treatment of high blood cholesterol

B. M. Rifkind

A recent editorial (Dargie 1989) characterized coronary heart disease (CHD) as Scotland's national disease and placed Scotland at the very top of the international league for its rates of this condition. It was noted that for men aged 35–65 coronary mortality is 30–40% higher than in England, that the differences were even more striking for women and that, in 1988, nearly 4000 men and women in Scotland died from CHD before the age of 65, it being by far the single most common cause of premature death.

Although much has been achieved by treating the clinical consequences of CHD it is much more desirable to prevent the onset of CHD in the first instance. This is especially so when one considers that a high proportion of all CHD deaths occur suddenly and before any medical care can be brought to bear.

Several major and potentially substantially modifiable risk factors for CHD have been established. The higher the level of plasma cholesterol or blood pressure or smoking or the lower the levels of high density lipo-protein (HDL) the greater the risk of various clinical manifestations of CHD. When two or more risk factors coexist the risk is especially high. Cholesterol has received particular attention. It is thought to play a primary role in CHD and that other risk factors only operate when the cholesterol level is sufficiently high to lead to the development of atherosclerotic lesions.

The evidence that cholesterol plays a causal role in CHD comes from many research approaches. Cholesterol was first suspected when it was noted that it was a prominent component of both the early and the advanced atherosclerotic lesion. A detailed picture of how cholesterol enters the arterial wall and accumulates, and how the atherosclerotic lesion develops is being assembled gradually (Ross 1986). In many animal species including primates, experimentation has shown that the induction of hypercholester-olaemia through dietary fat manipulation, leads to severe atherosclerosis and, sometimes, to myocardial ischaemia. When hypercholesterolaemia occurs as a result of a genetic defect, as in the WHIL rabbit, severe atherosclerosis also occurs. Many human clinical genetic disorders, each due to a specific mutation of a particular gene, develop raised levels of cholesterol-rich lipoproteins. These include familial hypercholester-olaemia, familial defective apo B100, familial dysbetalipoproteinaemia, and familial combined hyperlipidaemia. All exhibit the early onset of athero-sclerosis and premature CHD. Thus, when atherogenic lipoproteins increase in concentration either due to dietary and/or genetic causes atherosclerosis and CHD may ensue.

Another fruitful approach has been through detailed studies of lipo-protein structure and function which have been performed over the past several decades. These have provided considerable insight into the processes that deliver and remove cholesterol from the artery (Brown & Goldstein 1986).

Epidemiological studies have been particularly important in incriminating cholesterol in atherogenesis and have taken different forms. They include cross-cultural, migrant, and case-control studies as well as prospective studies such as Framingham, the British Regional Heart Study and the Multiple Risk Factor Intervention Trial screenees (Stamler 1979, Castelli et al 1986). They have consistently shown that a high cholesterol level predicts the onset of future coronary events in individuals with or without prior manifestations of CHD up to 30 years later.

Consequently clinical trials of cholesterol-lowering have been conducted to assess its impact on CHD morbidity and mortality. These show conclusively that reduction of plasma cholesterol levels, whether by diet or drug and either in individuals with or without clinical CHD, reduces the incidence of fatal and non-fatal coronary events (Lipid Research Clinics Program 1984a, Yusuf et al 1988). The risk reduction is proportional to the degree of cholesterol reduction so that each 1% reduction in cholesterol has led to an approximate 2% reduction in CHD risk (Lipid Research Clinics Program 1984b).

The reductions in CHD mortality have not been accompanied by corresponding reductions in total mortality. This has been generally attributed to inadequate sample size, insufficient period of follow-up or an increase in certain causes of non-coronary mortality. The last possibility cannot be ruled out, but has been doubted in view of the small number of cases involved, and the variations in the causes of non-coronary deaths reported from study to study. It should be emphasized, however, that even if overall mortality were not reduced, a reduced cardiac morbidity remains as a net gain and is a sufficient goal with evident health benefits and a potential to substantially reduce medical costs.

This impressive range of evidence ranging from basic science studies at the molecular level to applied studies in large populations has led to recommendations from many bodies that high-risk and population-based cholesterol-lowering strategies be implemented with the ultimate aim of markedly reducing CHD rates. For example, the report of the British Cardiac Society Working Group on Coronary Disease Prevention emphasizes the complementarity of population and high-risk approaches and recommends that they should be implemented simultaneously (British Cardiac Society 1987).

REPORT OF THE EXPERT PANEL

High-risk strategies have the aim of detecting individuals with especially high blood cholesterol levels who are at greatest risk for CHD and are most in need of detailed clinical guidance and monitoring. The US National Cholesterol Education Program's Expert Panel on Detection, Evaluation and Treatment of High Blood Cholesterol in Adults has recently developed a report for physicians which offers practical recommendations for the detection, evaluation and treatment of such individuals (Report of the National Cholesterol Education Program Expert Panel on Detection, Evaluation and Treatment of High Blood Cholesterol in Adults 1988). The report deals with three principal topics, namely the classification of blood cholesterol and patient evaluation, dietary treatment, and drug treatment. The report addresses only patients age 20 and over. Its treatment approach is the same for adults of both sexes and all ages. However, it emphasizes that there is room for modification based on the judgement of the physician and the preference of the patient, particularly when treating young adults (20–29 yrs), the elderly ($>$ 60), and women. The Expert Panel describes its approach as a patient-based one that seeks to identify individuals at high risk who will benefit from intensive intervention efforts. The goal was to establish criteria that define the candidates for medical intervention and to provide guidelines on how to detect, set goals for treatment and monitor these patients over time.

The Expert Panel initially classifies individuals by their total blood cholesterol level. The serum total cholesterol level should be measured in all adults 20 years and over, at least once every five years. To this end the National Cholesterol Education Program (NCEP) has adopted the slogan 'know your cholesterol level' for every adult American. Cholesterol is best measured in a conventional clinical laboratory. However, as increasing numbers of subjects are being screened this is frequently done using various portable chemical analysers that determine cholesterol in capillary blood specimens. This allows cholesterol to be measured quickly, conveniently, near painlessly, and cheaply. The patient does not have to be fasting; this is only required for concomitant triglyceride measurement.

Classification by total cholesterol

The best place to screen is in the doctor's surgery. Appropriate patients attending for various reasons can have their cholesterol checked at the same time (opportunistic screening). This can be conveniently combined with blood pressure and body weight measurements and cigarette smoking evaluation to provide a quick and easy assessment of cardiovascular risk.

Table 2.1

Initial classification based on total cholesterol	
< 5.2 mmol/l (< 200 mg/dl)	Desirable blood cholesterol
5.2–6.1 mmol/l (200–239 mg/dl)	Borderline–high blood cholesterol
⩾ 6.2 mmol/l (⩾ 240 mg/dl)	High blood cholesterol
Classification based on LDL-cholesterol	
< 3.4 mmol/l (< 130 mg/dl)	Desirable LDL-cholesterol
3.4–4.0 mmol/l (130–159 mg/dl)	Borderline high-risk LDL-cholesterol
⩾ 4.1 mmol/l (⩾ 160 mg/dl)	High-risk LDL-cholesterol

Cholesterol can also be measured in a public ('mass') screening setting as is becoming common. Public screening is acceptable provided that it is conducted with attention to several important considerations. The screenee should be provided with information to allow interpretation of his/her cholesterol level and whether he/she ought to see a physician for further evaluation and possible treatment. The Expert Panel designated levels below 5.2 mmol/l (200 mg/dl) as 'desirable blood cholesterol', between 5.2–6.1 mmol/l (200–239 mg/dl) as 'borderline high blood cholesterol' and 6.2 mmol/l (240 mg/dl) and above as 'high blood cholesterol' (Table 2.1). The cutpoint that defines high blood cholesterol is a value above which the risk of CHD rises steeply. It approximates the 75th percentile for the US adult population. The cutpoints recommended are uniform for adult men and women of all ages. Different cutpoints may be preferred for the UK population given its higher average cholesterol levels, as they are semi-arbitrary and can be adjusted, within limits, to influence the patient load that will flow from screening.

The Expert Panel report emphasizes the importance of other CHD risk factors (Table 2.2); along with cholesterol testing all adults should be evaluated for the presence of hypertension, cigarette smoking, diabetes mellitus, severe obesity, and a history of CHD in the patient, or of premature CHD in the family members. Being a male is also considered to be a risk factor for the purpose of estimating risk status. Patients with other risk factors should be given other forms of preventive care as appropriate.

Patients with a level below 5.2 mmol/l (200 mg/dl) are already in the desirable range (see Table 2.1). They should be given general dietary information designed to maintain them in this range. They should also receive risk reduction educational materials and should be advised to have another cholesterol test within five years given that cholesterol levels gradually rise through adult life. Patients with cholesterol levels 5.2 mmol/l (200 mg/dl) or greater should have their value confirmed by repeating the test; the average of the two test results then guide the subsequent decisions.

Patients with high blood cholesterol above 6.2 mmol/l (240 mg/dl) should undergo a lipoprotein analysis mainly to see whether the high total cholesterol is due to a high level of low density lipoprotein (LDL) cholesterol.

Table 2.2

The patient is considered to have a high risk status if he or she has one of the following:
Either:
Definite CHD: the characteristic clinical picture and objective laboratory findings of either
- Definite prior myocardial infarction, or
- Definite myocardial ischaemia, such as angina pectoris

Or: Two other CHD risk factors:
- Male sex*
- Family history of premature CHD (definite myocardial infarction or sudden death before age 55 in a parent or sibling)
- Cigarette smoking (currently smokes more than 10 cigarettes per day)
- Hypertension
- Low HDL-cholesterol concentration [below 0.91 mmol/l (35 mg/dl) confirmed by repeat measurement]
- Diabetes mellitus
- History of definite cerebrovascular or occlusive peripheral vascular disease
- Severe obesity ($\geqslant$ 30% overweight)

---

* Male sex is considered a risk factor in this scheme because the rates of CHD are three to four times higher in men than in women in the middle decades of life and roughly two times higher in the elderly. Hence, a man with one other CHD risk factor is considered to have a high risk status, whereas a woman is not so considered unless she has two other CHD risk factors.

Those with borderline high blood cholesterol 5.2–6.1 mmol/l (200–239 mg/dl) who already have definite CHD or two other risk factors for CHD should also be similarly evaluated. Patients in the borderline category without CHD or two other risk factors do not require further evaluation or active medical therapy; they should be given cholesterol-lowering diet information as is also appropriate for the general population and re-evaluated at one year (Table 2.3).

Classification by LDL-cholesterol

The ultimate objective of case-finding and screening is to identify individuals with elevated LDL-cholesterol levels. Once someone is identified as requiring lipoprotein analysis the focus of attention should shift from total cholesterol to LDL-cholesterol. It would be inappropriate to treat an individual whose high cholesterol is due to a high HDL-cholesterol as sometimes occurs in women especially in those receiving postmenopausal oestrogens. The specific goal of treatment is to lower LDL-cholesterol levels. Hence **the level of LDL-cholesterol serves as a key index for clinical decision-making about cholesterol-lowering therapy**. Lipoprotein analysis is simply performed and involves measurement of the fasting levels of total cholesterol, total triglyceride and HDL-cholesterol. From these values LDL-cholesterol is calculated as follows:

$$\text{LDL-cholesterol} = \text{total cholesterol} - \text{HDL-cholesterol} - \frac{\text{triglyceride}}{5}.$$

Table 2.3 Recommended follow-up

Total cholesterol < 5.2 mmol/l (< 200 mg/dl)	Repeat within 5 years
Total cholesterol 5.2–6.1 mmol/l (200–239 mg/dl)	
Without definite CHD or two other CHD risk factors (one of which can be male sex)	Dietary information and recheck annually
With definite CHD or two other CHD risk factors (one of which can be male sex)	Lipoprotein analysis; further action based on LDL-cholesterol level
Total cholesterol ⩾ 6.2 mmol/l (⩾ 240 mg/dl)	

When all concentrations in mg/dl (when expressed in mmol/l) VLDL cholesterol is estimated as triglyceride/2.17.

The Expert Panel classified LDL-cholesterol levels of 4.1 mmol/l (160 mg/dl) or greater as 'high-risk LDL-cholesterol' and those 3.4–4.0 mmol/l (130–159 mg/dl) as 'borderline high-risk LDL-cholesterol'. Patients with high-risk LDL-cholesterol levels and those with borderline high-risk LDL who have definite CHD or two other risk factors (one of which can be male sex) should have a complete clinical evaluation and then begin cholesterol-lowering treatment.

The clinical evaluation includes a complete history, physical examination, and basic laboratory tests. This assessment aims to determine whether the high LDL-cholesterol level is secondary to another disease or a drug and whether or not a familial lipid disorder is present. **The patient's total CHD risk and clinical status as well as age and sex should be considered in developing a cholesterol-lowering treatment programme.**

Dietary treatment

Treatment always begins with dietary therapy. Most elevations of cholesterol are dietary induced. Even under the occasional circumstances where a drug is necessary, diet should be maintained since the effects of diet and drug are usually additive. The minimal goals of therapy are to lower LDL-cholesterol to levels below the cutpoints for initiating therapy, that is to below 4.1 mmol/l (160 mg/dl) or to below 3.4 mmol/l (130 mg/dl) when definite CHD or two other CHD risk factors are present. However, even lower levels of LDL-cholesterol should ideally be obtained to achieve a further reduction in risk. The LDL-cholesterol level that is necessary to promote substantial or maximal atherosclerotic regression has not been established, but some investigators believe that an LDL-cholesterol as low as 2.6 mmol/l (100 mg/dl) may be considered an ideal goal. Thus, it may be desirable to strive for an LDL-cholesterol considerably below the minimal target goals of 4.1 mmol/l (160 mg/dl) or 3.4 mmol/l (130 mg/dl), particularly in patients with definite CHD or with other major risk factors, once

Table 2.4   Dietary therapy of high blood cholesterol

Nutrient	Recommended intake	
	Step-One Diet	Step-Two Diet
Total fat	Less than 30% of total calories	
Saturated fatty acids	Less than 10% of total calories	Less than 7% of total calories
Polyunsaturated fatty acids	Up to 10% of total calories	
Mono-unsaturated fatty acids	10 to 15% of total calories	
Carbohydrates	50 to 60% of total calories	
Protein	10 to 20% of total calories	
Cholesterol	Less than 300 mg/day	Less than 200 mg/day
Total calories	To achieve and maintain desirable weight	

the decision to institute therapy, particularly drug therapy, has been made.

Although the goal of therapy is to lower LDL-cholesterol most patients can be managed during dietary therapy on the basis of their total cholesterol levels avoiding additional costs and the need for fasting blood. Minimum goals during dietary therapy are to lower serum cholesterol level to below 6.2 mmol/l (240 mg/dl) for patients with an LDL-cholesterol goal below 4.1 mmol/l (160 mg/dl), and to below 5.2 mmol/l (200 mg/dl) for patients with an LDL-cholesterol goal of below 3.4 mmol/l (130 mg/dl).

Dietary therapy is designed to progressively reduce the intake of saturated fatty acids and cholesterol, which are not essential nutrients. The body can make these lipids in abundance. Therapy also aims to promote weight loss in overweight patients by eliminating excess total calories. It commences with the Step-One Diet which restricts total fat to less than 30% of calories, saturated fatty acids to less than 10% of total calories and cholesterol to less than 300 mg/day (Table 2.4). If the response to the Step-One Diet is insufficient, the Step-Two Diet is used which further reduces saturated fatty acid intake to less than 7% of total calories and cholesterol to less than 200 mg/day (Table 2.4). The involvement of a dietitian is very useful particularly when dietary therapy involves the Step-One Diet. The Step-Two Diet can be achieved by many patients without a radical alteration in dietary habits.

While a serum cholesterol-lowering diet requires modification of fat, it should be nutritious and palatable and include a variety of foods. Special attention has to be given to those foods which are the major sources of saturated fat and cholesterol in the diet (Table 2.5). The total fat intake should not exceed 30% of total calories; the typical western diet exceeds 40% of fat calories. For most saturated fatty acids intake will have to be reduced by about one-third to meet the requirements of the Step-One Diet and another third for the Step-Two Diet. Saturated fatty acids are found predominantly in animal fats and include butter fat contained in butter itself, whole milk, cream, ice cream and cheese, beef fat and pork fat. In addition, three oils, palm oil, palm kernel oil and coconut oil are especially

Table 2.5   Recommended diet modifications to lower blood cholesterol: the Step-One Diet

	Choose	Decrease
Fish, chicken, turkey, lean meats	Fish, poultry without skin, lean cuts of beef, lamb, pork, or shellfish	Fatty cuts of beef, lamb, pork; spare ribs, organ meats, regular cold cuts, sausage, hot dogs, bacon, sardines, roe
Skim and low-fat milk cheese, yogurt, and dairy substitutes	Skim or 1% fat milk (liquid evaporated) Buttermilk	Whole milk (4% fat): regular, evaporated, condensed; cream, half and half, 2% milk, imitation milk products, most non-dairy creamers, whipped toppings.
	Non-fat (0% fat) or low-fat yogurt	Whole-milk yogurt
	Low-fat cottage cheese (1% or 2% fat)	Whole-milk cottage cheese (4% fat)
	Low-fat cheeses, farmer or pot cheeses (all of these should be labelled no more than 2–6 g fat/ounce	All natural cheeses, (e.g. blue, roquefort, camembert, cheddar, swiss)
		Low-fat or 'light' cream cheese, low-fat or 'light' sour cream
		Cream cheeses, sour cream
	Sherbert Sorbet	Ice cream
Eggs	Egg whites (2 whites = 1 whole egg in recipes), cholesterol-free egg substitutes	Egg yolks
Fruits and vegetables	Fresh, frozen, canned, or dried fruits and vegetables	Vegetables prepared in butter, cream, or other sauces
Breads and cereals	Home-made baked goods using unsaturated oils sparingly, angel food cake, low-fat crackers, low-fat cookies	Commercial baked goods: pies, cakes, doughnuts, croissants, pastries, muffins, biscuits, high-fat crackers, high-fat cookies
	Rice, pasta	Egg noodles
	Whole-grain breads and cereals (oatmeal, whole wheat, rye, bran, multigrain, etc.)	Breads in which eggs are major ingredient
Fats and oils	Baking cocoa	Chocolate
	Unsaturated vegetable oils; corn, olive, rape seed (canola oil), safflower, sesame, soybean, sunflower	Butter, coconut oil, palm oil, palm kernel oil, lard bacon fat
	Margarine or shortening made from one of the unsaturated oils listed above	

Table 2.5—*continued*

	Choose	Decrease
	Diet margarine	
	Mayonnaise, salad dressings made with unsaturated oils listed above	Dressings made with egg yolk
	Low-fat dressings	
	Seeds and nuts	Coconut

rich in saturated fatty acids. They are sometimes referred to as tropical oils and together they have been estimated to contribute up to 8% of the intake of saturated fats of the US diet. Tropical oils appear in the ingredient list of many processed foods.

Dietary saturated fatty acids can be partly replaced by polyunsaturated fatty acids which can be increased to 10% of calories but not more. Very high intakes of polyunsaturated fatty acids were once but are no longer advocated for cholesterol lowering partly because there are no large human populations that habitually consume very high intakes of polyunsaturated fats. Vegetable oils rich in linoleic acid include safflower oil, sunflower seed oil, soybean oil, and corn oil. Fish oils are another source of polyunsaturated fatty acids. They have been found to lower triglyceride levels when given in high dosage, but there is little evidence that they are useful for reducing LDL-cholesterol levels. The use of fish oils capsules as a supplement in a therapeutic diet for high cholesterol levels is not recommended. However, fish can serve as a useful substitute for meats that are richer in saturated fatty acids.

In the Step-One or Step-Two Diets mono-unsaturated fatty acids, mainly oleic acids, should comprise 10–15% of total calories. Oleic acid is a major fatty acid found in olive oil, rape seed (canola oil), and high oleic acid forms of sunflower seed oil and safflower oil. The main use of polyunsaturated acids and mono-unsaturated fatty acids are to replace the cholesterol-raising saturated fatty acids. It is uncertain as to whether they have cholesterol-lowering properties per se.

Dietary cholesterol is derived exclusively from animal sources. It causes marked hypercholesterolaemia and atherosclerosis in many laboratory animals, including non-human primates. Although high intakes of cholesterol in humans rarely cause striking rises in the plasma cholesterol level, controlled metabolic studies show that dietary cholesterol usually raises the plasma cholesterol level. The degree of the rise varies from person to person. Overall, excess dietary cholesterol appears to contribute to the high LDL-cholesterol levels seen in high-risk patients and thus may add to CHD risk. Furthermore, concern about dietary cholesterol extends beyond its effects in raising the LDL-cholesterol level. Newly-absorbed cholesterol enters the circulation with chylomicrons, which are degraded to cholesterol-rich chylomicron remnants; the latter may be atherogenic. Dietary cholesterol is not required for normal body function. For practical purposes a cholesterol intake of less than 300 mg/day is reasonable as part of the first step in dietary management of high-risk LDL-cholesterol. However, further restriction, as recommended in the Step-Two Diet, is justified for patients who do not achieve the goals of therapy on the Step-One Diet despite adherence.

Cholesterol comes from animal products; particularly rich sources are egg yolk and organ meats (liver, sweetbreads, and brain), some shellfish such as shrimp are moderately high in cholesterol but not to the extent of egg yolk or organ meats. The flesh of all animals (beef, pork, lamb, chicken, and fish) contains cholesterol. Dairy products containing butterfat contribute cholesterol to the diet.

Drug treatment

The Expert Panel recommended that drug therapy should be considered for an adult patient who, despite dietary therapy, has an LDL-cholesterol level of 4.9 mmol/l (190 mg/dl) or higher (corresponding to an approximate total cholesterol level of 7.0 mmol/l [270 mg/dl or above]), if the patient does not have definite CHD or two other risk factors (one of which can be male sex). If the patient does have definite CHD or two other risk factors, then drug therapy should be considered when LDL-cholesterol levels are 160 mg/dl or higher. The goals of drug therapy are the same as those of dietary therapy, namely to lower LDL-cholesterol to below 4.1 mmol/l (160 mg/dl) or to below 3.4 mmol/l (130 mg/dl) if definite CHD or two other risk factors are present. Again it should be stressed that these are minimal goals; if possible considerably lower levels of LDL-cholesterol should be obtained.

It should be noted that the Expert Panel scheme does not advocate drug therapy for individuals who are below the levels for considering drug therapy but who have not yet achieved their target level through diet. This deliberate 'window' was introduced to avoid encouraging the overuse of drug therapy. In general, maximal efforts should be made in this intermediate group to achieve lower cholesterol levels and lower CHD risk by means of non-pharmacological approaches. Consideration can also be given to low doses of bile acid sequestrants in these patients, especially males. It was pointed out that many experts feel that patients with definite CHD should receive drug therapy if a minimal LDL-cholesterol goal of under 3.4 mmol/l (< 130 mg/dl) has not been reached.

The Expert Panel classified drugs which have been approved by the Food and Drug Administration (FDA) for lipid-lowering into three categories:

1. Drugs of first choice
2. New drugs: inhibitors of HMG CoA reductase
3. Other drugs

Drugs of first choice

To be classified as a drug of first choice an agent had to have been shown to be effective in reducing LDL-cholesterol levels (Table 2.6), to be acceptably safe over the long term and to have lowered CHD risk in clinical trials. The drugs which fulfilled these requirements are the bile acid sequestrants (cholestyramine, colestipol) and nicotinic acid.

The major effect of the bile acid sequestrants is a lowering of the level of LDL-cholesterol. They also produce a slight rise in HDL. They may further raise triglyceride levels when they are already elevated. The sequestrants are not absorbed in the gastrointestinal tract and lack systemic toxicity. The disadvantages of the sequestrants are related to the method of administration and the frequency of gastrointestinal side effects. The primary action is to bind bile acids in the intestinal lumen interrupting the intrahepatic circulation of bile acids and leading to an increased hepatic synthesis of bile acids from cholesterol. Depletion of the hepatic pool of cholesterol results in an increase in LDL receptor activity in the liver. This, in turn, stimulates removal of LDL from plasma lowering the concentration of LDL-cholesterol.

Cholestyramine and colestipol are both powders and must be mixed with

Table 2.6 Drugs highly effective in lowering LDL-cholesterol

Drug	Starting dose	Maximum dose	Usual time and frequency	Side effects	Monitoring
Cholestyramine	4 g twice daily	24 g/day	Twice daily within an hour of major meals	Dose-dependent upper and lower gastrointestinal	Dosing schedules of co-administered drugs
Colestipol	5 g twice daily	30 g/day			
Nicotinic acid	100–250 mg as single dose	3 g/day. Rarely, doses up to 6 g are used	Three times a day with meals to minimize flushing	Flushing, upper gastrointestinal and hepatic	Uric acid, liver function, glucose
Lovastatin*	20 mg once daily with evening meal	80 mg/day	Once (evening) or twice daily with meals	Gastrointestinal and hepatic, miscellaneous including muscle pain	Liver function, CPK, lens

* Other HMG-CoA reductase inhibitors also appear to be highly effective in lowering LDL-cholesterol using appropriate doses.

water or fruit juice. The cholesterol-lowering effects of 4 g of cholestyramine are equivalent to those obtained with 5 g of colestipol. Decreases in LDL-cholesterol of 10–15% may be achieved with the initial suggested starting dosage schedule of 5 g of colestipol (or 4 g of cholestyramine) taken twice daily. In patients who do not respond adequately, the dose is increased gradually. Generally the benefits of daily doses exceeding the equivalent of 16 g of cholestyramine are offset by poorer patient adherence and a greater incidence of gastrointestinal side effects. Reductions of 15–30% in the level of LDL-cholesterol may often be achieved with 16–24 g/day of cholestyramine or an equivalent dose of colestipol.

The most common side effects associated with sequestrant therapy are gastrointestinal, and include constipation, bloating, gastric fullness, nausea, and flatulence. Although not absorbed they may interfere with the absorption of other anionic drugs such as digoxin, warfarin, thyroxine, thiazide diuretics, beta blockers and others. It is generally advisable to take other medications at least one hour before or four hours after the bile acid sequestrants.

Nicotinic acid lowers total and LDL-cholesterol and triglycerides and raises HDL levels. It decreases hepatic production of VLDL and ultimately the production of LDL-cholesterol. It is a very effective drug which requires considerable physician and patient education. Its frequent side effects are generally reversible by reducing the dose or discontinuing the drug. Because of its proven efficacy and safety the Expert Panel regarded the efforts required to use this agent as justified. It has the added advantage of being the least costly of all the currently available agents. Side effects, especially flushing of the skin, often limit acceptance by patients, this can be significantly decreased by treatment with aspirin or non-steroidal anti-inflammatory drugs. Tolerance to this flushing develops rapidly over several weeks. Flushing is greatly reduced by slowly increasing nicotinic acid to its full dose and by avoiding administration on an empty stomach. Nicotinic acid therapy is generally initiated with a single dose of 100–250 mg/day. The frequency of dose and total daily dose is slowly increased every 4–7 days until the first-level therapeutic dose of 1.5–2 g/day is reached. If the LDL-cholesterol is not lowered sufficiently the dose should be increased to 3 g/day (1 g three times/day). In patients with marked elevation of plasma cholesterol a higher daily dose of up to 6 g/day is occasionally used.

Hyperuricaemia and abnormalities in liver function tests are other common adverse effects, but are more likely with higher doses of nicotinic acid. Hyperglycaemia and a number of gastrointestinal side effects occasionally occur. Liver function, blood glucose and uric acid levels should be evaluated before beginning nicotinic acid and after reaching therapeutic dosage or increasing the dose level. Contraindications to nicotinic acid therapy include peptic ulcer, hepatic disease and gouty arthritis or significant hyperuricaemia.

New drugs: inhibitors of HMG CoA reductase

This new class of cholesterol-lowering drugs is opening up a new era in cholesterol-lowering (Grundy 1988). They are very effective in reducing cholesterol levels and appear to have a low incidence of side effects as assessed in several thousand patients over several years. However, more time will be required before one can be certain regarding their long-term safety and there has also been insufficient time to assess the efficacy of these drugs in preventing CHD. One of these drugs, lovastatin, has been approved for prescription use in the US, others have been approved in the UK and elsewhere.

Most forms of hypercholesterolaemia respond to lovastatin treatment with reductions in LDL-cholesterol of 25–45%. Cholesterol-lowering results from these drugs increasing LDL receptor activity in the liver and thereby increasing the rate of receptor mediated removal of LDL from the plasma. Patients are generally started on 20 mg/day of lovastatin with the evening meal. The dose may be increased to 40 mg and then 80 mg/day as a single evening dose or divided doses with meals. The reported side effects to date have included changes in bowel function, headaches, nausea, fatigue, insomnia, skin rashes and myositis (myalgia associated with markedly elevated CPK levels) which collectively have occurred in less than 5% of treated patients. Biochemical changes have included increases in transaminases and CPK. About 2% of patients have developed persistent increases in transaminase levels of greater than three times normal after 3–16 months of therapy requiring discontinuance of therapy. Careful monitoring of liver function studies is essential. Lovastatin does not impair steroid hormone production. There is a concern that the drug may have effects on the formation of lens opacities but this has not been confirmed in human studies so far.

Other drugs

A. Gemfibrozil. Gemfibrozil is one of the two fibric acid derivatives approved by the FDA primarily for triglyceride-lowering to reduce the risk of pancreatitis and not for routine use for lowering cholesterol to reduce the risk of CHD. Gemfibrozil is highly effective in reducing triglycerides with an associated increase in HDL-cholesterol.

Gemfibrozil was used in the recently reported Helsinki Heart Study in which it reduced the incidence of CHD by 34% (Frick et al 1987). This finding prompted a footnote to be added to the Expert Panel report that, in view of the findings demonstrating the clinical efficacy and safety of gemfibrozil in reducing coronary risk in patients with high cholesterol levels, it would be reasonable for physicians to consider the use of gemfibrozil more readily when selecting drugs for patients with high cholesterol levels who meet the criteria for drug treatment. Gemfibrozil may be particularly useful, as an alternative to nicotinic acid, in patients with high LDL-cholesterol levels who also have borderline hypertriglyceridaemia (triglyceride levels 2.82–5.65 mmol/l or 250–500 mg/dl) and low HDL cholesterol levels.

Other fibric acid derivatives have been approved in several European and other countries but not yet in the US. They include fenofibrate, beza-fibrate, and ciprofibrate. Some of them are more effective cholesterol-reducing agents than gemfibrozil but have not yet been assessed in large-scale, long-term clinical trials of CHD prevention.

A hazard with fibric acid derivatives is their tendency to increase biliary lithogenicity so that they should be used cautiously by patients with gallstones.

B. Probucol. This drug reduces total cholesterol levels by moderate amounts but some of this is attributable to a marked reduction in HDL-cholesterol. It causes prolongation of the QT interval and is thus contrain-dicated in patients with ECG findings suggestive of ventricular irritability, with an initially prolonged QT interval or who are taking other drugs that prolong the QT interval.

In general its limited cholesterol-lowering ability, its HDL-lowering effects and the ECG changes, together with an absence of long-term clinical trial assessment of its CHD prevention efficacy, suggest that probucol should be used on a very limited basis. The tantalizing clinical observation that probucol use may lead to xanthoma regression in patients who have homozygous familial hypercholesterolaemia suggests that it may have other properties which merit further evaluation.

C. Clofibrate. This, too, is a fibric acid derivative approved by the FDA primarily for triglyceride-lowering to reduce the risk of pancreatitis and not for routine use in lowering cholesterol to reduce the risk of CHD. Its effect on lipids and lipoproteins and its side effects are generally similar to those described for gemfibrozil. Because of reports of long-term toxicity in clinical trials, particularly the WHO Clofibrate Study, it is used less frequently than gemfibrozil.

Combination drug therapy

The use of combination drug therapy is being increasingly explored. Combinations of two or three drugs used simultaneously have been very effective in producing marked reductions in total and LDL-cholesterol in severely hypercholesterolaemic patients. Thus the combination of a bile acid sequestrant with either nicotinic acid or lovastatin has the potential of lowering LDL-cholesterol by 45–60%. Combination drug therapy has been especially used in angiographic studies in which marked LDL lower-ing, together with different degrees of HDL elevation, have been found to stabilize coronary lesions, slow their progression and sometimes induce their regression. An increase risk of myositis, occasionally progressing to rhabdomyolysis, has been sometimes observed when lovastatin has been used in combination with nicotinic acid or gemfibrozil.

In summary it is possible using either diet or diet plus drug therapy to reduce cholesterol levels toward the desirable range in most patients in whom they are elevated. A dilemma still exists for those patients who maintain moderately elevated cholesterol levels despite dietary therapy but who have insufficient justification for drug therapy. In general we are moving into an era of much more aggressive and extensive cholesterol-lowering in an attempt to reduce CHD risk to as low a level as possible, compatible with safety and the avoidance of the overuse of drug therapy. Patients with coexisting CHD should be especially considered for cholesterol-lowering therapy.

REFERENCES

British Cardiac Society 1987 Report of British Cardiac Society working group on coronary disease prevention British Cardiac Society. British Medical Journal 299: 1475–1476

Brown M S, Goldstein J L 1986 A receptor-mediated pathway for cholesterol homeostasis. Science 232: 34–47

Castelli W P, Garrison R J, Wilson P W F, Abbott R D, Kalousdian S, Kannel W B 1986 Incidence of coronary heart disease and lipoprotein cholesterol levels. The Framingham Study. Journal of the American Medical Association 256: 2835–2838

Dargie H J 1989 Scottish hearts but British habits. British Medical Journal 299: 1475–1476

Frick M H, Elo O, Haapa K et al 1987 Helsinki Heart Study: Primary-Prevention Trial with gemfibrozil in middle-aged men with dyslipidemia. Safety of treatment, changes in risk factors, and incidence of coronary heart disease. New England Journal of Medicine 317: 1237–1245

Grundy S M 1988 HMG-CoA reductase inhibitors for treatment of hypercholesterolemia. New England Journal of Medicine 319: 24–33

Lipid Research Clinics Program 1984a The Lipid Research Clinics Coronary Primary Prevention Trial Results I. Reduction in incidence of coronary heart disease. Journal of the American Medical Association 251: 351–364

Lipid Research Clinics Program 1984b The Lipid Research Clinics Coronary Primary Prevention Trial Results II. The relationship of reduction in incidence of coronary heart disease to cholesterol lowering. Journal of the American Medical Association 251: 365–374

Report of the National Cholesterol Education Program Expert Panel on Detection, Evaluation, and Treatment of High Blood Cholesterol in Adults 1988. Archives of Internal Medicine 148: 36–69

Ross R 1986 The pathogenesis of atherosclerosis. New England Journal of Medicine 314: 488–500

Stamler J 1979 Population Studies. In: Levy R I, Rifkind B M, Dennis B H, Ernst N D (eds) Nutrition, lipids, and coronary heart disease: a global view. Raven Press, New York, pp 25–88

Yusuf S, Wittes J, Friedman L 1988 Overview of results of randomized clinical trials in heart disease II. Unstable angina, heart failure, primary prevention with aspirin and risk factor modification. Journal of the American Medical Association 260: 2259–2263

FURTHER READING

Consensus Conference Statement on lowering blood cholesterol to prevent heart disease 1985. Journal of the American Medical Association 253: 2080–2086

Havel R J 1988 Lowering cholesterol. Rationale, mechanisms and means. Journal of Clinical Investigation 81: 1653–1660

Rose, G 1985 Sick individuals and sick populations. International Journal of Epidemiology 14: 32–38

Study Group, European Atherosclerosis Society 1987 Strategy for the prevention of coronary heart disease: A policy statement for the European Atherosclerosis Society. European Heart Journal 8: 77–88

3. Dilemmas in the management of thromboembolic disease

C. D. Forbes

Thrombosis, both arterial and venous, remains the most important cause of death in all developed countries. Despite the major advances in knowledge about the mechanisms of thrombus formation there are still great areas of ignorance and uncertainty. Venous thrombi differ from arterial thrombi in that there is little or no platelet activation and histologically the main structure is a fibrin meshwork which has entrapped red cells, platelets and white cells.

Venous thrombosis is probably as common as arterial thrombosis but due to the difficulties in establishing a diagnosis it has been poorly documented and it is often only diagnosed when major life-threatening pulmonary embolism occurs. Numerous autopsy studies confirm how common undiagnosed venous thrombosis is, as in up to half of all patients dying in hospital, venous thrombi may be detected in the deep veins of the calf or thigh (Berquist & Lindblad 1985). In addition, between 10–30% of these cases have detectable pulmonary emboli and in 3–10% of cases embolism has been a major contributing factor to death. Implicit in these recorded figures is the knowledge that venous thrombosis and subsequent pulmonary embolism is associated in some cases with terminal events and irreversible disease. Such figures are difficult to quantify from the literature but a conservative estimate from the USA suggests a death rate of about 200 000 patients per year from pulmonary embolism—about half of whom have incurable disease. The implication is that about 100 000 patients per year die of a potentially preventable disease. Knowing that this figure represents only about 2–5% of those who had developed deep vein thrombosis (DVT) in the first place it will be appreciated how common venous thrombosis is. Also it will be appreciated how expensive it is to health care systems to prevent or treat and at a national level how expensive it is in productive-years-lost from those dying prematurely.

PATHOGENESIS OF DVT

The initial trigger to the development of DVT is unknown but it is clear that the condition never occurs when the venous endothelium is normal. The vast majority of DVTs occur in the deep veins of the leg, especially in the venous plexuses of the calf. For over 100 years it has been suggested (Virchow 1856) that three factors are implicated, i.e.

1. Changes in the vessel wall.
2. Alteration of the constituents of the blood.
3. Alteration of blood flow.

It is only recently, with advances in the understanding of the physiology of blood coagulation and related haemostatic parameters and further understanding of endothelial function and rheology that we now can attempt to postulate the sequence of events which have altered the normal protective mechanisms.

From animal experiments it is well established that a combination of venous stasis and activation of the blood coagulation cascade will induce thrombosis on the venous wall (Wessler et al 1959). This is probably the situation in man as DVT occurs in situations of venous stasis, such as paraplegia or hemiplegia or prolonged immobilization in a plaster cast. Normal venous flow depends on the action of the muscle pump and also on the viscosity of the blood. Viscosity may be increased in conditions such as primary proliferative polycythaemia as well as in conditions associated with a high fibrinogen level. Further evidence of the importance of venous return may be found therapeutically where it can be shown that intermittent leg compression by inflatable cuffs can significantly reduce the incidence of DVT. Also reduction of blood viscosity, e.g. by dilution, can be shown to have a similar action.

In association with stasis, activation of coagulation plays a key role in the development of thrombosis. How this occurs is unknown but there are situations where it can be proven, for example following the infusion of activated factor II, VII, IX, X concentrates in the management of bleeding in Christmas disease when deep vein thrombosis or disseminated intravascular coagulation (DIC) has been shown to occur. In addition we know both that patients lacking either antithrombin III or proteins C and S have a high probability of developing DVT, and that activation of coagulation following the release of endogenous thromboplastins, e.g. following burns, extensive tissue injury, surgery for cancer, etc. leads to DVT (Verstraete & Vermylen 1984).

There is little evidence that activation of platelets plays a key role in venous thrombosis. Histologically venous thrombi do not contain a 'white' platelet head as do arterial thrombi. Tests for platelet release factors are however often elevated during the acute illness and this presumably is a secondary phenomenon of platelet adhesion and aggregation to the surface of the developing thrombus. This can be shown using 'indium-labelled platelets' and may be used as a method of imaging the forming thrombi.

There is also evidence of down-regulation of fibrinolysis during the acute events which may be an important factor in allowing accumulation of fibrin with resulting extension of the growing thrombus.

Table 3.1   Risk factors for deep vein thrombosis and pulmonary thromboembolism

---

Clinical and laboratory factors
Advancing age (> 40 years)
Obesity (BMI > 25)
Trauma/surgery, especially orthopaedic
Immobility, especially paralysis of lower limbs
Malignancy
Previous DVT/PTE
Heart failure
Infection
Varicose veins
Pregnancy
Puerperium
Oestrogen therapy (high dose)
Presence of anticardiolipin antibody
A spectrum of medical conditions such as:
    nephrotic syndrome, myeloproliferative diseases, Behçet's disease, paroxysmal nocturnal haemoglobinuria, homocystinaemia
Deficiency of protective plasmaproteins i.e.
    antithrombin III, protein C and S., abnormal plasminogen, fibrinogen

---

Unfortunately, even with the explosion of knowledge of all these haemostatic systems there is as yet no available biochemical test which can be used diagnostically.

DIAGNOSIS OF DVT

Diagnosis of DVT remains a major clinical and investigative difficulty. The only way to establish with reasonable certainty that DVT is present is to undertake venography which remains the gold-standard test. This is clearly totally impossible in any population to be studied and even in major centres cannot be undertaken routinely. This throws the clinician back on old-fashioned clinical skills aided by some screening investigations. It is critical to a correct diagnosis to have knowledge of the background risk factors for DVT (Table 3.1) and a suspicious mind.

CLINICAL PRESENTATION

With the advent of specialist centres for the investigation and treatment of DVT it is now clear that only about 50% of patients with the disease have any clinical signs at all. This means that studies in the past which have used the onset of clinical signs to activate specialist investigations have grossly underestimated the incidence of this condition. For a review of the pitfalls of clinical diagnosis see Forbes & Lowe (1987).

Symptoms which may cause the patient to present include a sensation of pain, intermittent cramps and tenderness on touching or attempting to weight bear. The patient may occasionally be aware of a colour change which can range from redness through waxy whiteness to a mottled blue.

Table 3.2   Conditions mimicking deep vein thrombosis

Muscular strain	—usually obvious from the history
Popliteal cyst (Bakers cyst)	—usually associated with arthropathy of the knee
Haematoma of muscle	—often a history of injury
Leg swelling due to hemiplegia	
Cellulitis	
Lymphatic obstruction	
Lymphangitis	
Post-phlebitic leg	
Oedema due to heart failure, cirrhosis or nephrotic syndrome	
Arteriovenous fistula	

There may also be associated swelling and a systemic upset with fever and tachycardia. These symptoms may be present in any combination, however the first presentation may be acute pulmonary embolism (PTE).

The signs which may be present include swelling, with or without pitting oedema, increased temperature of the whole or part of the limb, tenderness over the deep veins, venous dilatation, change in colour (red, white, blue), superficial thrombophlebitis, varicose veins or ulceration. No signs may be present at all in the leg even when the patient has acute PTE.

An additional clinical dilemma occurs in patients who are known to have had a previous venous thrombosis and who present with recurrence of pain or swelling in the affected limb. In this situation oedema is to be expected as venous valves will have been damaged by the prior event, and there may also be early varicose veins. Clinical features are almost always unhelpful and investigations are mandatory because of the need for continuation of anticoagulant therapy.

The major additional problem is that none of the above symptoms and signs are specific to DVT and in half of the patients presenting in this way an alternate diagnosis requires to be considered (Table 3.2). These conditions, in their own right, require separate appropriate investigation.

Where does all this leave the worried clinician? He must maintain a high index of suspicion because the condition is so common. He must realize the major limitations of clinical features. Every hospital should have access to investigative facilities so that patients under suspicion can be rapidly and effectively screened and the presence or absence of DVT rapidly determined. This means a same-day service with all the administrative and economic implications.

WHAT INVESTIGATIONS SHOULD BE AVAILABLE

As has already been said clinical symptoms and signs of DVT are low in sensitivity and specificity. A diagnosis based solely on such symptoms and signs which leads to a patient receiving a course of anticoagulants is medical malpractice and certainly in the USA has involved doctors being sued. The same will happen elsewhere as patients become better informed. A range of invasive and non-invasive techniques are now available and the pros and cons of these have recently been discussed (Whitehouse 1990).

Venography

Venography remains the accepted reference standard for the diagnosis of DVT. This is not a difficult technique and can be rapidly mastered by a competent registrar. It is best done by injection of the contrast medium via a vein on the dorsum of the foot so that the deep venous system is outlined. With good technique, care and modern contrast medium it should be possible to outline all the leg veins as well as the veins in the pelvis and the inferior vena cava. The technique may be associated with local discomfort especially if DVT is indeed present. With all contrast media there is still a risk of allergy to iodine, local tissue injury if the contrast is extravasated and possibly a very small incidence of irritation to the veins locally. It is, however, a reasonably safe technique which should be readily available and should provide a rapid answer. It can also be repeated at a later date if further signs develop and if the patient will allow it (Hull et al 1981).

Non-invasive tests

There are a large number of non-invasive tests which immediately indicates that none are totally satisfactory. They include ^{125}I-fibrinogen leg scanning, impedance plethysmography (IPG), Doppler ultrasound, thermography, radio-isotope venography, strain gauge plethysmography and ultrasonic imaging. Perhaps the most widely used has been ^{125}I-fibrinogen scanning. A huge literature has developed round this but a major safety scare about the source of the fibrinogen and the question of freedom from HIV has cast major doubts over its future use. Also IPG has had doubts cast on its specificity as it has recently been shown to be insensitive to non-occluding thrombi. Thermography and current isotope techniques are of little value. The best hope is ultrasound as it is cheap, readily available, easily repeatable, non-invasive and gives a rapid answer in the proximal venous system—the part in which thrombi form and embolize. It probably will become the screening method of choice despite its deficiencies. Recent studies with magnetic resonance imaging suggest that if available it will be a useful tool in DVT diagnosis and also in the diagnosis of other pathologies which mimic DVT (Erdman et al 1990).

PULMONARY EMBOLISM

Despite programmes aimed at prevention of DVT, pulmonary embolism (PTE) remains a significant clinical event. Non-fatal PTE will be found in approximately 12–15/1000 inpatients and fatal PTE in about 1–2/1000 inpatients in hospitals with acute medical and surgical services, especially

Table 3.3   Background problems often found in patients who develop PTE (Sasahara et al 1973)

Associated risk	(%)
Enforced bed rest	59
Coexistent DVT	45
Prior heart/lung disease (especially failure)	35
Miscellaneous disorders (vascular, collagen, etc.)	18
Cancer	6
Oral contraceptive use	24*

* This figure is now historical and was associated with the use of oral contraceptives containing 100 μg of oestrogen. The figure now is insignificant.

orthopaedics. The vast majority of pulmonary emboli arise from thrombi in the proximal leg veins which become dislodged. The majority of deaths from pulmonary emboli (80%) occur within a few hours of the acute event, i.e. the majority die before acute interventional thoracic surgery can be done. Therefore prevention of death from PTE should be wholly aimed at DVT prevention.

There is good evidence that early diagnosis of PTE and early treatment can significantly reduce mortality by up to four-fold. So how can the doctor make an early diagnosis? The difficulties are similar to those of DVT. The classical 'textbook' symptoms and signs may be minimal or totally absent and the presentation may be protean, so that the best test is clinical suspicion and the use of rapid effective screening investigations. Pulmonary embolism rarely occurs in people who have been previously totally well and free of any prior risk factor. The most important background factor is enforced bed rest usually in someone recovering from a surgical operation, or with immobilized long bone fractures or bed bound with another disease such as heart failure or cancer. Such a scenario is found in over 90% of proven PTE cases. Coexistent deep vein thrombosis is found in about 50% of such cases. The other background problems are listed in Table 3.3. It is often the development of an acute PTE in someone with the above background that alerts the clinician (Sasahara et al 1987).

The clinical symptoms are often non-specific when they do occur at all and it is clear that most small pulmonary emboli are missed because they produce no symptoms or trivial ones. Larger emboli may produce one of three distinct syndromes: (a) acute cor pulmonale, (b) pulmonary infarction, (c) acute pulmonary embolism.

Acute cor pulmonale is due to a large sized embolism suddenly obstructing the outflow tract of the right ventricle and this is often associated with acute onset dyspnoea, cyanosis, signs of acute right ventricular failure with severe hypertension and shock. Pulmonary infarction symptoms tend to occur somewhat later after an acute event and the dominant feature is acute pleuritic chest pain which is often associated with haemoptysis. They will

Table 3.4 Symptoms and signs of pulmonary embolism (Sasahara et al 1973)

	% of patients
Symptoms	
Dyspnoea	83
Pleuritic chest pain	78
Cough	60
Apprehension	59
Haemoptysis	30
Signs	
Tachypnoea (> 20/min)	85
Accentuated P_2	55
Rales	55
Tachycardia (> 100/min)	51
Fever ($> 37.8°C$)	45
Phlebitis	35
$S_3 S_4$ gallop	34
Sweating	34
Pleural rub	20
Cyanosis	18

often have signs of pleural friction and may develop a pleural effusion. Acute pulmonary embolism may be associated with dyspnoea and pain with signs of tachypnoea, tachycardia and fever (Table 3.4).

As already emphasized all these clinical symptoms and signs are non-specific and may be found in the other clinical conditions which beset the population at risk, e.g. acute myocardial infarction, heart failure, pneumonia, pneumothorax, septic shock, etc. A battery of simple bedside tests are usually done but they are of little value in confirming the diagnosis. The ECG, chest X-ray and blood gases may be normal or if abnormal any changes are not diagnostic. A range of ECG changes were found in the National Cooperative Trial (NHLBI) (Table 3.5). Similarly the X-ray of chest may show a range of non-specific changes (Table 3.6). Perhaps the two most important radiological features which should raise suspicion of

Table 3.5 Incidence of abnormalities in the ECG after acute PTE (modified Sasahara et al 1973)

ECG changes	(%)
Arrhythmias	11
QRS abnormalities	44*
T-wave abnormalities	40
ST segment abnormalities	35
P pulmonale	4

* The $S_1Q_3T_3$ abnormality originally described by Paul Wood as being diagnostic of PTE was found in 11%.

Table 3.6 Chest X-ray abnormalities in patients with the diagnosis of acute PTE confirmed (after Sasahara et al 1973 and NHLBI)

X-ray changes	(%)
Infiltrate or consolidation	41
Elevated hemidiaphragm	41
Pleural effusion	28
Increased pulmonary artery diameter	23
Atelectasis	20
Left ventricular enlargment	16
Focal oligaemia	15
Right ventricular enlargement	5

PTE are infiltration or consolidation associated with a raised hemidiaphragm on the affected side. Blood gases often show evidence of a drop in po_2 values, the extent of this often parallels the size of the embolism. This is abnormal in 90% of patients but is of course not specific for the diagnosis. Other tests may be of some value when considering the differential diagnosis, e.g. the white cell count is often normal initially as PTE is not an inflammatory disease. Enzyme levels in plasma are not particularly helpful, creatine phosphokinase (CPK) may be slightly elevated (it can be in pneumonia as well); AST, LDH and bilirubin measurements were once thought to be helpful as in pulmonary infarction LDH and bilirubin were elevated due to release from damaged red cells and AST was normal (urobilinogen is also elevated); measurement of products of coagulation and fibrinolysis can be shown to have elevated levels but are not specific for PTE.

Once the suspicion has formed in the medical attendant's mind it is important to proceed rapidly to an appropriate screening test to prove the diagnosis. It is bad medical practice to sentence a patient to a course of anticoagulants without a definite diagnosis. Having said that the problem is to know which test to do: lung scanning or angiography. Pulmonary angiography is said to be the gold standard reference test for the diagnosis of PTE. The problem is that it is not *routinely* available except in a few specialized centres. The diagnosis of PTE is made if there are constant intraluminal filling defects and if there are sharp cut offs in vessels of reasonable size (> 2.5 mm diameter). Angiography carries a small mortality which can be further reduced by selective angiography. There remains, however, a small mortality and a modest morbidity which when added to the expense of the technique means that it is rarely used outside specialist centres staffed by enthusiasts.

The more widely used technique is that of pulmonary scanning using both a perfusion and ventilation phase (i.e. V/Q scanning—Hull et al 1985). This has now become the routine screening test for PTE in the UK. Perfusion scanning is carried out after injection of ^{99m}Tc-labelled macroaggregates of albumin into a forearm vein. These particles, which are about

100 µ in size, embolize into capillaries in the lung and demonstrate relatively the current state of lung perfusion. Pulmonary emboli cause a defect in perfusion and this shows on the γ camera image as a 'cold' area. This must of course be interpreted in conjunction with the known clinical history and X-rays, as perfusion defects may be found in a range of conditions such as pneumonia, emphysema, atelectasis, bronchial carcinoma, pleural effusion, heart failure, post-radiotherapy and following lung surgery. For the ventilation scan the patient inhales ^{133}Xe or ^{127}Xe in air from a spirometer and the distribution is imaged at a separate time on the γ-camera. Defects in *perfusion* are usually associated with normal *ventilation* in that area, i.e. there is mismatching of perfusion and ventilation. These features are not absolute but they allow patients to be allocated into a series of management groups:

1. Normal perfusion scan/normal ventilation scan which virtually excludes PTE.
2. Perfusion defect matched by a ventilation defect in a person with a normal chest X-ray signifies a very low probability and probably no specific anticoagulant therapy is indicated.
3. Multiple lobar or segmental defects in perfusion associated with a normal ventilation scan and a normal X-ray of chest suggests a high probability and indicates the need for appropriate antithrombotic treatment.
4. Perfusion defects are present but correspond with lesions seen on the chest X-ray or are mismatched with the ventilation scan. This group is a diagnostic problem and may account for 10–20% of the patients seen. In this group a search should be made for a source of emboli, i.e. by venography, IPG or leg scanning with ultrasound. If positive they should then be treated with appropriate antithrombotic treatment. In specialist centres this subgroup would be considered for pulmonary angiography.

PREVENTION OF VENOUS THROMBOSIS AND PULMONARY EMBOLISM

As in every disease state it is logical to attempt to prevent the onset of the disease rather than attempt to reverse the ravages—a much more difficult problem. The most cost-efficient way to proceed is to identify patients who are at risk of DVT and give all of them prophylaxis (Hirsh et al 1981). There is now a huge literature on this subject which clearly indicates the value of this course of action and it is a source of disappointment that only a minority of doctors use effective methods which have been clearly proven to reduce the incidence of DVT, subsequent PTE and probably in the long term, the post-phlebitic limb. The groups of patients at risk have been well documented from hundreds of studies using a variety of screening techniques such as ^{125}I-fibrinogen scanning, IPG, ultrasound and venography. Most studies have focused on surgical patients, i.e. general abdominal, orthopaedics, urology and cardiovascular surgery and there has been less interest in medical cases. Medical studies show a high incidence of DVT/ PTE in hemiplegic stroke, paraplegia, heart failure and cancer. Review of these studies using meta-analysis techniques has at last produced reliable figures of DVT and PTE incidence, and the value of prevention regimes (Collins et al 1988). The evidence from these meta-analyses is that in a wide range of surgery the incidence of DVT is from 20–40% and that this can be significantly *reduced* by a half to a quarter with a simple regime of low dose subcutaneous heparin. In a range of orthopaedic operations (hip fractures and replacement) DVT incidence is 45–65% and the risk of DVT can be reduced by a half to two-thirds with low dose heparin. Figures for pulmonary embolism are more difficult to obtain but for fatal pulmonary embolism deaths may be reduced by a half to two-thirds as can the figures for total mortality. Earlier studies suggest the same reduction can be achieved with oral anticoagulants (Morris & Mitchell 1976). International guidelines on prevention have already been published—National Institutes of Health Consensus Development Conference Statement 1986 and an updated and modified document is currently in production for the UK (*Thr*ombembolic *Ri*sk *Fa*ctors (THRIFT) Consensus Group 1991). Patients at risk should be allocated into a mild, moderate and high risk group according to the published criteria and should have an appropriate prevention regime which may involve graduated compression stockings, intermittent pneumatic compression devices, dextran 70, heparin (unfractionated or low molecular weight) or oral anticoagulants.

Pregnancy and the puerperium have very specialized problems and the reader is referred to the excellent review of this topic by Greer (1989).

TREATMENT OF ESTABLISHED DVT/PTE

The treatment of choice is anticoagulation which is aimed at preventing the extension of the thrombus or embolus while allowing the normal process of fibrinolysis to reduce it in size and also permit the normal healing process to proceed. The agents most commonly used are standard unfractionated heparin and warfarin. Before starting these drugs it is important to ensure that no bleeding risk is present (Table 3.7).

Heparin is a mixture of glycosaminoglycans of a range of molecular weights from 2000–50 000 daltons. It acts in conjunction with anti-thrombin III with which it forms a complex. This combination is then potently anti-Xa and anti-IIa but with minor actions on other activated factors (IXa, XIa and XIIa). Because heparin is sensitive to digestion in the alimentary tract it should be given by intravenous infusion after a loading dose. Subcutaneous injection may also be used but most authors prefer the intravenous route which produces better long term anticoagulant control.

Table 3.7 Contraindications to the use of anticoagulants

Subarachnoid or recent cerebral haemorrhage (6/12)
Active bleeding from any site
Recent surgery, trauma, or delivery
Any bleeding tendency (genetic or acquired)
Bacterial endocarditis
Renal or hepatic failure
Recent arterial puncture
Diabetic retinopathy
Malignant hypertension
Known allergy to heparin

Enough heparin should be given to control the activated partial thrombo-plastin time at 1.5 to 2 times the control. A reasonable starting dose of heparin is 20 000 units per 12 hours after a bolus loading dose of 5000 units. Heparin requires to be continued for five days. There is little evidence that there is any benefit in giving it for longer and indeed this policy seems to be associated with a proportionately greater incidence of bleeding.

The administration of heparin may be associated with thrombocyto-penia, allergic reactions, alopecia and in the long term may produce osteoporosis. The incidence of thrombocytopenia is reported in from 0–30% of patients, particularly from North America. In the UK it is reported in well under 5% of patients. There are two recognized causes, the first occurs soon after the start of the infusion, is associated with a modest fall in platelet count and is due to a heparin/platelet interaction. The second type is more severe producing a major fall in platelet count and occurs later in heparin therapy. A heparin-dependent IgG antibody has been identified in this type and it may be due to an immune based reaction. Osteoporosis is only seen with prolonged administration. Bleeding which occurs during heparin therapy can be easily reversed using protamine sulphate.

An exciting advance in heparin therapy both for prevention and also treatment is the production of low molecular weight heparins either by filtration or degradation of the larger molecules. These have a molecular weight of 3000–10 000 daltons and have a greater anti-Xa than anti-IIa activity and thus retain their antithrombotic potential without the risk of inducing bleeding by acting as anticoagulants. They also do not have an antiplatelet action and thus may reduce the risk of inducing bleeding.

Oral anticoagulant therapy

Warfarin is the oral anticoagulant of choice in the UK and is usually started at the same time as the heparin infusion in a dose of 10 mg/day for two days and on the third day the prothrombin time (or equivalent test) is performed using a standard thromboplastin reagent. Warfarin requires this period for its action because it works by interfering with the hepatic production of biologically active molecules of factors II, VII, IX and X by virtue of inhibition of the enzyme, vitamin K epoxide reductase. Its action starts in about 12 hours after warfarin administration and is optimal at 48 hours. Tests should be reported by the laboratory as the International Normalized Ratio (INR) and should be maintained at 2–4.5 using a sliding scale nomogram (Fergusson et al 1987). Such therapy should be continued for 12 weeks. There is little evidence that there is benefit from a longer period of administration especially when the chances of bleeding are considered. Bleeding is the major risk as so many drug interactions may occur. The reader is referred to the Standing Advisory Committee 1982 for further details of these drug effects. Bleeding should be managed by stopping the warfarin and giving vitamin K, intravenously. In severe life-threatening bleeding a decision to use fresh frozen plasma or factor concentrates should be considered but these carry the risk of virus transmission and are not to be used lightly.

In addition to conventional anticoagulants fibrinolytics have been used both in DVT and PTE. There is little evidence they produce a better end result than anticoagulants.

Surgery has little or no place in the routine management of DVT or in PTE except for the emplacement of vena caval 'filters'. The decision to do this is very difficult and has usually been based on the finding of large free-floating proximal vein thrombi. However, recent studies with repeated imaging show that these thrombi are not as dangerous as were predicted. Most lyse spontaneously and do not break off and embolize (Baldridge et al 1990). Further studies are required to define the criteria necessary for this potentially life-saving but extremely expensive procedure.

Recurrent venous thromboembolism

Despite the optimal management outlined, up to 10% of patients will have recurrent venous thrombosis or pulmonary emboli. These require to be confirmed objectively as aches and pains and swelling of the legs are commonly seen for some years after a DVT. The adequacy of the anti-coagulant regime (if still applicable) should be reviewed and a search made for any underlying disorder which may be pro-thrombotic, i.e. latent cancer, deficiency of protein C and S and antithrombin III or an abnormal fibrinogen or plasminogen.

SUMMARY

Deep vein thrombosis and pulmonary embolism remain a major source of morbidity and mortality in the Western world. Despite clear evidence that a significant amount of this disease can be prevented by relatively safe means, there has been a general failure so to do. Part of the problem is education of doctors whose views on the risks v benefits of antithrombotic therapy may be outdated, and another is failure of patients to educate themselves and demand modern prophylaxis. Various groups, e.g. THRIFT have been set up to remedy the knowledge gap but they face an uphill struggle. It is clear that doctors change attitudes only slowly and may need strong incentives so to do. Such incentives have now appeared in the form of court cases in which actions are being raised against doctors who have not offered any form of prophylaxis to patients in an 'at-risk' situation.

REFERENCES

Baldridge E D, Martin M A, Welling R B 1990 Clinical significance of free-floating thrombi. Journal of Vascular Surgery 11: 62–69
Berquist D, Lindblad B 1985 A thirty-year survey of pulmonary embolism verified at autopsy: an analysis of 1274 surgical patients. British Journal of Surgery 72: 105–108
Collins R, Scrimgeour A, Yusuf S et al 1988 Reduction in fatal pulmonary embolism and venous thrombosis by perioperative administration of subcutaneous heparin. New England Journal of Medicine 318: 1162–1173
Erdman W A, Jayson H T, Redman H C et al 1990 Deep venous thrombosis of extremities: role of MR imaging in the diagnosis. Radiology 174: 425–431
Fergusson R J, Eade O E, Logie A W et al 1987 A flexible loading dose schedule for warfarin therapy. Scottish Medical Journal 32: 169–171
Forbes C D, Lowe G D O 1987 In Hirsh J (ed) Clinical diagnosis in venous thrombosis and pulmonary embolism. Churchill Livingstone, Edinburgh, pp 9–20
Greer I A 1989 Thromboembolic problems in pregnancy. Fetal Medicine Review 1: 79–103
Hirsh J, Genton E, Hull R 1981 Venous thromboembolism. Grune & Stratton, New York, p 1–5
Hull R, Hirsh J, Carter C et al 1985 Diagnostic value of ventilation-perfusion lung. Scanning in patients with suspected pulmonary embolism. Chest 88: 819–828
Hull R, Hirsh J, Sacket D L et al 1981 Cost-effectiveness of clinical diagnosis, venography and non-invasive testing in patients with symptomatic deep-vein thrombosis. New England Journal of Medicine 304: 1551–1567
Morris G K, Mitchell J R A 1976 Warfarin sodium in prevention of deep vein thrombosis and pulmonary embolism in patients with fractured neck of femur. Lancet 2: 869–872
National Cooperative Trial (NHLBI) 1974 Urokinase—streptokinase pulmonary embolism trial Phase 2 results. Journal of the American Medical Association 229: 1606–1613
National Institutes of Health Consensus Development Conference Statement 1986 Prevention of venous thrombosis and pulmonary embolism. NIH Consensus Development 6 (No. 2), 1–7
Sasahara A A, Hyers T M, Cole C M et al 1973 Urokinase pulmonary embolism trial: a national cooperative trial. Circulation 47 (suppl II): 1–108
Sasahara A A, Sharma G V R K, Pietro D A 1987 In: Hirsh J (ed) The clinical diagnosis of acute pulmonary embolism in venous thrombosis and pulmonary embolism. Churchill Livingstone, Edinburgh, pp 123–133
Standing Advisory Committee for Haematology of the Royal College of Pathologists 1982 Drug interaction with coumarin derivative anticoagulants. British Medical Journal 285: 274–275
Thromboembolic Risk Factors (THRIFT) Consensus Group 1991. To be published— personal communication
Verstraete M, Vermylen J 1984 Thrombosis. Pergamon Press, Oxford pp 1–54
Virchow R 1856 Gessammelte Abhandlungen zur. Wissenschaftlichen Medizin. Von Meidlinger Sohn, Frankfurt-am-Main
Wessler S, Reiner L, Freiman D G et al 1959 Serum induced thrombosis. Circulation 20: 864–874
Whitehouse G H 1990 Venous thrombosis and thromboembolism. Clinical Radiology 41: 77–80

FURTHER READING

Browse N L, Burnand K G, Thomas M L 1988 Diseases of the veins. Pathology diagnosis and treatment. Edward Arnold, London

Hirsh J, Genton E, Hull R 1981 Venous thrombo-embolism. Grune & Stratton, New York

Lane D A, Lundahl U I 1989 Heparin. Chemical and biological properties and clinical application. Edward Arnold, London

Ogston D 1987 Venous thrombosis: causation and prediction. Wiley, Chichester

4. The sleep apnoea/hypopnoea syndrome

N. J. Douglas

INTRODUCTION

The importance of the sleep apnoea/hypopnoea syndrome in causing morbidity and mortality is only slowly being realized by many physicians in both Britain and the developing world. The condition is characterized by daytime sleepiness and impaired daytime function in loud snorers and may occur in around 1% of the population. In the 30 years since it was first described, understanding of the mechanisms, consequences and treatment has grown considerably. Nevertheless, many physicians still fail to make this important diagnosis.

DEFINITION

The best definition in young or middle-age patients is the presence of more than 15 apnoeas plus hypopnoeas per hour of sleep in conjunction with at least two major symptoms (Gould et al 1988). In adults, an apnoea is defined as cessation of airflow for at least 10 seconds and a hypopnoea as a 50% reduction in thoracoabdominal movement for at least 10 seconds (Fig. 4.1). Many other definitions have been used, but these have been

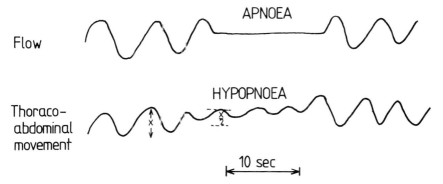

Fig. 4.1 Definitions of apnoeas and hypopnoeas indicating that an apnoea is a 10 second cessation of airflow and a hypopnoea a 10-second period where thoracoabdominal movement is reduced by 50%.

more lax, and it is now recognized that many normal subjects fulfil such criteria (Gould et al 1988). There are few good population-based studies to indicate the prevalence of the sleep apnoea/hypopnoea syndrome. The largest studies currently available would indicate a likely prevalence of around 1% of the adult population (Lavie 1983). Although other small studies suggest prevalences of up to 10%, this seems inherently unlikely.

MECHANISMS

Almost all apnoeas result from airway occlusion around the level of the soft palate or the back of the tongue (Fig. 4.2) and hypopnoeas result from severe narrowing without occlusion at the same level. The pressure within the upper airway on inspiration is subatmospheric and airway patency depends upon the contraction of upper airway opening muscles. These muscles, including genioglossus, geniohyoid and omohyoid, contract actively with each inspiration. During sleep, muscle tone drops throughout the body and the upper airway opening muscles are no exception. Thus, there is a greater tendency for the upper airway to narrow on inspiration during sleep. If the airway narrows subcritically, turbulent flow occurs resulting in the vibration of snoring. If the airway occludes almost totally, hypopnoeas occur and occlusion results in apnoeas.

The intraluminal pressure sucking the airway closed will depend on the

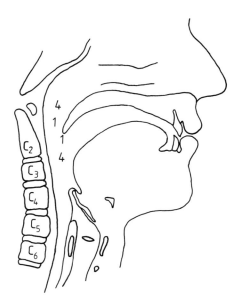

Fig. 4.2 Location of upper airways obstruction in 10 patients with sleep apnoea/hypopnoea syndrome. The numbers in the upper airway indicate the number of patients obstructing at that level (from Chaban et al 1988).

resistance of the upstream airway (nose and nasopharynx) and on flow rate. Patients with the sleep apnoea/hypopnoea syndrome have increased pharyngeal resistance and narrower upper airways when awake. The upper airways of patients with the syndrome are not only narrow but they narrow further when lung volume falls, as occurs during apnoeas. Patients with the syndrome have smaller mandibles than controls and this may contribute to the narrowing of their upper airways. Obesity also contributes to narrowing of the upper airway, due to submucosal fat deposition around the nasopharynx (Horner et al 1989).

Almost all apnoeas in patients with the sleep apnoea/hypopnoea syndrome are obstructive, but so-called mixed and central apnoeas also occur. I do not think that this classification of apnoeas is either clinically or aetiologically valuable as:

1. Many patients have all three types of apnoeas.
2. The treatment of central apnoeas with diaphragm pacing and of obstructive apnoeas by tracheostomy may increase the alternate type of apnoea.
3. Patients with central apnoeas have abnormal upper airways.
4. Positive airway pressure therapy abolishes mixed apnoeas and most central apnoeas.

It is more useful to divide apnoeas into those which are responsive to continuous positive airway pressure (CPAP) and those which are not (CPAP resistant). CPAP resistant apnoeas are rare and as yet remain poorly understood.

Once airway occlusion or near occlusion has occurred in patients with the sleep apnoea/hypopnoea syndrome, normal breathing is only restored by a brief (1–5 seconds) awakening which is not recalled by the patient. The arousal is not directly caused by hypoxaemia but results from the negative intrapleural pressure generated as the patient struggles to breathe. After the arousal the patient rapidly falls back to sleep, his upper airway narrows, he snores, and with further upper airway narrowing becomes apnoeic or hypopnoeic. This cycle of arousal followed by apnoea followed by arousal recurs all night and the patient may have up to 100 arousals per hour. This disrupted sleep results in the characteristic daytime sleepiness.

CLINICAL FEATURES

Daytime sleepiness and loud snoring are the hallmarks of the sleep apnoea/hypopnoea syndrome (Whyte et al 1989; Table 4.1).

The extent of daytime sleepiness varies markedly from patient to patient. The most severely affected patients may be unable to complete a sentence without falling asleep. However, most find that they fall asleep only when idle or performing monotonous tasks, such as driving on motorways. Patients with the sleep apnoea/hypopnoea syndrome have more accidents

Table 4.1 Clinical features of sleep apnoea/ hypopnoea syndrome

	% with feature
Loud snoring	97
Daytime sleepiness	88
Restless sleep	36
Unsatisfying sleep	35
Nocturnal choking	26
Morning headache	24
Irritability	11
Nocturia	10
Decreased libido	6
Ankle swelling	33
Respiratory failure	13
Polycythaemia	10

than controls, and their driving skills improve with therapy (Findley et al 1989). I have patients who have fallen asleep whilst driving buses and lorries and even when flying planes. In addition to such hazardous consequences, daytime sleepiness frequently causes major problems and embarrassment at work. I have patients who fall asleep chairing meetings, interviewing job applicants and when on security duties. Even when awake, the work performance of sufferers is impaired with poor concentration and impaired learning skills. One of the commoner presentations for children is failing to achieve potential in education.

The snoring of the sleep apnoea/hypopnoea syndrome is extremely loud and intermittent. The absence of a history of snoring is a strong pointer against the presence of the sleep apnoea/hypopnoea syndrome but does not exclude it. Some patients do not have a bed partner, some bed partners seem either extremely unobservant or are themselves somnolent and miss very marked snoring! A history of snoring in those without bed partners should be sought from other family members—the snoring is so loud that patients have occasionally been referred by their neighbours! When interviewing potential patients, it is important to speak to the bed partner where possible, both to get a clear picture of the snoring but also to ascertain whether apnoeas have been witnessed. Often the spouse becomes so concerned about the frequent apnoeas that their own sleep is disrupted as they anxiously await the termination of the apnoeas, or repeatedly prod the patients to stimulate resumption of breathing. It is all too easy to see how individuals who keep their bed partners awake each night by snoring and by thrashing about in bed, who have job difficulties and who fall asleep in mid-conversation when their spouse remonstrates during the daytime, become unpopular at home.

Patients usually find nocturnal sleep unsatisfying, awaking most mornings feeling that they have not been refreshed by their sleep. Many patients have occasional episodes of nocturnal choking, presumed to be due to the upper airway opening muscle tone returning after the patient has awoken. These extremely frightening episodes seem to last up to a minute in duration. Many patients experience nocturia which appears to be due to excess salt and water excretion due to atrial natriuretic peptide secretion being stimulated by the apnoeas. Enuresis may occur, particularly in young patients. Decreased libido is a common problem in North American and Australasian patients but less common in our own experience. This may reflect different aspirations in the different cultures.

Around 85% of patients with the sleep apnoea/hypopnoea syndrome are male. The explanation for this is not known but testosterone is important as the syndrome has been induced by testosterone administration both in hypogonadal males and in females. It seems likely that testosterone promotes fat deposition in the neck, thus narrowing the upper airway.

While most patients with the sleep apnoea/hypopnoea syndrome are overweight, obesity is by no means a prerequisite. Between one-half and one-third of patients are within 30% of ideal body weight and around 20% of patients within 15% of ideal body weight. Thus, it is important to consider this diagnosis in the thin as well as in the obese.

Patients with severe longstanding sleep apnoea may develop the hypoxaemic complications of cor pulmonale and secondary polycythaemia and also daytime carbon dioxide retention, particularly if they have coexisting lung disease (Bradley et al 1985). The combination of these features in a patient with the sleep apnoea/hypopnoea syndrome comprises the 'Pickwickian Syndrome' so called because of Dickens' description of Joe the fat boy in the Pickwick Papers. The 'Pickwickian Syndrome' is apparently declining in frequency in the USA as the sleep apnoea/hypopnoea syndrome is being diagnosed at an earlier stage before the nightly recurrent hypoxia and hypercapnia results in sustained pulmonary hypertension and blunted daytime ventilatory responses.

Patients with the sleep apnoea/hypopnoea syndrome often have systemic hypertension. However, such patients are often obese and frequently consume excess alcohol, and both predispose to hypertension. Early studies suggesting an increase in apnoea frequency in patients with essential hypertension were performed on patients who are either taking or had recently been taking antihypertensive medication. In addition, in these studies, the increase in apnoeas in hypertensives was small and few patients qualified for a diagnosis of the sleep apnoea/hypopnoea syndrome. The slight increase in apnoeas may be a consequence either of the drug therapy or of mild central nervous system damage due to the hypertension. While there is epidemiological evidence that loud snoring is associated with systemic hypertension, with ischaemic heart disease and with cerebrovascular accidents (Partinen & Palomaki 1985), a recent study indicates that the sleep apnoea/hypopnoea syndrome is not an independent risk factor for hypertension (Stradling & Crosby 1990).

DIAGNOSIS

Physical examination

The extent of obesity should be noted and retrognathia sought. The nose and oropharynx should be examined both by the physician and preferably by an Ear, Nose & Throat (ENT) Surgeon. The point of the ENT opinion is to exclude major abnormalities such as pharyngeal tumours or major restrictions to nasopharyngeal airflow. As a rule, correction of minor ENT abnormalities, such as nasal septal deviation and minor nasal polyps has little effect on the extent of the sleep apnoea/hypopnoea syndrome. Each patient should be assessed for predisposing factors such as hypothyroidism or acromegaly and also for complications, such as right heart failure or cyanosis.

Diagnostic techniques

The sleep apnoea/hypopnoea syndrome can only rarely be diagnosed confidently from the history alone. A recent study of our own and also one from Australia (Crocker et al 1990) have both shown that the most useful question which differentiated patients with the syndrome from others referred for investigation was whether apnoeas had been reported by bed partners. However, apnoeas were reported in about 55% who proved not to have the sleep apnoea syndrome as well as in around 85% of those with the syndrome. Thus, the presence of apnoeas on history is not a clinically useful pointer.

The next easiest method of diagnosing the sleep apnoea/hypopnoea syndrome would be to visually observe a patient at night. However, even experienced observers will miss around a third of patients with the sleep apnoea/hypopnoea syndrome. Various screening tests have been proposed. Holter monitoring of the ECG can be used to detect the characteristic bradycardia of the apnoeas and post-apnoeic tachycardia. However, the sensitivity and specificity of this technique has not yet been examined rigorously. Recently it has been suggested that such monitoring could be improved by the use of microphones to detect snoring or apnoeas but again this technique has not been validated.

Oximetry alone will often allow diagnosis of the sleep apnoea/hypopnoea syndrome from the characteristic pattern of recurrent desaturation (Fig. 4.3). In a recent study, I was able to make a confident diagnosis of the sleep apnoea/hypopnoea syndrome from oximetry traces alone in 37 out of 63 patients with the condition and I found no false positive diagnosis. Sixteen of the remaining 26 patients with the syndrome had questionable oxygen saturation traces as did 12 of the patients without the sleep apnoea/hypopnoea syndrome. Thus, visual scoring of the oxygen saturation trace alone is of considerable diagnostic value, although some patients with mild forms of the condition will have visually normal oxygen saturation traces.

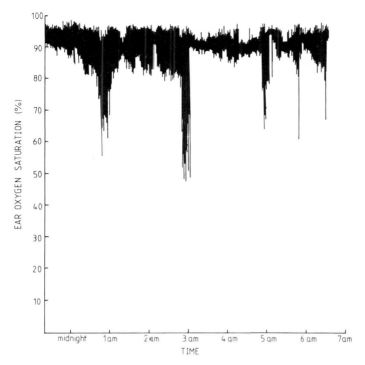

Fig. 4.3 Overnight oxygen saturation trace in a patient with the sleep apnoea/hypopnoea syndrome.

In our experience, existing computer programs to examine desaturation frequencies are less accurate than visual scoring of the saturation trace. One of the problems with the use of oximetry alone to investigate patients with the sleep apnoea/hypopnoea syndrome is that those patients with suggestive symptoms who have normal oximetry traces will need further investigation to exclude alternative treatable causes (see below).

The ideal diagnostic technique for the sleep apnoea/hypopnoea syndrome is overnight polysomnography, recording at least oxygen saturation by an oximeter, thoracoabdominal movement by surface techniques, airflow by temperature or carbon-dioxide sensors, and electroencephalogram, electromyogram and electro-oculogram. This allows quantification of the frequency of apnoeas, hypopnoeas and arousals and of the frequency and extent of desaturation. Such monitoring has built-in cross checks in case of instrumental failure or artefects. Polysomnography allows identification of sleep disruption due to other causes (for example, nocturnal myoclonus) and of abnormally rapid sleep onset or of abnormally early rapid eye movement (REM) sleep (which often occurs in narcolepsy). However, such polysomnography is expensive and in our laboratory costs around £350 per night exclusive of medical staff time.

Differential diagnosis

Alternative diagnoses to be considered in the somnolent patient include narcolepsy which seems to be around a tenth as common as the sleep apnoea/hypopnoea syndrome. The clinical tetrad of narcolepsy—somnolence, cataplexy, sleep paralysis and hypnogogic hallucinations—should always be sought in all patients referred. Hypnogogic hallucinations can occur in the sleep apnoea/hypopnoea syndrome although this is rare in our own experience, but when cataplexy, or sleep paralysis are present in a somnolent patient, the diagnosis of narcolepsy can be made with confidence. Confirmatory evidence of narcolepsy includes the occurrence of sleep onset REM sleep (REM sleep occurring within 15 minutes of sleep onset) or at least 2 of 5 sleeps, and the presence of HLA DR2.

Nocturnal myoclonus is a condition in which there is regular leg twitching during non-REM sleep often associated with recurrent arousals. This is best diagnosed by the use of anterior tibial EMG recording which is standard during our polysomnography. Idiopathic hypersomnolence is a condition with rapid sleep onset and long nocturnal sleeps (8–12 + hours) but without associated cataplexy, sleep paralysis or sleep onset REM. Depression may present with daytime sleepiness as may central nervous system stimulant abuse.

The Kleine–Levin syndrome is an uncommon condition characterized by periodic somnolence sometimes associated with increased appetite and bizarre behaviour. During attacks, the patients often sleep for 20 of the 24 hours and the attacks last for a few days or even a few weeks.

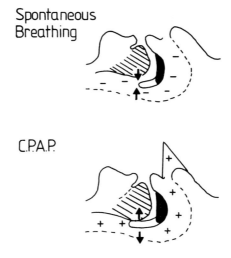

Fig. 4.4 Schematic diagram showing (above) the mechanics of upper airways obstruction during spontaneous breathing and (below) the principle of continuous positive airway pressure (CPAP) therapy in which positive pressure is applied via the nose to blow the throat open at night.

TREATMENT

All patients with the sleep apnoea/hypopnoea syndrome should be encouraged to lose weight, to avoid alcohol in the evenings and to avoid sedative use. These measures alone will suffice in some patients with mild forms of the condition. Patients with any underlying predisposing causes such as myxoedema, acromegaly, retrognathia or major abnormalities of the nose or pharynx should be treated appropriately.

Despite earlier optimistic reports, it appears that there is no role for drug therapy in the sleep apnoea/hypopnoea syndrome. Protriptyline gives rise to more side effects than benefits (Whyte et al 1988) and the same is true of both acetazolamide and progesterone. Thus, in the majority of patients who fail to respond to the simple measures above, the choice is between continuous positive airway pressure therapy or upper airway surgery.

CPAP therapy works by physically blowing the back of the throat open using a positive pressure of usually between 5 and 17.5 cm of water (Figs 4.4, 4.5). The level of therapy required is assessed by an overnight study in a sleep laboratory and the patient must then use the machine nightly thereafter. Initiation of CPAP requires careful explanation and coaching both of the patient and the spouse, the latter being particularly important if

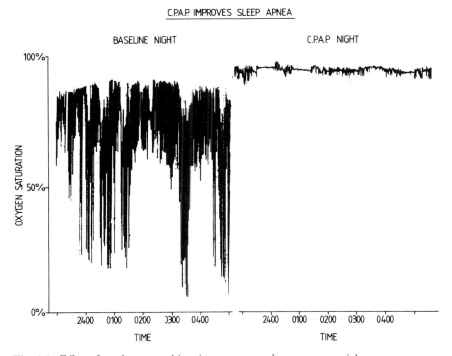

Fig. 4.5   Effect of continuous positive airway pressure therapy on overnight oxygen saturation.

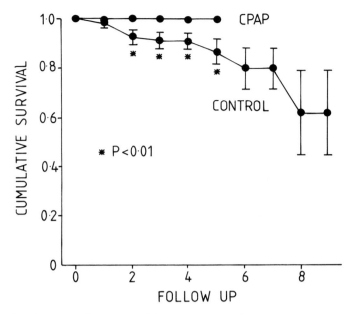

Fig. 4.6   Survival curves for patients with the sleep apnoea/hypopnoea syndrome who either received CPAP therapy or did not (controls) (from He et al 1988.)

the patient is not enthusiastic. The educational process involves explanation of the mechanisms of both upper airways obstruction and CPAP
therapy. The beneficial effect of CPAP on survival must also be explained
(He et al 1988; Fig. 4.6). In most patients, little further encouragment is
required as they feel so much better symptomatically following initiation of
therapy but in some, CPAP is an uphill battle. Many patients who get a
good initial response with CPAP find after several months or years of CPAP
use that the use of the machine is beginning to pall. However, at present,
continued encouragement is the best one can offer.

The role for surgery in the sleep apnoea/hypopnoea syndrome is controversial. Uvulopalatopharyngoplasty is an operation in which the uvula and
part of the soft palate are removed and the lateral pharyngeal wall tensed.
This operation is extremely effective in preventing snoring but less effective in treating the sleep apnoea/hypopnoea syndrome. Three recent studies
have shown only 15% of patients improve in terms of symptoms and
apnoeas after this procedure: an extremely low success rate for an operation
which has caused several perioperative deaths. In addition, around half of
the patients with the syndrome obstruct at a lower level than the soft palate
(Chaban et al 1988; Fig. 4.2) and at least until these patients can be
accurately excluded preoperatively, the success rate of the operation is
unlikely to improve. In addition, there is no evidence that uvulopalatopharyngoplasty affects survival (He et al 1988) whereas CPAP undoubtedly

does. Finally, some patients who fail to benefit from uvulopalatopharyngo-plasty subsequently find that CPAP therapy is intolerable as there is no longer a seal between the soft palate and the tongue and air blown in through the nose leaks out through the mouth rather than dilating the retroglossal airway where the obstruction is occurring. Thus, I do not advocate uvulopalatopharyngoplasty for the sleep apnoea/hypopnoea syndrome.

Various operations are being developed which produce anterior move-ment of the tongue by mandibular surgery or affect hyoid position but their use is experimental. Tracheostomy should only be performed in an emer-gency situation in which CPAP is unsuccessful or unavailable or to provide a safe airway in the perioperative period. All patients with the sleep apnoea/hypopnoea syndrome are high risk surgical cases as their upper airway not only tends to obstruct when given sedatives but also they are very difficult patients to intubate.

A recent study has suggested electrical stimulation of the tongue might be a possible form of therapy of the sleep apnoea/hypopnoea syndrome (Miki et al 1989). However, this technique is only at the experimental stage.

PROGNOSIS

The prognosis of the sleep apnoea/hypopnoea syndrome is relatively good, 5-year survivals being in excess of 80% even in untreated patients. Two recent studies have shown that survival can be improved with either CPAP (He et al 1988) or with longstanding tracheostomy (Partinen et al 1988). However, these studies were carried out on patients with severe forms of the syndrome and it is not yet known whether patients with minor sleep apnoea/hypopnoea receive major benefits from therapy.

WHO TO STUDY

Any patient who complains of going to sleep in an unplanned fashion at least once per day when not in bed should be referred for evaluation for the sleep apnoea/hypopnoea syndrome. Referral is also indicated in patients who are reported to have frequent apnoeas. Patients who are merely loud snorers should not be referred for study. Other situations in which sleep studies are indicated include unexplained polycythaemia or unexplained cor pulmonale.

HOW TO STUDY

When access to a full sleep laboratory is impracticable, the best simple diagnostic technique is overnight oximetry alone, but it is important that the continuous oximetry trace is recorded for visual or computer analysis. It is perfectly possible to institute CPAP therapy under oximetry guidance alone provided one can ascertain that the patient is asleep as failure to sleep on CPAP will normalize the oxygenation trace. However, any patient whose CPAP was commenced on the basis of oximetry alone whose symptoms remain while on CPAP should be referred for polysomnography lest there is a coexisting alternative cause for his symptoms.

CONCLUSION

The sleep apnoea/hypopnoea syndrome is a common clinical problem but one which will continue to be missed until physicians include in their standard history taking two additional questions: 'How often do you fall asleep when not in bed' and 'Do you snore'. Once these questions are adopted into standard clinical practice, many patients who are presently sleepy, dangerous and failing to achieve their full potential may be able to lead a normal, safe and longer life.

REFERENCES

Bradley T D, Rutherford R, Grossman R F et al 1985 Role of daytime hypoxemia in the pathogenesis of right heart failure in the obstructive sleep apnea syndrome. American Review of Respiratory Disease 131: 835–839

Chaban R, Cole P, Hoffstein V 1988 Site of upper airway obstruction with idiopathic obstructive sleep apnoea. Laryngoscope 98: 641–647

Crocker B D, Olson L G, Saunders N A et al 1990 Estimation of the probability of disturbed breathing during sleep before a sleep study. American Review of Respiratory Disease 142: 14–18

Findley L J, Fabrizio M J, Knight H, Norcross B B, Laforte A J, Suratt P M 1989 Driving simulator performance in patients with sleep apnea. American Review of Respiratory Disease 140: 529–530

Gould G A, Whyte K F, Rhind G B, Airlie M A A et al 1988 The sleep hypopnea syndrome. American Review of Respiratory Disease 137: 895–898

He J, Kryger M H, Zorick F J, Conway W, Roth T 1988 Mortality and apnea index in obstructive sleep apnea: Experience in 385 male patients. Chest 94: 9–14

Horner R L, Mohiaddin R H, Lowell D G et al 1989 Sites and sizes of fat deposits around the pharynx in obese patients with obstructive sleep apnoea and weight matched controls. European Respiratory Journal 2: 613–622

Lavie P 1983 Incidence of sleep apnea in a presumably healthy working population: A significant relationship with excessive daytime sleepiness. Sleep 6(4): 312–318

Miki H, Hida W, Chonan T, Kikuchi Y, Takishima T 1989 Effects of submental electrical stimulation during sleep on upper airway patency in patients with obstructive sleep apnea. American Review of Respiratory Disease 140: 1285–1289

Partinen M, Palomaki H 1985 Snoring and cerebral infarction. Lancet 2: 1325–1326

Partinen M, Jamieson A, Guilleminault C 1988 Long-term outcome for obstructive sleep apnea syndrome patients: Mortality. Chest 94: 1200–1204

Stradling J R, Crosby J H 1990: Relation between systemic hypertension and sleep hypoxaemia or snoring: analysis in 748 men drawn from general practice. British Medical Journal 300: 75–78

Whyte K F, Allen M B, Jeffrey A A, Gould G A, Douglas N J 1989 Clinical features of the sleep apnoea/hypopnoea syndrome. Quarterly Journal of Medicine 72: 659–666

Whyte K F, Gould G A, Airlie M A A, Shapiro C M, Douglas N J 1988 Role of protriptyline and acetazolamide in the sleep apnea/hypopnea syndrome. Sleep 11(5): 463–742

FURTHER READING

Guilleminault C, Partinen M (eds) 1990 Obstructive sleep apnea syndrome: Clinical research and treatment. Raven Press, New York

5. Acute liver failure

A. Forbes, I. Murray-Lyon

INTRODUCTION

Acute hepatitis of whatever cause is usually a self-limiting condition which does not require specific medical intervention, and many cases, particularly those of viral origin in childhood, are subclinical. Only a small proportion of patients develop fulminant hepatic failure (FHF), defined by the presence of severe liver failure with encephalopathy, occurring within 8 weeks of the first symptom, and with no pre-existing chronic liver disease. It is not the intention of this review to consider the very much more common occurrence of acute liver failure superimposed on chronic liver disease; the management of this complication is well covered in standard texts.

AETIOLOGY

The aetiology of FHF in the UK (O'Grady et al 1989) is predominantly (about 55%) from paracetamol poisoning and about three-quarters of these cases are female. Viral causes account for about two-fifths of cases, with hepatitis A (HAV) responsible for about 15% of these, hepatitis B (HBV) for about 35%, and non-A, non-B infection for over 50%. Idiosyncratic drug reactions, including halothane toxicity, are responsible for between 5 and 10% of cases (Table 5.1). For all aetiologies there is an observed excess of females, which has been attributed to a generally more pronounced antibody response to immunological challenge compared to that in males. A link with oestrogens was supported by a study in which the clinical expression of HBV infection in adult females was examined in relation to

Table 5.1 Fulminant hepatic failure in UK

Aetiology		%
Paracetamol poisoning		55
Viral hepatitis		40
Non A, non B	20	
Hepatitis B	14	
Hepatitis A	6	
Drug reactions		5

their circulating sex hormone binding globulin (SHBG) concentrations (Forbes et al 1988). Higher levels of SHBG effectively increase the expression of oestrogens [by causing a marked shift in the ratio of serum free (unbound/active) oestrogen to free androgen]. Women with fulminant hepatitis B had significantly higher SHBG concentrations at presentation than those whose acute hepatitis was not as severe but who subsequently failed to clear the virus and became chronic HBV carriers. Fortunately pregnancy, in which SHBG levels are very high, is rarely associated with FHF, except when the third trimester is complicated by epidemic food/water-borne non-A, non-B hepatitis (hepatitis E) which is often accompanied by severe liver failure and a mortality in excess of 50% (Zuckerman 1990). Hepatic complications of pregnancy otherwise account for a small proportion of cases of FHF in most series; both acute fatty liver of pregnancy and pre-eclampsia can be responsible. Fortunately, prompt delivery is usually associated with a good prognosis for mother and child. Hepatic manifestations of these two conditions sometimes occur only in the first few days after parturition, but the prognosis appears similarly good.

DIAGNOSIS

In the jaundiced patient the diagnosis of acute liver failure is usually obvious, particularly when there is a clear history of late presentation after paracetamol overdose. However, in some cases the diagnosis is not immediately apparent and we have learnt to maintain a high index of suspicion in sick patients in whom an underlying diagnosis is lacking, particularly when coma or metabolic acidosis are features. The best screening test for an hepatic aetiology in such cases is the prothrombin time, or international normalized ratio (INR), and many delays in diagnosis would be avoided were INRs performed as readily as a full blood count or chest radiograph. FHF is a multisystem disorder, and attention may be drawn to the possibility of occult paracetamol poisoning by the combination of unexplained metabolic acidosis and marked oliguria with a normal (or near normal) plasma urea concentration: a greater readiness to estimate plasma creatinine levels would help to avoid confusion.

Following the recognition of acute hepatic failure it is important to establish the aetiology as quickly as possible. There may be epidemiological implications, particularly for the viral causes which are notifiable diseases in the UK, but an accurate diagnosis is also important for the patient. Specific therapy is rarely applicable, but a substantial proportion of patients have such a poor prognosis that urgent liver transplantation should be considered. Since the patient with poor-prognosis FHF may deteriorate very rapidly, and there is inevitably delay between the identification of a potential transplant recipient and the earliest time of operation, early recognition of the probable need for transplantation is crucial.

Paracetamol levels are usually unhelpful (i.e. in the low therapeutic range or negative) by the time the patient presents with liver failure, but detectable levels in a patient who has specifically denied paracetamol ingestion may point to subterfuge. The history (from patient or relatives) may indicate a likely drug or risk factors for a viral cause, and it should be noted that the likelihood of viral hepatitis running a fulminant course appears to increase with increasing age (perhaps even exponentially so in the case of hepatitis A) (Forbes & Williams 1988). From a prognostic viewpoint the most important distinctions to be drawn are between patients with paracetamol- or pregnancy-related liver disease, hepatitis A and hepatitis B, on the one hand, and the whole group of non-A, non-B hepatitides and idiosyncratic drug reactions on the other. The serological tests for viral infection are fortunately adequate to this challenge, since the estimation of IgM antibody to HAV, and IgM antibody to HBV core antigen (HBcAb), are readily available, and have very high sensitivity and specificity for acute infection with these two viruses. There is now a commercially available assay for antibody to hepatitis C, but this is not helpful in acute liver failure as it is rarely positive in the early stages of the disease; it usually becomes positive for the first time only 3 to 6 months after the onset. Assessment in the special case of acute hepatitis E virus infection—generally good outlook except for the appalling prognosis in late pregnancy—will be easier when the serological tests currently being developed become generally available.

Paracetamol poisoning

In paracetamol poisoning the normal conjugation pathways become saturated leading to the formation of the toxic metabolite, N-acetyl-p-benzoquinone imine (NAPQI), which binds covalently to protein thiol groups, particularly on hepatocyte and renal tubular cell membranes (Davis 1986). Tissue damage can be prevented by stopping the formation of NAPQI by the early use of methionine—a thiol group donor which increases glutathione (GSH) synthesis (five enzyme steps)—or N-acetyl cysteine (NAC)—a thiol group donor which increases hepatic GSH (two enzyme steps) and also increases paracetamol conjugation. Other cytochrome p450 inhibitors which are effective (at least experimentally) at high dose include cimetidine, the acute administration of ethanol, and certain antithyroid drugs.

When a patient presents with established acute liver failure the above manoeuvres cease to be strictly relevant, but it may none the less be possible to prevent further damage from NAPQI. NAC can be shown to increase reduction of NAPQI to paracetamol, increase NAPQI conjugation, decrease lipid peroxidation, and decrease free radical release. Other antioxidants such as vitamins B, C and E, and selenium may also have value. A recent well-matched placebo-controlled trial evaluated NAC in paracetamol-related FHF (Keays et al 1989a). All patients had presented more than 36 hours after drug ingestion and had had no prior therapy. NAC was given by standard protocol but the infusion was continued beyond 20 hours at 100 mg/kg/20 hours, until patients were no longer encephalopathic (or died). Treated patients had a significantly improved outcome, with a 64% survival rate compared to 20% in the controls ($P < 0.05$). Use of NAC later than is currently recommended in the British National Formulary (but before the onset of FHF) is also supported by North American data (Smilkstein et al 1988), and more strongly by a recent Lancet paper (Harrison et al 1990), which suggests benefit when NAC is given at anything up to 36 hours from the time of overdose.

MANAGEMENT

General supportive management of FHF

The management of the patient with FHF in whom paracetamol is not implicated, turns on careful attentive nursing and general supportive measures. The prompt recognition and treatment of hypoglycaemia consequent on depletion of hepatic glycogen are important, but should preferably be pre-empted by prophylactic infusions of glucose. Intravenous H_2 blockade plays a major role in reducing the risk of upper gastrointestinal bleeding in these patients (MacDougall & Williams 1978). The administration of Parentrovite, vitamin K, folate, and possibly other antioxidants, amongst which NAC may be included, are of probable but unproven value. The place of charcoal haemoperfusion in severely encephalopathic patients had been debated for some years, but it is no longer regularly employed since it failed to benefit patients in a major controlled trial (O'Grady et al 1988a). Intravenous prostaglandin E1, sometimes followed by oral prostaglandin E2, had been advocated as a valuable hepato-protective agent in viral FHF (Sinclair et al 1989); controlled studies are awaited with interest.

Infection and sepsis

Sepsis is a major source of morbidity and mortality in FHF. In a prospective study of 50 consecutive patients with FHF, 40 patients had 53 confirmed bacterial infections, and there was a strong suspicion of infection (but repeatedly negative cultures) in a further 5 patients (Rolando et al 1990). Pyrexia and leucocytosis were often absent (neither present in 30% of cases with confirmed infection), but infection was significantly more frequent in patients with renal failure than in those with normal renal function. Most of the infections were of respiratory (47%) or urinary tract (23%) origin, and surprisingly 70% of the organisms were Gram-positive bacteria, approximately half of which were *Staphylococcus aureus*. Although 70% of documented infections were found within 3 days of admission, in all 9 patients who died more than 7 days after admission, death was directly attributable to infection. Fungal infection was confirmed in 16 patients including 9 late deaths; diagnosis in life remains difficult even with the newer immunological techniques.

Whether or not encouragement of the prophylactic use of antibiotics in FHF is wise, it is clear that frequent samples should be taken from multiple sites for microbiological examination, and that a very low threshold for the use of broad-spectrum antibiotics (including anti-staphylococcal cover) is required. Similarly, the disturbing fatality rate from fungal infections can only be combated by early treatment with amphotericin, based on clinical suspicion (unexplained pyrexia, general deterioration, or late rises in INR), without waiting for laboratory results.

Cardiovascular management

Fluid balance and haemodynamics in FHF are unusually difficult to judge clinically. Sinus tachycardia is usual but some patients with a viral aetiology have a relative or absolute bradycardia which may reflect myocardial involvement by the virus; fortunately this is rarely a management problem. Because patients with FHF have profound but variable vasodilatation associated with a very low peripheral vascular resistance (PVR), hypotensive crises are a frequent problem, and especially so at times of medical or nursing intervention. Continuous arterial monitoring is accordingly essential. The central venous pressure (CVP) is often misleading—probably because of raised portal venous pressure—and a Swan–Ganz flotation catheter for estimation of left-sided cardiac filling pressure is therefore invaluable, not least because the incorporation of a thermister at its tip also allows calculation of cardiac output/index and peripheral vascular resistance. The insertion and subsequent management of these intravascular devices do not appear to be accompanied by noticeably greater morbidity than in other groups of patients despite the presence of coagulopathy, but experienced operators are mandatory.

Fluid administration should consist of 5–20% glucose solutions, plasma expanders or blood as determined by standard intensive care practice. Fresh frozen plasma (FFP) and platelet concentrates are not often necessary and should be reserved for the occasional patient with spontaneous bleeding ($< 5\%$); avoidance of FFP has the additional advantage that the prothrombin ratio (INR) then remains a valid and a very useful prognostic marker. Fluid overload is not unusual in patients with FHF and renal impairment, and may be unavoidable when several intravenous antimicrobial agents are indicated. This situation is best dealt with by passive ultrafiltration across a flat-bed dialysis membrane or ultrafiltration hollow-fibre system (see below), as these patients do not generally respond to diuretics.

Hypotension despite adequate left-sided filling pressures ($> 5\,\mathrm{mmHg}$) is an indication for inotropes; the vasodilatation predicts a poor response to dopamine and dobutamine which is confirmed in practice. Noradrenaline and adrenaline (at times in massively high dosage) will usually succeed in raising systemic arterial pressure, but at some cost. Pulmonary arteriovenous shunting, which is generally present in FHF, is usually minor and of little or no clinical significance prior to the use of inotropes. Exogenous catecholamines, however, tend to increase shunting and may render this a major problem. If the increase in oxidative metabolism they initiate is not balanced by a correspondingly significant increase in oxygen delivery, a net deterioration in tissue oxygen extraction results. These effects have now been examined systematically (Wendon et al 1990), and although improved perfusion pressure and oxygen delivery can be achieved by both adrenaline and noradrenaline, this may indeed be at the cost of impaired oxygen extraction ratio and oxygen consumption. There is support for a beneficial role for prostacyclin—probably from focal vasodilatation—and it is clear that monitoring of oxygen handling should become standard practice in FHF if inotropes are employed.

Respiratory management

Respiratory management in FHF is usually straightforward, but there should be a very low threshold for endotracheal intubation and mechanical ventilation. Hepatic encephalopathy is conventionally graded on a five-point scale where 0 represents normality and IV indicates coma (with or without response to painful stimuli) (Table 5.2). Particularly in the paracetamol-related case there may be a very rapid transition from Grade I or II, through aggression and hyperactivity (Grade III encephalopathy) to Grade IV and sudden respiratory arrest. It is almost always safest to paralyse and intubate the patient with acute liver failure if there is any concern about the airway or if the conscious level is deteriorating rapidly; this is especially important when considering the transfer of patients between hospitals (and even within a hospital), since transfer is frequently associated with a worsening of encephalopathy. The continuing debate between anaesthetists and hepatologists on the question of sedation is perhaps unnecessarily acrimonious; a patient ventilated because of aggressive and potentially self-harming behaviour clearly needs sedation as well as paralysis, while a patient in deep coma will not need sedation, and may not need paralysis except for its role in the controlled management of cerebral oedema. It is good practice, if sedation is thought appropriate, to use short-

Table 5.2   Grading of hepatic encephalopathy (after Trey et al 1966)

Grade 0	Normal
Grade I	Mild drowsiness: reversal of sleep/wake pattern; occasional confusion; may have asterixis alone
Grade II	Moderate drowsiness; mild confusion: possible to hold conversation
Grade III	Very drowsy: sleeping most of time; marked confusion; unable to converse coherently; may be manifest as extreme agitation/irritability with violence to self/others
Grade IV	Comatose: may or may not respond to painful stimuli

acting agents which are not prone to accumulation: midazolam and propofol have been used effectively and apparently safely. The use of sedation in patients with acute liver failure who are not intubated is, however, to be deprecated.

Positive pressure ventilation is often complicated by bronchial mucus plugs, recognized by sudden deterioration in blood gases, and not infrequently by obvious and lateralized reduction in chest expansion. Sometimes physiotherapy and bronchial lavage are sufficient to clear the airways, but facilities for immediate bedside fibreoptic bronchoscopy should be available. Adult respiratory distress syndrome occurs only rarely in FHF but is almost inevitably a preterminal event.

Management of renal failure

Renal failure requiring intervention is seen mainly but not exclusively in patients with FHF secondary to paracetamol intoxication. It is usually suspected from progressive oliguria and justifies urinary catheterization despite the potential for sepsis. The catheter may be removed if the patient becomes anuric. It should not be necessary to comment that the plasma urea is an almost valueless investigation in patients with acute liver failure, but there is too often a lack of appreciation of the significance of its hepatic synthesis amongst junior medical staff, and in a disturbingly high proportion of UK hospitals it is difficult, or even impossible, to obtain urgent creatinine estimations. Plasma creatinine usually rises very rapidly once a value of around 400 µmol/l is reached, and this has led to most liver units using this level as a criterion for dialysis (not normally considered a strong indication by general renal units). Hyperkalaemia is rarely a problem (presumably because of the high circulating concentrations of endogenous catecholamines), and when present usually indicates concurrent rhabdomyolysis with the attendant risks to the kidneys of additional damage from myoglobin. Although acidosis (pH ≤ 7.2) is an important indication for renal support therapy, it rarely exists without a substantially elevated plasma creatinine.

The haemodynamic instability of patients with FHF frequently necessitates haemodialysis (HD) being conducted at a suboptimal rate of blood flow through the dialysis circuit, and premature curtailment is often inevitable because of hypotension or cerebral oedema. These factors lend support to a policy of early renal intervention. Although not yet subjected to controlled trial, it is almost certain that there is a major place for continuous arteriovenous haemodialysis (CAVHD) in FHF. This technique (Miller et al 1990) relies on passive ultrafiltration across a flatbed dialysis membrane, but achieves substantially greater clearance of small and middle molecules than filtration alone, by virtue of counter-current flow of solute across the opposite side of the membrane. CAVHD has been found to be remarkably safe and effective in numerous general intensive care units, as in addition to its freedom from the need for expensive, cumbersome, technically-demanding dialysis machines, it causes very much less haemodynamic disturbance. The ability to run CAVHD continuously allows almost as efficient renal support as 3 hours of conventional haemodialysis daily; supplementary HD has been found necessary in a few patients with extreme hypercatabolism, but it is unlikely that more than a small proportion of FHF patients would fall into this category.

Vascular access for dialysis may be achieved from a forearm Scribner arteriovenous shunt inserted under local anaesthesia at the bedside, the use of large arterial and venous lines, or (in the case of HD) from a veno-venous route such as the VasCath. Decisions as to which route to use will depend on local expertise and manpower: a shunt is the most difficult to create but the easiest to manage once inserted, and probably least likely to malfunction or become infected.

When dialysis is complicated by hypotension, adequate perfusion pressures (which may drop on commencing dialysis despite an initial 'priming' infusion) should be ensured. If the pulmonary wedge pressure is satisfactory then the flow of blood through the HD circuit should be reduced to the minimal effective rate for the equipment in use, and if hypotension persists inotropes should be infused as outlined above. If hypotension is not readily controlled, dialysis must be abandoned, at least temporarily. Cerebral oedema not infrequently recurs or presents for the first time during dialysis: dialysis should be suspended and the cerebral oedema treated as below. This can be something of a 'Catch 22 situation', since it is usually the patients with severe acidosis who most need dialysis, and who have the highest frequency of cerebral oedema! Despite the profound coagulopathy in patients with FHF, all forms of extracorporeal circulation remain very prone to thrombosis, and anticoagulation for dialysis/haemofiltration is almost always necessary. Fortunately even with full heparinization for HD (e.g. activated clotting time of 250 seconds) frank bleeding is rare. When problems do emerge, it is more often at the completion of dialysis when the thrombogenic effects of contact with extravascular materials have ceased, than during intervention. Patients with FHF have profoundly low circulating levels of anti-thrombin III (ATIII), and it has recently been shown that its replacement (to control concentrations) dramatically reduces the amount of heparin required for effective dialysis, with a possible concurrent reduction in bleeding episodes (Langley et al 1990). This appears an appropriate manoeuvre for problem cases, but the expense of ATIII militates against its routine use. Prostacyclin was found effective in allowing heparin-free dialysis some years ago, but was difficult to use and very unpopular with conscious patients because of unpleasant sensations due to intense vasodilatation. The important beneficial effects on oxygen delivery suggest that its place should now be re-evaluated.

Whichever methods are employed for the control of renal failure, the aim should be to keep plasma creatinine at or below 500 µmol/l; if conventional

HD is being used this may require daily dialysis for the first 3 or 4 days. Once established on dialysis, most patients will need renal support for 2 to 3 weeks.

Cerebral oedema

Cerebral oedema is a serious complication that accounts for between quarter and half of all deaths from FHF, the figure depending not so much on its presence or absence but on whether it is judged to be the final mode of death. It is seen always in association with advanced encephalopathy and would not be expected unless the patient has deteriorated to at least Grade III (Table 5.2); the proviso that cerebral oedema may be the first evidence of such deterioration emphasizes the vigilance with which patients with FHF must be monitored. Especially when paracetamol is the cause of FHF, the development of cerebral oedema, unless promptly recognized and treated, may be associated with (or shortly followed by) respiratory arrest. The clinical distinction between cerebral oedema and conditions warranting sedation is critical for the correct handling of these patients, and remains perhaps the cause of the most serious management errors in non-specialist centres. The keys to recognition of cerebral oedema are hypertension (bursts of systolic pressure above 200 mmHg, or a sustained systolic pressure above 150 mmHg), rarely bradycardia, any pupil changes including sluggishness, and cerebral 'posturing' (usually extensor movements of the spine and limbs, with pronation of the forearms). It will be plain that early diagnosis is dependent on excellent nursing, with very frequent neurological observations—it is not excessive to advise examination of the pupil responses every 10 minutes.

Patients with FHF complicated by cerebral oedema should be nursed semi-recumbent (as if for a cardiac diagnosis), as this will lower intracerebral pressure (ICP) by up to 10 mmHg (Ede & Williams 1986). It is similarly crucial to keep such patients as static as possible, as all forms of nursing and medical intervention significantly raise ICP—by as much as 40 mmHg once oedema has developed. It is accepted that this may entail a serious risk of pressure sores, especially since these are often the very patients who will be receiving vasoconstrictor inotropes which further reduce skin blood flow. Fortunately, most are relatively young, and even the most extensive pressure sores heal well once recovery has occurred, whereas inadequately controlled cerebral oedema is usually rapidly fatal. The controversy over paralysis has already been commented on, but as a means of immobilizing the patient with a labile ICP who might otherwise be moving around uncontrollably, it is essential. As patients with cerebral oedema inevitable have advanced encephalopathy, the need for sedation is minimal (but also see below). Controlled hyperventilation to yield an arterial pCO_2 of between 3.5 and 4 kPa will, through its regulatory effects on cerebral blood flow, help to control raised ICP: as the volume of the cranial contents is fixed there is an, otherwise unusual, positive correlation between blood pressure and blood flow. Even after prolonged periods of unresponsiveness of the pupils and absence of other brain-stem reflexes, full recovery may be seen; continued active management is mandatory while there is a cardiac output. Brain death is not diagnosable in this multisystem metabolic disturbance. The cerebral oedema of FHF is unresponsive to steroids, but intravenous mannitol (e.g. 100 ml of a 20% solution administered as a bolus) is highly effective (Canalese et al 1982). There is inevitably a problem in patients with oliguric renal failure, which must be overcome by concurrent ultrafiltration; a 'diuresis' of 300 ml ultrafiltrate is recommended for each 100 ml mannitol given. The value of early establishment of comprehensive vascular access for renal intervention is reinforced, since once cerebral oedema has occurred the manipulations necessary to achieve arteriovenous cannulations may be harmful.

Intracranial pressure measurement is of theoretical value since it is known that the earliest clinical signs of intracranial hypertension lag some minutes behind raised pressure measurements; the insertion of an ICP probe and transducer allows monitoring not only of ICP, but also of cerebral perfusion pressure (CPP). CPP (the ICP less the perfusion 'head' represented by the mean systemic arterial pressure) is physiologically the more relevant measure since a normal ICP is of no value if there is profound systemic hypotension, and conversely, an elevated ICP may not necessarily be harmful if there is systemic hypertension. The safety of insertion of an intracranial pressure monitoring system in FHF has, however, naturally been questioned.

A recent evaluation of the Ladd extradural transducer inserted at the bedside under local anaesthetic included 36 (of 95) Grade IV FHF patients with cerebral oedema (Keays et al 1989b). There was no major morbidity, although one patient developed a small area of cerebral infarction adjacent to the probe with no detectable long-term sequelae, and another had a superficial haematoma. A similarly excellent safety profile is described by a group using the subarachnoid screw in FHF (Le Roux et al 1990), but in the absence of data showing greater or more reliable diagnostic yield, this potentially more hazardous technique (one epidural haematoma amongst 14 patients in another series (Schafer & Shaw 1989)) should perhaps not be recommended. In the former study 25% of patients were found to have considerable increases in ICP (> 25 mmHg) and reduced CPP, without the development of clinical signs, the significance of this observation is uncertain however, as a rising ICP was assumed to indicate the initiation of therapy for cerebral oedema. It appeared that the peak ICP was discriminant for the eventual prognosis, as the peak recorded ICP was 35 mmHg (median) in survivors, compared to 46 mmHg in non-survivors ($P < 0.01$). There was an apparently better survival in patients who were monitored than in those who were not (44% versus 29%), but this is difficult to interpret since not only does it fail to reach statistical significance, but also may reflect patient selection.

Some patients with FHF develop intractable cerebral oedema, which has been defined as cerebral oedema in the presence of renal failure unresponsive to 3 cycles of mannitol and ultrafiltration. It has an expected mortality of greater than 95%. Alternative or additional therapeutic strategies have therefore been sought. Barbiturates have a prophylactic effect on cerebral oedema both in animal models and in human head injury, and can have a therapeutic effect in cerebral oedema following head injury. They also have a possible beneficial effect in the cerebral oedema of Reye's syndrome. A cautious and carefully restricted study of thiopentone was therefore conducted in 13 patients with FHF who fell into this appalling prognostic group (Forbes et al 1989). All had failed to respond to standard therapy. Continuous monitoring included the measurement of ICP, mean arterial pressure (MAP), and cerebral perfusion pressure. Thiopentone was administered as a 15 minute infusion to a median dose of 250 mg (range 185–500 mg). ICP improved in all 13, and a normal CPP with resolution of clinical signs was achieved in 11 cases. Continued infusion achieved long-term control of cerebral oedema in 8 of the patients, 5 of whom made a complete recovery, and 3 of whom died of causes unrelated to cerebral oedema. Only 3 of the 13 patients died from cerebral oedema, and the overall survival of 38% is impressive. No serious toxicity from thiopentone was identified but it would clearly be inappropriate at this juncture to use such agents other than as a last resort.

Pancreatitis

Pancreatitis rarely presents a clinical problem in FHF, but is a common complication. Many patients—especially those with a paracetamol overdose—have significantly elevated serum amylase levels, and ultrasound scans of the pancreas are often diffusely abnormal. It has been suggested (Mallory & Kern 1980) that many examples of drug-related acute pancreatitis are the result primarily of systemic acidosis. Although acidosis does not necessarily coexist in the covert cases, our experience of FHF patients in whom pancreatitis is clinically significant indicates that acidosis is indeed associated. As patients frequently have other problems (sepsis/renal failure etc.) clinically overt cases of pancreatitis have a very poor prognosis.

Nutrition in FHF

Nutrition has never been a major consideration in the management of FHF since the patients are (by definition) healthy and well-nourished prior to the illness: indeed protein/calorie withdrawal has been thought appropriate. However, patients with acute liver failure are known to exhibit anergy and behave in many ways like the immunosuppressed. Sepsis in particular is a frequent and often fatal complication (see above). Little was known about the true energy or nitrogen requirements in FHF prior to a small study in which indirect calorimetry was combined with comprehensive nitrogen balance data and serial anthropometry in 16 patients with advanced encephalopathy receiving conventional nutritional support (effectively none) (Forbes & Wick 1989). The resting energy expenditure was calculated as a modest 1700 kcal/day, with a nitrogen loss of 7 g/day (but heavily dependent on whether or not dialysis was employed). By 72 hours the patients' median energy debt was 4500 kcal, with a nitrogen deficit of 20 g. Slight deteriorations in the anthropometrical measurements were claimed even at this early stage. Interim data indicate that provision of nutrients is practicable and safe, despite the many constraints that operate in FHF; the same constraints combine, however, to ensure that it is unlikely that a double blind randomized controlled clinical trial will follow to clarify whether the feasible is actually of benefit.

OUTCOME

The patient who survives FHF is most unlikely to suffer long-term sequelae. There appear to be no reports of subsequent chronic liver disease. When hepatitis B, hepatitis C, or non-A, non-B, non-C hepatitis have caused FHF, recovery from the acute illness is almost always coupled with complete viral clearance. Careful review of the literature reveals as few as 4 reported cases of long-term morbidity after survival of FHF, which in each case was manifest as permanent neurological deficit remaining after the treatment of severe cerebral oedema (O'Brien et al 1987). One individual was left with dysphasia, 1 with optic atrophy and decreased visual fields, and 2 had residual pyramidal weakness which was significantly disabling in 1. Interestingly, the future suicide and attempted-suicide rate in survivors of paracetamol-related FHF approaches zero.

The likelihood of survival from FHF is firmly dependent on its underlying aetiology, but is also heavily dependent on management in an experienced centre. The data from King's College Hospital and Birmingham suggest that treatment in a designated liver failure unit is preferable to that in a general intensive care unit.

The prognosis of FHF from paracetamol intoxication should be relatively good, and even when deterioration to Grade III encephalopathy has occurred, at least 60% of patients should recover. Pregnancy-related cases are relatively unusual and firm figures cannot be given, but an expectation of at least 60% survival from Grade III/IV encephalopathy is reasonable. More than 60% of patients with Grade III/IV encephalopathy from hepatitis A should survive with intensive medical management, and about one-third of those with hepatitis B. However the non-A, non-B group (including hepatitis C) and those with idiosyncratic drug reactions have a survival of less than 20% despite full medical management. Liver trans-

Table 5.3   Criteria for transplantation in fulminant hepatic failure (after O'Grady et al 1989)

Aetiology other than hepatitis A, hepatitis B, paracetamol related, or pregnancy-related
Plus TWO of these:
  Age < 10 years or > 40 years
  Jaundice for more than 7 days prior to development of encephalopathy
  Serum bilirubin > 300 μmol/l
  INR > 3.8 (or prothrombin time > 50 seconds)

---

plantation has naturally been considered for these individuals, and prognostic markers have been sought to identify the patients with other aetiologies (such as hepatitis B) with a bad prognosis.

TRANSPLANTATION IN FHF

Criteria

The criteria for transplantation in FHF advocated by the King's College Hospital group (O'Grady et al 1989) are broadly in line with those from other centres apart from a greater reluctance to transplant paracetamol-related cases (because of the rather better results for their medical management at King's than elsewhere). It is recommended that any patient with FHF where the aetiology is other than paracetamol-related, pregnancy-related or from hepatitis A or B is considered for urgent liver transplantation if any two of the criteria summarized in Table 5.3 are satisfied, or if the INR is greater than 7.0. In paracetamol-related cases an INR greater than 7.0 (prothrombin time > 100 seconds) and acidosis (pH < 7.3) are required. Patients with hepatitis A and B will need to be considered on their individual merits, and it is probable that exhibition of several (i.e. more than two) of the criteria given in Table 5.3 would indicate a poor outcome from medical intensive care alone. A number of other discriminant prognostic factors have been identified, particularly amongst the specific co-agulation factors, but although well represented in the literature, the tests required are unavailable on a routine basis to most clinicians in the UK.

Outcome of transplantation in FHF

Liver transplantation is being performed increasingly for poor prognosis patients with FHF. The surgical aspects of the operation have proved relatively straightforward, as the dissection to remove the recipient liver is not complicated by the leash of collateral vessels found in patients with chronic liver disease and portal hypertension. The results of transplantation in FHF are none the less among the worst for any underlying diagnosis, with reported in-hospital mortalities of between 30 and 40% in most early reports (e.g. Schafer & Shaw 1989)—when an equivalent overall mortality figure for transplant programmes was nearer 10%. This reflects not only the haemodynamic instability of the patients, and the tendency to develop intractable cerebral oedema during the operation, but also the frequent deterioration occurring between the decision to transplant and the availability of a donor liver, by which time surgery may be barely justifiable. The excess mortality resides accordingly largely in the perioperative period. However, improved preoperative monitoring, particularly the inclusion of routine ICP measurement, and the greater appreciation of the risk factors for sudden cardiac death (O'Grady et al 1988b) are beginning to be reflected in improved outcome figures, with up to 80% one-year survival reported (Bismuth & Samuel 1989). Better results are probably not an effect of transplanting patients who might have been saved by intensive medical means. This remains a somewhat controversial topic (Chapman et al 1990) in the current (and probably future) absence of controlled trials. There have not been well-documented cases of disease recurrence in the transplanted liver, as early graft failure is more probably of vascular origin or from hyperacute rejection, but this spectre remains in patients transplanted for viral causes.

There has been a recent resurgence of interest in heterotopic liver grafting, where the donor liver is placed in an ectopic site (such as the right iliac fossa) and the patient's own liver is left in situ. This approach has not yet been widely applied in the patient needing transplantation for acute liver failure. As it is firmly believed that the liver affected by FHF will recover fully if the patient survives the acute illness, there is considerable logic in preserving it. It is therefore to be expected that the provisional report from Metselaar et al (1990) describing the successful use of this technique in a single patient with subacute autoimmune hepatic failure will be followed by a more general application in the management of severe FHF. The possibility exists that a heterotopic graft providing short- to medium-term substitution while the host liver recovers, could then be removed electively, thus freeing the patient from a lifetime of immunosuppression.

Finding a donor liver sufficiently quickly for the patient rapidly deteriorating with FHF is often a major difficulty; the use of a partial graft from a live donor is becoming accepted in paediatric practice and could be a viable option in FHF also. This could be applied equally well in the case of heterotopic grafting, and indeed Metselaar et al (1990) used a reduced (non-live) donor liver.

TRANSFER OF PATIENTS WITH FHF

If it is accepted that fulminant hepatic failure is best managed by the experienced, it follows that the transfer of patients within or, more often, between hospitals will frequently be required. Equally there is no doubt that those with advanced disease tolerate transfer poorly, and the following

Table 5.4   Aids to safe transport of patients with FHF

1 Continuous oxygen
2 Endotracheal tube if *any* doubt as to adequacy of respiratory reserve
3 At least one reliable venous access site
4 Sitting posture
5 Monitor pupils and (if possible) blood pressure
6 Monitor blood glucose
7 Medical escort (usually an anaesthetist) capable of performing endotracheal intubation in suboptimal circumstances
8 Concentrated glucose and mannitol solutions available

Note: The coma grade often deteriorates by about one point per hour during transit.

is intended as a guide to minimize the hazards (summarized in Table 5.4). All patients should receive oxygen and if there is any doubt as to the adequacy of their respiratory reserve, an endotracheal tube should be placed before leaving the referring centre. The patient should have at least one reliable venous access site, and should travel sitting up. During transit, pupils, blood glucose, and (if possible) blood pressure should be monitored frequently. Concentrated glucose solutions and mannitol should be available, and the patient should be escorted by a doctor (usually an anaesthetist) who is used not only to dealing with sick patients but who is capable of performing endotracheal intubation in suboptimal circumstances. The coma grade can be expected to deteriorate by at least one point in a typical journey of 1 to 2 hours.

Whether a patient with apparently severe paracetamol intoxication but who is not obviously encephalopathic should be transferred is not always clear. The following criteria (summarized in Table 5.5) are suggested as guidelines for onward referral but should not be considered as a substitute for telephone consultation between the originating hospital and the regional liver centre. Parenthetically it may be worth noting that the development of coma within 36 hours of the overdose is never from paracetamol: other drugs or incorrect timing should be suspected. Coagulopathy is rarely markedly abnormal before 36 hours, but has often peaked by 48 hours and is a very valuable pointer to what can be expected thereafter. An INR greater than 4.0 at 48 hours is almost always followed by hepatic and/or renal failure requiring intervention. Acidosis—a pH < 7.3—should prompt

Table 5.5   Guidelines for referral of patients with paracetamol poisoning to specialist liver centres

1 INR > 4.0 at 48 hours from time of overdose
2 Arterial pH < 7.3
3 Plasma creatinine > 200 µmol/l
4 Encephalopathy

Notes
(a) Coma within 36 hours of overdose almost certainly indicates non-paracetamol cause.
(b) Even extreme elevations of aminotransferases of no appreciable prognostic significance.

transfer, as should a plasma creatinine $> 200\,\mu\text{mol/l}$, since both presage later problems. Elevations, even to astronomic levels, of the aminotransferases merely indicate liver damage and have no appreciable prognostic significance: any patient with sufficient hepatic necrosis to raise the INR (even to 1.5 or 2) will have transaminases in the thousands but will have a good prognosis with conventional non-specialist supportive care if there are none of the adverse features listed above.

COMMON ERRORS IN THE MANAGEMENT OF FHF

Many of the errors made in the management of patients with fulminant hepatic failure could be avoided with a little more general awareness of the condition, but even in expert hands mistakes occur. The following notes are intended as a guide to spotting trouble, and are arranged in an order roughly corresponding to the order in which they might be expected to occur: reference should be made in each case to the relevant section of the main text.

The failure to recognize the presence of FHF can be overcome best by experience and by the continued maintenance of a high index of suspicion; a lower threshold for measuring coagulation in ill patients would certainly help to draw appropriate attention to the liver. It should not be necessary to quote a failure to treat hypoglycaemia adequately, but too often a severe episode is treated and not then followed by hypertonic glucose infusion to prevent recurrence. More serious is the failure to recognize renal failure, and the reliance of clinicians on plasma urea estimations (especially when liver disease is yet to be thought of) has obvious serious implications. There is a widespread reluctance to intubate and ventilate patients with rapidly progressing liver failure; this leads to semi-elective procedures being done as emergencies, and in extreme cases to irreversible cardiorespiratory arrest. Part of the blame must be laid on the physician's reluctance to surrender aspects of care to the intensive care team, but we have also seen intubation, and more commonly the use of central venous and arterial cannulation, falsely considered contra-indicated on grounds of hypocoagulability. The failure to recognize early signs of cerebral oedema is understandable in the inexperienced, but the use of sedation in the aggressive phase of Grade III encephalopathy (if not coupled with ventilation) is certainly the most serious error of commission and may prove fatal. Positive evidence of systemic infection (and certainly its microbiological confirmation), often emerges only when the patient is moribund: a very low threshold for administration of antibiotics is appropriate. A late rise in INR is usually a pointer to uncontrolled sepsis, and antifungal treatment should be introduced if a comprehensive regime of antibacterials is already employed. Delayed treatment of renal failure and acidosis arises from the reliance on criteria for dialysis too stringent for the patient with acute liver injury, but the wider availability of CAVHD will, with luck, begin to make this a thing of the past; as with ventilation interdisciplinary barriers must not be allowed to compromise the optimal care of the patient. The patient with cerebral oedema really must be treated statically with minimal intervention, and the natural zeal of nursing staff for frequent turning of the comatose patient will need to be curbed! There can still be a tendency to 'give up too soon'; the long-term prognosis is so good (even in patients with an initial suicidal intent) that 'everything' should be tried.

REFERENCES

Bismuth H, Samuel D 1989 Liver transplantation in fulminant and subfulminant hepatitis. Transplantation Reviews 3: 47–58

Canalese J, Gimson A E S, Davis C, Mellon P J, Davis M, Williams R 1982 Controlled trial of dexamethasone and mannitol for the cerebral oedema of fulminant hepatic failure. Gut 23: 625–629

Chapman R W, Forman D, Peto R, Smallwood R 1990 Liver transplantation for acute hepatic failure? Lancet 335: 32–35

Davis M 1986 Protective agents for acetaminophen overdose. Seminars in Liver Disease 6: 138–147

Ede R J, Williams R 1986 Hepatic encephalopathy and cerebral oedema. Seminars in Liver Disease 6: 107–118

Forbes A, Williams R 1988 Increasing age—an important adverse prognostic factor in hepatitis A virus infection. Journal of the Royal College of Physicians of London 22: 237–239

Forbes A, Alexander G J M, Smith H, Williams R 1988 Elevation of serum sex hormone-binding globulin in females with fulminant hepatitis B virus infection. Journal of Medical Virology 26: 93–98

Forbes A, Wicks C 1989 Fulminant hepatic failure, nutrition and fat clearance. Recent Advances in Nutriology 1: 67–69

Forbes A, Alexander G J M, O'Grady J G et al 1989 Thiopental infusion in the treatment of intracranial hypertension complicating fulminant hepatic failure. Hepatology 10: 306–310

Harrison P M, Keays R, Bray G P, Alexander G J M, Williams R 1990 Improved outcome of paracetamol-induced fulminant hepatic failure by late administration of acetylcysteine. Lancet 335: 1572–1573

Keays R, Gove C, Forbes A, Alexander G J M, Williams R 1989a Use of late N-acetyl cysteine in severe paracetamol overdose. Gut 30: A1512

Keays R, Alexander G J M, Darkins A, Gullen R, Williams R 1989b Safety of extradural intracranial pressure monitors in fulminant hepatic failure. Gut 30: A745–746

Langley P G, Keays R, Hughes R D, Forbes A, Delvos U, Williams R 1990 Controlled trial of antithrombin III supplementation to improve biocompatibility of haemodialysis in fulminant hepatic failure. British Association for the Study of the Liver, Spring Meeting, London

Le Roux P D, Elliott J P, Perkins J D, Winn H R 1990 Intracranial pressure monitoring in fulminant hepatic failure and liver transplantation. Lancet 335: 1291

MacDougall B R D, Williams R 1978 H2-receptor antagonist in the prevention of acute upper gastrointestinal hemorrhage in fulminant hepatic failure. Gastroenterology 74: 164–165

Mallory A, Kern F Jr 1980 Drug-induced pancreatitis: a critical review. Gastroenterology 78: 813–820

Metselaar H J, Hesselink E J, De Rave S et al 1990 Recovery of failing liver after auxiliary heterotopic transplantation. Lancet 335: 1156–1157

Miller R, Kingswood C, Bullen C, Cohen S 1990 Renal replacement therapy in the ICU: continuous arteriovenous haemodialysis. British Journal of Hospital Medicine 43: 354–361

O'Brien C J, Wise R J S, O'Grady J G, Williams R 1987 Neurological sequelae in patients recovered from fulminant hepatic failure. Gut 28: 93–95

O'Grady J G, Gimson A E S, O'Brien C J et al 1988a Controlled trials of charcoal haemoperfusion and prognostic factors in fulminant hepatic failure. Gastroenterology 94: 1186–1192

O'Grady J G, Alexander G J, Thick M, Potter D, Calne R Y, Williams R 1988b Outcome of orthotopic liver transplantation in the aetiological and clinical variants of acute liver failure. Quarterly Journal of Medicine 68: 817–824

O'Grady J G, Alexander G J, Hayllar K M, Williams R 1989 Early indicators of prognosis in fulminant hepatic failure. Gastroenterology 97: 439–445

Rolando N, Harvey F, Brahm J et al 1990 Prospective study of bacterial infection in acute liver failure: an analysis of fifty patients. Hepatology 11: 49–53

Schafer D F, Shaw B W Jr 1989 Fulminant hepatic failure and orthotopic liver transplantation. Seminars in Liver Disease 9: 189–194

Sinclair S B, Grieg P D, Blendis L M et al 1989 Biochemical and clinical response of fulminant viral hepatitis to administration of prostaglandin E. Journal of Clinical Investigation 84: 1063–1069

Smilkstein M J, Knapp G L, Kulig K W, Rumack B H 1988 Efficacy of oral N-acetylcysteine in the treatment of acetaminophen overdose. New England Journal of Medicine 319: 1557–1562

Trey C, Burns D G, Saunders S J 1966 Treatment of hepatic coma by exchange blood transfusions. New England Journal of Medicine 274: 473–481

Wendon J, Keays R, Harrison P M, Alexander G J M, Williams R 1990 The effect of vasopressor agents and prostacyclin on oxygen transport variables in fulminant hepatic failure. British Association for the Study of the Liver, Spring Meeting, London

Zuckerman A J 1990 Hepatitis E virus. British Medical Journal 300: 1475–1476

6. The spondylarthropathies

A. Calin

INTRODUCTION

The seronegative spondylarthr.tides (Fig. 6.1) are a group of disorders characterized by involvement of the sacroiliac joints, by peripheral inflam-

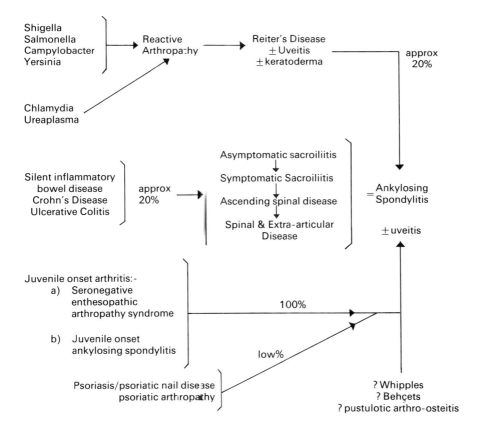

Fig. 6.1 The interrelated conditions making up the spondylarthropathy group.

Table 6.1   Distribution of HLA B27 among different healthy and diseased groups

	HLA B27 (%)
Healthy Caucasians	6–14
British	6
Northern Scandinavian	14
Healthy Blacks	< 1–4
African Black	< 1
USA Black	4
Japanese	1–2
Chinese	5–10
Haida Indians	50
Caucasians	
Primary ankylosing spondylitis	95
Reactive arthropathy/Reiter's	80
Enteropathic spondylarthropathy	50
Uveitis	40–50
Psoriatic spondylitis	50–60
Blacks	
Primary ankylosing spondylitis	50
Reactive arthropathy	50

matory arthropathy, insertional tendinitis (enthesopathy) and by the absence of rheumatoid factor (Calin 1989).

There are serveral other important features:

1. Pathological changes are concentrated at the site of insertion of ligaments or tendons rather than the synovium. Further pathological changes may also develop in the eye, the aortic valve, lung parenchyma and skin.
2. There is clinical evidence of overlap between the various seronegative spondylarthritides. Thus, a patient with psoriatic arthropathy may develop uveitis or sacroiliitis and a patient with inflammatory bowel disease may develop ankylosing spondylitis or mouth ulcers.
3. There is a tendency towards familial aggregation, suggesting that these disorders 'breed true' within families.
4. There is an association with HLA B27, ranging from about 50% (psoriatic and enteropathic spondylitis) to over 95% (primary ankylosing spondylitis). The specific frequency depends on ethnic group and disease type (Table 6.1).

CLINICAL SUBSETS

The interrelated group of conditions constituting the spondylarthropathies have a variety of signs and symptoms (Table 6.2). They are categorized according to the specific articular or extra-articular pattern. Depending on the associated clinical features (i.e. urethritis, eye disease, skin involvement) and the way the disease progresses (i.e. remission, relapse) a specific

Table 6.2 Features of the spondylarthropathies

	Ankylosing spondylitis	Reiter's syndrome	Psoriatic arthropathy	Enteropathic spondylitis	Juvenile arthropathy (JAS* subset)	Reactive arthropathy
Sex	Male > Female	Male = Female	Female > Male	Female = Male	Male > Female	Male = Female
Age at onset	20	Any age	Any age	Any age	< 16	Any age
Uveitis	− −	++	+	+	+	+
Conjunctivitis	−	+	−	−	−	+
Peripheral joints	Lower > Upper	Lower usually	Upper > Lower	Lower > Upper	Lower > Upper	Lower > Upper
Sacroiliitis	Always	Often	Often	Often	Often	Often
HLA B27	95%	80%	20% (50% with sacroiliitis)	50%	90%	80%
Enthesopathy	+	+	+	+	+	+
Aortic regurgitation	+	+	?+	?	?	+
Familial aggregation	+	+	+	+	+	+
Risk for HLA B27 positive individual	5–20%	20%	?	?	?	20%
Onset	Gradual	Sudden	Variable	Gradual	Variable	Sudden
Urethritis	−	+	−	−	−	±
Skin involvement	−	+	++	−	−	−
Mucous membrane involvement		+	−	++	+	−
Symmetry (spinal)	+	−	−	±	±	±
Self-limiting	−	±	±	±	±	±
Remission, relapses	−	±	±	−	±	±

*JAS = Juvenile ankylosing spondylitis.

diagnostic label is given. However, it is readily apparent to the student of these diseases that clearly defined criteria are frequently absent and one often meets patients who have a spondylarthropathy but in whom the symptoms and signs are such that one is left with an undifferentiated picture. Family and epidemiological studies confirm this clinical finding. For example, a patient may appear with unilateral sacroiliitis and little else, or chest wall symptoms due to intercostal muscle insertional tendinitis and, for example, uveitis. Clearly, the specific phenotypic expression is the end product of a variety of interrelating genetic and environmental factors.

DIAGNOSTIC CRITERIA AND CLASSIFICATION

Classification criteria for most of the disorders already exist. However, the spectrum of spondylarthropathy is wider than the sum of these disorders suggest. For example, seronegative oligoarthropathy with or without dactylitis, heel pain due to an enthesopathy perhaps with some spinal syndesmophytes, and other undifferentiated phenomena (e.g. uveitis and calcaneodynia) are typically ignored in epidemiological studies due to an inadequacy of existing criteria. Given that the current criteria for ankylosing spondylitis, reactive arthropathy, psoriatic spondylarthritis and the other members are too restricted to include all the entities forming the disease spectrum, we and others have attempted to provide diagnostic criteria for the spondylarthropathy group as a whole. In essence, patients with inflammatory spinal pain or asymmetric synovitis predominantly of the lower limb, together with at least one of the following—family history positivity, psoriasis, inflammatory bowel disease, enthesopathic lesions or asymmetric sacroiliitis, have 'undifferentiated spondylarthropathy' with acceptable sensitivity and specificity. The proposed classification criteria known as the 'European seronegative study group criteria for spondylarthropathy', will help broaden our acceptance and understanding of the entire spondyloarthropathic disorders.

PATHOGENESIS

Even in the reactive arthropathies where the infective trigger is recognized (e.g. yersinia, shigella, salmonella, campylobacter, chlamydia) and the genetic background (HLA B27) clearly defined, the precise pathogenesis is not well understood (Yu 1989). The various steps may include some low-grade inflammatory change in the bowel, the absorption of micro-organisms or parts thereof, endocytosis of the inciting fragments by antigen-presenting cells, degrading of the material followed by linking of the putative antigenic peptide with the HLA molecule. These are expressed on the cell surface as a binary product. Finally this HLA/antigenic peptide composite interacts with the T cell receptor determinant, the three forming a tertiary product. An acute arthropathy results and perhaps following further unknown environmental factors, and poorly defined genetic characteristics, the chronic disease state may develop (Schwartz 1990).

HLA B27

The HLA B27 molecule is a two-chain structure that consists of a polymorphic glycoprotein, termed the heavy, or alpha, chain. The alpha chain is encoded by the HLA complex and is non-covalently linked to a non-HLA-encoded non-polymorphic protein, Beta-2 microglobulin. The entire molecule is anchored to the cell membrane by the heavy chain. The extracellular portion of the heavy chain is divided into three domains, termed alpha-1, alpha-2 and alpha-3, each of which contains approximately 90 aminoacids. The alpha-1 and alpha-2 domains are distal to the cell membrane and it is these that demonstrate the greatest HLA polymorphism. The alpha-1 and alpha-2 domains each consist of four beta strands and an alpha helix. The eight beta strands of these two domains form a beta-pleated sheet or platform which in turn supports the two alpha helices. The alpha helices create a groove which serves as the antigen-binding site for the putative peptide fragment which has been processed from the larger antigen. The two alpha helices with the bound antigen fragment comprise a ligand which is recognized by the T cell receptor on a class 1 restricted CD8 positive T cell.

There are several hypotheses explaining the HLA B27 association with spondylarthropathy. In contrast to the situation with Reiter's disease where clearly defined organisms are known to be operative (e.g. chlamydia, shigella, salmonella, campylobacter and others) the trigger for ankylosing spondylitis (AS) remains unclear and could either be one of the above organisms or viruses or indeed other environmental phenomena.

The first hypothesis suggests that a particular B27 molecule can act as a receptor for the aetiological agent. Support for such a hypothesis comes from observations that other cell surface molecules can act as receptors for viruses, such as CD4 for the human immunodeficiency virus. Individuals with B27 who contact the putative trigger will develop disease.

The second hypothesis suggests that the antigen-binding groove of only certain HLA molecules can accept the processed antigenic fragment that is ultimately responsible for causing disease. Thus, when the AS-causing organism enters the cell the antigens are degraded to peptides and only certain B27 molecules accept the antigen, presented to the T cell and disease takes place.

The third hypothesis postulates that the T cell antigen receptor which recognizes the HLA molecule-peptide complex is responsible for disease but because the T cell recognition is restricted by an HLA molecule there is an association between the disease and B27. Finally, an hypothesis termed 'the molecular mimicry' phenomenon occurs. Here the peptide derived from the organism that causes disease is immunologically identical to HLA

B27. Therefore the peptide is not recognized as foreign—no immune response is mounted and the disease process develops. Alternatively, the peptide is recognized as foreign and a vigorous immune response is mounted against the organism but the response cross-reacts with self tissue causing disease.

In 1991 we still do not know which of these many possibilities—if any—is correct. Interestingly, certain strains of shigella which contain a plasmid (an extrachromosomal piece of DNA) are known to be arthritogenic, causing Reiter's syndrome. Recent data suggest that B27 positive individuals share structural and immunological homology with a sequence of five aminoacids present in the plasmid.

At least six variants of the HLA B27 molecule exist but disease predisposition does not appear to be restricted to a particular variant. Using monoclonal anti-HLA B27 antibodies, several bacterial components have been recognized. The relevance of this cross-reaction remains unclear. Through a computerized search, a klebsiella protein has been identified that carries a stretch of six aminoacids identical to residue 72 to 77 of two of the HLA B27 variants. Moreover a synthetic peptide carrying the six aminoacids of the HLA B27 protein is reactive with serum antibodies in some patients with disease. These recent developments need confirmation in other groups of patients and only then will their significance, or lack thereof, be established.

Regardless of the putative klebsiella link, there is still no certainty that this organism is arthritogenic in ankylosing spondylitis. It may well be that numerous bacteria (and indeed viruses) can induce disease in genetically susceptible individuals.

Recently, transgenic mice have been created that express HLA B27 and it is possible that this model will help clarify the above issues (Taurog 1989).

Reactive arthropathy or intra-articular 'infection'?

Reactive arthropathy is defined as an inflammatory joint disease that relates to an infective organism that is distant in both time and place from the arthropathy. For example, chlamydia inducing a urethritis may be followed 2 weeks later by uveitis, arthropathy and other stigmata of Reiter's disease. A similar situation can follow dysenteric infection with campylobacter, yersinia or other organism. However, there have been recent studies demonstrating both chlamydia, yersinia and salmonella antigenic components within the synovial tissues (Granfors et al 1990). Whether these represent an epiphenomenon or whether they are central to disease pathogenesis remains unclear but at least at the moment it is not considered that viable organisms are found in the joint space. Moreover, we have described post-salmonella vaccination arthropathy—a rheumatic condition related to the inoculation of dead organisms.

Interestingly, Lyme disease, which is known to be a multisystem disorder related to *Borrelia burgdorferi* may produce a 'reactive' phenomenon in addition to the direct infective process.

Epidemiological studies tell us that reactive arthropathy is more common in the epidemic situation than where the organism is endemic. Adults are more at risk than are children in contradistinction to the situation with acute rheumatic fever. In post-dysenteric arthropathy patients frequently suffer only minimal gastrointestinal symptoms. As mentioned, post-vaccination (salmonella) Reiter's disease can occur. Ankylosing spondylitis is seen in both the developing and developed world with an increased age of onset in the latter. Other epidemiological studies demonstrate that ankylosing spondylitis occurs predominantly in the Haida and Pima Indians and the relatives of white patients with ankylosing spondylitis, while Reiter's syndrome occurs among the Navaho Indians and Inupiat Eskimo in addition to white family members of probands with Reiter's disease. Presumably B27 is not sufficient and, as stated, additional gene or genes modify the phenotypic expression (i.e. HLA B27 plus appropriate environmental trigger, plus the ankylosing spondylitis gene results in ankylosing spondylitis while HLA B27 plus environmental trigger plus the Reiter's syndrome gene leads to Reiter's syndrome).

The risk for the HLA B27 positive individual depends on the nature of that individual. For example, if related to an HLA B27 positive patient with ankylosing spondylitis the chance of developing that same disease is approximately 1 in 3. HLA B27 positive relatives of healthy B27 positive subjects appear to be at much less risk of developing spondylarthropathy. Interplay between different chromosomes almost certainly occurs. Chromosome 6 is clearly important with HLA B27, BW60 and CW6 all relevant. In addition, recent interest focuses on the tumour necrosis factor and class III genes (complement) on the same sixth chromosome. Other possible genetic factors relate to the T cell receptor beta gene (defined by a locus on the seventh chromosome) and the TCR alpha gene, alpha 1 antitrypsin gene and the IgG heavy chain gene products related to loci on the fourteenth chromosome. Additional gene loci and products thereof include the IgG light kappa chain (chromosome 2), ABO secretor status gene (chromosome 19) and the IgG light lambda chain (chromosome 22).

Reactive arthropathy appears to be mediated by HLA Class 1 restricted CD8 positive T cells, given that both psoriatic arthropathy and Reiter's disease thrive in the presence of human immunodeficiency virus infection. This is in contrast to the CD4 positive T cell-maintained arthropathy of rheumatoid arthritis, which appears to remit in the presence of human immunodeficiency virus infection.

ANKYLOSING SPONDYLITIS

Symptomatic sacroiliitis (ankylosing spondylitis; AS) may occur in up to 1% of the white population. It is often undiagnosed and sufferers may well be inappropriately managed (e.g. an erroneous diagnosis of mechanical back pain disease is made and bed rest prescribed). The sex distribution in population studies suggests a male predominance of approximately 3:1 in favour of males, although men tend to have more ascending spinal disease while woman have more peripheral joint involvement.

The criteria for diagnosing AS have evolved over recent years. The characteristic features of inflammatory spinal disease include:

Insidious onset
Age less than 40 years at onset
Persistence for more than 3 months
Association with morning stiffness
Improvement with exercise

If several of these features are present, a radiograph may confirm sacroiliitis. Additional studies including radionuclide scans, computed tomography and other investigations are of little value and are certainly expensive.

Physical examination may reveal muscle spasm and decreased mobility of the spine and to varying degree, there may be extra-articular features as mentioned above. HLA B27 testing should not be used as a routine test given the relatively high background frequency (some 6–8% of the normal population in the UK).

The extra-skeletal involvement

General. Fatigue, weight loss, and low-grade fever may occur. Cord compression due to spinal fractures (the brittle fused spine can snap following minimal trauma), and the cauda equina syndrome (a bizarre inflammation of the nerve roots in the lumbar regions) may cause neurological symptoms.

Eye involvement. Uveitis develops in up to 40% of patients during their illness.

Pulmonary disease. Patients with severe disease may exhibit chronic infiltrative and fibrotic changes in the upper lung fields that mimic tuberculosis.

Cardiovascular disease. Aortic incompetence, cardiomegaly and persistent conduction defects occur in up to 10% of patients with severe spondylitis.

Cardiac involvement may be clinically silent, or it may dominate the clinical picture.

Amyloidosis. Amyloid deposition is an occasional complication of AS, particularly in Europe. It appears to be of little clinical significance in most patients.

Renal disease. In contrast to patients with rheumatoid arthritis, who may show renal impairment as an expression of disease, glomerular function is usually unimpaired in AS, despite recognized pathological changes. An IgA nephropathy, however, has been described in patients with sero-negative spondylarthropathy.

The bone in AS (Will et al 1989)

Juxta-articular and generalized osteoporosis are well recognized in rheumatoid arthritis but the relative role of hormonal factors, immobility, drug therapy and the disease process is unclear. Ankylosing spondylitis (AS) is characterized by inflammation at the site of the enthesis in the spine and peripheral skeleton. This may lead to local bone erosion or juxta-insertional osteoporosis in early disease but subsequent new bone formation and ankylosis of the spine occurs.

Patients with severe AS may develop a dorsal kyphosis. Radiological assessment of patients with AS often reveals anterior wedging of vertebrae at the area of maximal spinal curvature of the dorsal spine. 'Codfish' vertebrae also occur suggesting a significant degree of vertebral osteoporosis.

Spinal osteoporosis in patients with severe AS has been attributed to immobility resulting from bony ankylosis. By contrast the status of the skeleton in early disease has not been defined. In a recent study we measured the bone mineral density of the lumbar spine, femoral neck and carpus in 25 patients with early ankylosing spondylitis who maintained normal spinal mobility and in 25 age-matched male controls.

Both the lumbar and femoral neck bone mineral density in the patient population was significantly lower than the control population. For the lumbar spine bone mineral density of patients was 0.82 against an expected value of 0.91 g/cm². For the femoral neck bone mineral density was 0.83 and 0.92%, respectively. The bone mineral density of the carpus was the same in patients and controls. The pattern of bone loss in this group of patients suggests loss of trabecular bone due to a systemic cause. Interestingly, biochemical indices of calcium turnover, including a fasting 2-hour urinary calcium/creatinine ratio were the same in patients with AS and healthy controls.

PROGNOSIS

Much can be accomplished towards meliorating symptoms if ankylosing spondylitis is discovered early. The primary objectives are to relieve pain, decrease inflammation and maintain good posture and function with an aggressive exercise programme. Why some individuals have relatively mild self-limiting disease while others have a persistent chronic multisystem involvement remains poorly defined. However, we do now recognize that the younger the age of onset the more likely there is to be hip and cervical spine involvement. For example, the risk of the former (requiring total hip replacement) reaches 20% in a 20-year follow-up of individuals with disease onset in their mid-teens, whereas with an onset beyond the mid-twenties hip involvement is extremely rare.

TREATMENT

General

Patient education (including patient groups and self-help). The patient must understand that the purpose of anti-inflammatory medication is to reduce pain and stiffness, so that an active exercise programme can be followed. The patient must have insight into the natural history of disease and understand something of the inflammatory process.

Family education. Unless family members understand the nature of the disease, it is difficult for them to give appropriate encouragement to the patient.

Genetic counselling. Most patients with ankylosing spondylitis are HLA-B27 positive. They should know that the risk of transmitting the same antigen to their offspring is 50%. Thereafter, if HLA-B27 positive, a son or daughter has a 1 in 3 chance of developing ankylosing spondylitis. The only advice that need be given is that the overall risk for the son or daughter is 1 in 6 and that they should seek specialist help if he or she develops symptoms such as swollen joints or painful eyes.

Specific

Pain relief. Non-steroidal anti-inflammatory drugs are indicated (e.g. ibuprofen or indomethacin).

Disease modification. A debate continues as to whether sulphasalazine can alter the course of the disease. There is no doubt that laboratory variables improve and peripheral joint involvement may benefit. The effect on the spine remains less clear.

Improve posture. Advice regarding day and night posture must be given. A firm bed with one pillow is appropriate at night, as are straight-back chairs and regular walking and swimming during the day.

Stop smoking.

Encourage exercises. Swimming is best (the patient must exercise the muscles and protect the joints). Extension exercises are useful. The disease tends to cause spinal flexion and so anything the patient can do to extend upwards is appropriate.

Referral for surgery. Surgical intervention is most often carried out for hip involvement. Rarely, spinal osteotomy is used for severe spinal curvature.

Physiotherapy. The patient should be taught exercises which can be performed daily at home.

Occupational therapy. The use of appropriate wing mirrors for the car, together with other gadgets to aid daily living, are useful.

Treatment of complications and extraskeletal problems. For example, intra-articular corticosteroid injections may be helpful for extra-spinal joint disease. A patient with severe uveitis should be referred to an ophthalmologist.

THE CHANGING EPIDEMIOLOGY OF RHEUMATIC DISEASES (Will et al 1990)

There are many reasons why the pattern (perceived or real) of a disease may change. Increased interest and recognition by the medical profession and greater concern and pressure from patients may lead to more emphasis on a particular disease. For example, osteoporosis, until recently ignored by rheumatologists, has become a major focus of interest.

Chronic tophaceous gout, once the scourge of medical clinics, is an example of a rheumatic disorder which has all but disappeared, in part due to changing dietary habits and in part because of hypouricaemic agents. By contrast, a recent rise in prevalence of gout in older females relates to the greater use of diuretics.

Rheumatic fever, at least until recently, had become rare in the West. The decline in fatal rheumatic carditis accelerated after 1945 perhaps due to an alteration in the pathogenicty of the streptococcal group A M antigen induced by penicillin. Altered streptococcal antigenicity may also be responsible for the recent recognition of a post-streptococcal arthropathy.

Recent studies suggest that rheumatoid arthritis may be declining in frequency in the West, perhaps due to the advent of the contraceptive pill, but is becoming more prevalent and more severe in the developing world. For example, recent published data have demonstrated that as rural black Africans migrate to an urban environment, rheumatoid arthritis increases in frequency and becomes a more destructive disease. Hypothetical explanations for this phenomenon may include either exposure to new antigens present in an urban environment but uncommon in a less crowded rural setting or, conversely, a reduction in the antigenic load due to fewer parasitic infestations (which in turn could result in less immunosuppression).

There is increasing evidence accumulating from Western and developing countries suggesting that the pattern of AS may be changing. This relates to both the age of onset of the disease and the pattern of joint involvement. AS develops at an earlier age in countries with poor living conditions but as these improve the age of onset is delayed. We have recently suggested that the age of onset of the disease may also be increasing over time in Britain. The influence of potential left and right censoring biases on the UK data has been emphasized elsewhere, though the importance of this phenomenon is difficult to quantify. Can the conclusion of an increasing age of onset of AS in Britain be substantiated by data from other Western countries? The putative change may be due to a later age of exposure to the presumed 'infective trigger(s)' or altered pathogenicity of the trigger(s) perhaps due to modifying factor such as the widespread use of antibiotics.

Amor and colleagues in France recently noted that the age of onset of AS was influenced by the geographic background of their patients. They observed that 25% of patients from North Africa develop disease before the age of 15 whereas only 10% of patients in France did so. Moreover, 47 second generation North Africans with AS born and living in France (but whose parents were born in North Africa) were identified from a survey conducted by the French Society of Rheumatology in 1983. None of these 'Beur' as they are known, developed disease before the age of 15. Other studies have also noted a lower frequency of juvenile onset AS (age < 16) in white caucasian populations as compared to subjects in the developing world. In spite of the inevitable ascertainment biases, there are now a series of studies consistently demonstrating a greater frequency of patients with a lower age of disease onset from developing countries.

We have recently taken an entirely separate epidemiological route and studied the changing pattern of new patient referral to the London Hospital. Of interest, patients with non-specific mechanical back pain have become progressively younger over the last three decades whereas new patients with AS have become progressively older. We feel that these data, together with the Bath and the French data of Amor add further support for a changing pattern.

Family studies of sibling pairs with AS also suggest that the date of onset in each sib is similar while the age at onset is discordant suggesting exposure to the trigger at about the same time. This emphasizes the importance of the environmental trigger determining the time of onset of disease in sibling pairs who have a similar genetic predisposition (Calin 1989).

It has recently been noted that the age of disease onset influences the need for total hip replacement (THR). In a recent study we have shown that 16% of a juvenile cohort (10–15 years), 10% of an early onset (18–20 years) and 1% of a late onset cohort (30–40 years) had THRs performed. Amor et al also observed that the frequency of THR in a spondylitic population correlates well with the mean age of disease onset. A study of THRs performed in patients from four French hospitals between 1977–83 was undertaken: 22 of 71 patients (30%) who had THRs were born in North Africa as compared with only 8% of non-surgical patients treated in French hospitals during this same period. The explanation for more severe hip joint involvement in a juvenile cohort is unknown. The developing hip joint may be at greater risk of damage. Conversely, a more marked inflammatory response may result in greater joint destruction in juveniles compared with patients who develop the disease at an older age.

Of interest, a changing pattern in inflammatory bowel disease is now also recognized and we have noted that in many studies Crohn's disease, which became progressively more common until the mid-seventies, has now begun to be less prevalent. The intriguing interrelationship between the bowel and AS is, of course, well known.

In conclusion, chronic rheumatic diseases should not be considered immutable processes. A changing pattern of disease is to be expected given the interaction of genes and the environment. AS should now be considered as another example of a rheumatic disorder whose characteristics may be altering as a result of a changing environment. We might expect a diminished need for THR among patients as a consequence of an increasing age of onset of patients in the West and perhaps in developing countries as the environment changes. Physicians will need to be increasingly aware that patients may present with symptoms of disease in their 30s or later.

REITER'S SYNDROME AND THE REACTIVE ARTHROPATHIES

The commonest cause of an inflammatory oligoarthropathy in a young male is Reiter's syndrome or reactive arthropathy. These two terms should be used synonymously since the classical triad of urethritis, conjunctivitis and arthritis may not necessarily occur at the same time. Other terms used include enteropathic reactive arthritis and sexually acquired reactive arthritis. For the majority of patients there may not be an obvious bowel or urethral portal of entry for the infective trigger. Reiter's syndrome was once considered a self-limiting disease but this is not necessarily the case and the condition may progress relentlessly. The condition can be defined as an episode of arthropathy within one month of urethritis or cervicitis.

In many cases the distinction between urethritis as a precipitating factor and urethritis as an integral manifestation of the syndrome remains unclear. Both chlamydia and *Mycoplasma urealyticum* have been implicated in sexually acquired disease, while yersinia, campylobacter, shigella, salmonella and other organisms are precipitating agents in post-dysenteric disease.

The prevalence and incidence of Reiter's syndrome remain unknown but it is clear that at least 1% of patients with non-specific urethritis or dysentery and the appropriate arthritogenic agent will develop Reiter's syndrome. This equates to a 20% risk to the B27 positive individual who succumbs to the inciting infection.

The sex distribution is difficult to define because the syndrome is recognized with difficulty in females in whom urethritis or cervicitis may be inapparent. Nevertheless a woman presenting with an inflammatory arthropathy of the knee perhaps with a uveitis with or without B27 may well have a reactive arthropathy.

As intimated, the syndrome may present as the classical triad, or as a tetrad (i.e. with the addition of buccal ulceration or balanitis) or only two or even one of the cardinal features may be present. The urethritis is frequently mild, the discharge may be minimal and missed by both patient and clinician. Balanitis may not be in evidence unless the prepuce is retracted and the glans penis closely inspected. Buccal ulceration is usually painless and apparent only on close inspection. The rheumatological features include arthralgias, tenosynovitic episodes, plantar fasciitis and other enthesopathies as well as frank arthritis. The typical sausage-shaped digit (i.e. extra-articular swelling in addition to synovitis) is a common occurrence. Dactylitis may also be seen in psoriatic arthropathy. Some 20% of patients with Reiter's syndrome develop sacroiliitis and ascending spinal disease. Other radiological evidence of Reiter's can include plantar spurs and new bone formation.

Extra-articular complications similar to those of ankylosing spondylitis may occur late in the course of Reiter's syndrome.

HLA B27 is present in some 70–80% of cases and the ESR may be normal or high. There is little correlation with the disease severity.

JUVENILE CHRONIC ARTHROPATHY

Chronic arthritis in a child or teenager often persists into adulthood. One subset (in the spondylarthropathy group) consists largely of adolescent males (often positive for HLA B27) who predominantly exhibit oligoarthropathy of the large joints of the lower limbs and sacroiliitis. An HLA B27-related syndrome known as the seronegative enthesopathic arthropathy syndrome (SEA) is now recognized in children. The majority of such cases develop AS at a later date.

ENTEROPATHIC ARTHROPATHIES

There are two main clinical patterns of arthropathy associated with inflammatory bowel disease—ulcerative colitis and Crohn's disease. These include peripheral arthropathy (complication of severe disease) and spondylarthropathy (a manifestation of a similar genetic background). About 50% of individuals with enteropathic spondylitis are positive for HLA B27, a percentage which is lower than that found in patients with primary AS. The sex ratio is equal.

Table 6.3   Subsets of psoriatic arthropathy

Asymmetric oligoarthropathy—often associated with dactylitis
Symmetric polyarthropathy—resembles rheumatoid arthritis
Arthritis mutilans—a resorptive arthropathy, and the most severe form of destructive arthritis. The telescoping digits appear as the so-called 'opera-glass hand'
Psoriatic spondylitis—approximately 20% of subjects with psoriatic arthropathy have radiological sacroiliitis (ankylosing spondylitis)
Psoriatic nail disease and distal interphalangeal joint involvement—nail pitting, transverse depressions, and subungual hyperkeratosis often occur in association with distal interphalangeal joint disease

---

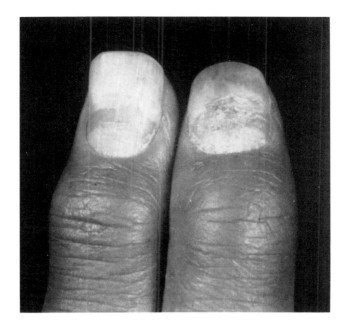

Fig. 6.2   Psoriatic arthropathy. Hand showing nail disease and DIP involvement.

PSORIATIC ARTHROPATHY

Different subsets of psoriatic arthropathy are recognized (Table 6.3), several forms of which appear to be enthesopathic in nature. Uveitis, sacroiliitis and ascending spinal disease occur in up to 20% of cases. Patients are seronegative for rheumatoid factor and exhibit dactylitis and characteristic radiological change. The disease can be very destructive.

Psoriatic arthropathy is a common disorder occurring in about 20% of individuals with psoriasis, particularly in those with psoriatic nail disease (Fig. 6.2). Women are affected slightly more frequently than are men, in contrast to the more marked sex distribution in rheumatoid disease. Psoriatic spondylitis occurs in a sex ratio of 3.5:1 in favour of men.

Radiological findings

Characteristic changes include the 'pencil-in-cup' appearance (the narrow distal end of the proximal bone fits into the splayed out proximal end of the distal bone (Fig. 6.3)), extensive bone resorption can result in an 'opera-glass hand' (the digits can be lengthened or shortened because of the collapsing nature of the underlying bony architecture). Erosions, ankylosis, periostitis, sacroiliitis and AS are the typical radiological findings.

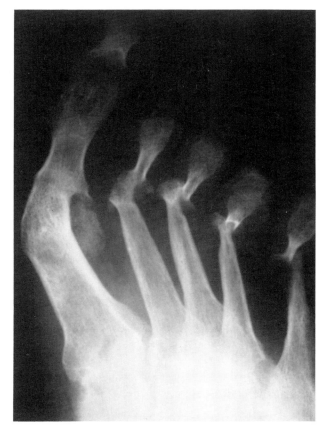

Fig. 6.3 Psoriatic arthropathy. Foot X-ray with 'pencil-in-cup' (acro-osteolysis).

TREATMENT OF THE SPONDYLARTHROPATHIES

Many of the principles outlined in the treatment of ankylosing spondylitis are important in the management approaches to the other spondylarthropathies. The specific points relating to the management of Reiter's disease are summarized in Table 6.4.

The non-steroidal anti-inflammatory drugs are helpful in the treatment of the spondylarthropathies, but probably do not have any major effect on the course of the disease. For this reason, trials with drugs such as sulphasalazine, methotrexate and azathioprine have been carried out. Whether any of these have a long lasting disease remittive effect remains unclear, although it is likely that all have some role to play in modifying disease activity. For the reactive arthropathies and psoriatic arthropathy, Methotrexate may be considered the drug of choice. Sulphasalazine provides theoretical grounds for optimism, but no consensus exists.

Table 6.4 Management approaches in Reiter's syndrome

General

Patient education—the patient is often bewildered about the nature of Reiter's syndrome. Undue concern regarding sexual activity should be allayed because most patients with Reiter's syndrome do not necessarily have sexually acquired disease. Feelings of guilt are common

Family education—frank discussion regarding the relationship of infection to the disease is important. Spouses are often concerned about 'catching' the disease from the patients. It should be stressed that this cannot occur

Avoidance of fragmented care—too often, patients seek help from dermatologists, ophthalmologists and others who may not be aware of the relationship between these various problems and the underlying rheumatological disease

Specific

Drug therapy—for most patients a non-steroidal anti-inflammatory drug, such as ibuprofen or indomethacin, is useful; if indomethacin is ineffective, phenylbutazone may be appropriate. In patients with severe intractable disease, methotrexate or azathioprine should be considered

Exercise—swimming is best

Attention to physical problems (e.g. spinal involvement, foot problems, eye care)—the rehabilitation programme should include a variety of exercises tailored to the needs of the patient

Selected referral for complications (e.g. eye and cardiovascular disease)—uveitis should be evaluated by an ophthalmologist unless it responds very rapidly to steroid eye drops

---

REFERENCES

Calin A 1989 Ankylosing spondylitis. In: Kelley W N, Harris E D, Ruddy S, Sledge C G (eds) Textbook of rheumatology, 3rd edn. Saunders, Philadelphia, pp 1021–1037

Calin A 1989 Reiter's syndrome. In: Kelley W N, Harris E D, Ruddy S, Sledge C G (eds) Textbook of rheumatology, 3rd edn. Saunders, Philadelphia, pp 1038–1052

Granfors K, Jalkanen S, Lindberg A A 1990 Salmonella lipopolysaccharide in synovial cells from patients' reactive arthritis. Lancet 335: 685–688

Schwartz B D 1990 Infectious agents, immunity, and rheumatic diseases. Arthritis and Rheumatism 33 (No. 4): 457–465

Taurog J D 1989 Genetics and immunology of the spondylarthropathies. Current Opinion in Rheumatology 1: 144–150

Will R, Palmer R, Bhalla A K, Ring F, Calin A 1989 Marked osteoporosis is present in early ankylosing spondylitis and may be a primary pathological event. Lancet 2: 1483–1484

Will R, Amor B, Calin A 1990 The changing epidemiology of rheumatic diseases: should ankylosing spondylitis now be included? British Journal of Rheumatology 29: 299–300

Yu D T Y 1989 Molecular mimicry in HLA-B27-related arthritis. Annals of Internal Medicine 111: 581–591

7. Bone marrow transplantation

A. K. Burnett

Current clinical bone marrow transplantation (BMT) has its origins in the experimental work of Jacobsen (Jacobsen et al 1952) and Lorenz (Lorenz et al 1957) in the early 1950s, who showed that lethally irradiated mice could be protected by shielding a limb, or the injection of suspension of spleen cells. It was soon accepted that it was the cellular component of the suspension that was responsible for restoring haemopoiesis.

The precise characterization of the cells responsible for reconstitution in man are still not known, since there is no way of identifying the haemo-poietic stem cell in man. The equivalent in the mouse is the so-called colony forming unit (spleen) (CFU-S), which can restore itself and is capable of differentiation into all haemopoietic lineages. It is the equivalent cellular component in man that is transferred in allogeneic, syngeneic or autologous BMT.

The potential clinical benefits of successfully transplanting haemo-poiesis, or replacing individual deficient haemopoietic lineages were soon realized, and during the 1950s and 60s sporadic attempts were made albeit usually unsuccessfully. Failure was most often due to graft rejection, the immunologically competent component of the graft causing a reaction against the host (graft-versus-host disease; GVHD) or failure of supportive care.

An additional incentive was the compelling experimental data suggesting that the graft itself has an immunological reactivity against leukaemic cells of the host. The possibilities of installing new marrow to take advantage of this 'graft-versus-leukaemia' (GVL) effect, were apparent to physicians treating leukaemia patients.

An initial problem was to devise a means of treating the patient (conditioning) to ensure that the donor marrow would reliably graft. Developmental work in dogs by Thomas and co-workers (Thomas et al 1959) established the reliability of high doses of cyclophosphamide and total body irradiation (TBI) to a dose of around 1000 cGy. This schedule was devised primarily to secure engraftment rather than to have any important anti-leukaemic effect. Indeed in early studies in twins with end-stage disease, substantially higher doses were given with anti-leukaemic intent, but failed to eradicate the disease. This conditioning protocol, or minor variations of it, has remained the standard approach to this day.

It was not until the development of a clearer understanding of the HLA system and the requirements to ensure engraftment that transplantation became anything more than a high risk experimental treatment. Most subsequent experience has been gained from transplantation between HLA matched mixed lymphocyte culture non-reactive sibling donors. In recent years the boundaries of HLA disparity that are compatible with a satisfactory clinical result have been explored but remain in an experimental phase.

CLINICAL AIMS OF TRANSPLANTATION

Allogeneic transplantation can be employed in three general categories of disease, which will have some influence on the justification for the procedure, and how it is carried out. The major complications and immuno-biological reasons for morbidity and mortality are common to any allograft whatever the clinical indication.

First, transplantation can replace a congenital or acquired deficiency of the haemopoietic system such as immune deficiency syndromes or severe aplastic anaemia, in which case the intention is to install a graft into what is functionally an empty space. Treatment of the host is required to condition acceptance of the graft, but there is no requirement to eliminate disease marrow.

Second, there may be a need to replace defective marrow products such as defective red cells in sickle cell anaemia or thalassaemia syndromes, or supply a source of enzyme for the large group of inborn errors of metabolism. In this situation, as well as ensuring engraftment, an element of space creation in the host marrow is required.

Finally, and so far the most widespread indication, is to eradicate haemopoietic malignancy from the patient—including in the bone marrow—and provide a source of haemopoietic rescue of all haemopoietic lineages. As well as safe engraftment this also presents the challenge of eradicating neoplastic cells, which may be quite resistant. This last approach is potentially applicable to non-haematological malignancies but in practice success is at present only achievable in sensitive diseases such as the haematological malignancies, and within these diseases success is less likely if the transplant is attempted at a late stage. By far the most common use of BMT has been in the treatment of haematological malignancies. Some of the diseases correctable by bone marrow transplantation are listed in Table 7.1.

COMPLICATIONS OF ALLOGENEIC TRANSPLANTATION

Over the past decade considerable clinical experience has been accumulated mostly of transplantation between HLA matched siblings for haemato-

Table 7.1 Disorders correctable by bone marrow transplantation

A *Congenital Defects*
Primary Immunodeficiencies
   Severe combined immunodeficiency (SCID)
   Wiskott–Aldrich syndrome
   Chronic granulomatous disease
   Kostmann's syndrome
   Chediak–Higashi syndrome
   Leucocyte adhesion deficiency
   Di George syndrome

Inborn Errors of Metabolism
   Gaucher's disease
   Hurler's syndrome

B *Marrow Failures*
   Severe aplastic anaemia
   Fanconi's anaemia
   Thalassaemia

C *Malignant Disease of Bone Marrow*
   Acute myeloid leukaemia
   Acute lymphoid leukaemia
   Chronic myeloid leukaemia
   Myelodysplastic syndromes
   Myeloma
   Non-Hodgkin's lymphoma
   Myelofibrosis

logical malignancy. It is clear that the procedure-related risk is about 30%. That is, 30% of patients undergoing transplant die directly from complications of the transplant, unrelated to whether the underlying disease is successfully corrected.

The major reasons for procedural failure are the consequences of immunosuppression, pneumonitis, and GVHD. For haematological malignancies the patients are prepared with combined chemotherapy and TBI designed to be lethal to the host marrow. The protocols are heavily immunosuppressive, therefore graft rejection has been unusual. Whether the preparative protocols truly eradicate the host's marrow has recently been questioned. With the recent availability of very sophisticated methods of detection of donor or host cells, persistence of host haemopoietic cells is seen regularly, indicating that the preparative protocol is not truly ablative.

SUPPORTIVE CARE

Within a few days of completing the TBI, which is now usually given over 3 or 4 days, the patient's marrow ceases to function. It will be about a month before the incoming marrow starts to repopulate the peripheral blood. The intervening time period represents a major challenge in supportive care. Of crucial importance is the delivery of very high standard of nursing. The preparative treatment is likely to result in a substantial amount of tissue damage particularly to the mouth and oropharynx. If the patient has previously been subject to herpes type I infections, reactivation will almost certainly take place, thus increasing the tissue damage and providing a portal of entry for opportunistic pathogens.

Most patients are nursed by reverse barrier techniques, in some form of isolation facility. To this is often added an oral non-absorbable antibiotic combination, designed to eradicate potentially fatal commensal organisms from the bowel. Most patients have an indwelling tunnelled venous catheter, which, although of great convenience for administration of drugs and fluids and monitoring of the patient, represents a further infective hazard to the patients. Every transplant unit has a very carefully worked out management policy for patients during the cytopenic period. This must include a set policy of promptly and empirically treating febrile incidents. Substantial blood product support, particularly platelets, is required on a daily basis. Since the patients are optimally prepared to accept a foreign graft, and since circulating peripheral blood cells can engraft, it is necessary to irradiate blood products for the first 8–10 weeks. Fatal bacterial infections or haemorrhage are rare in well organized units.

Following resolution of the neutropenia the risk of bacterial and fungal infections diminishes. It takes a further 3–6 months for lymphocyte function to return. This protracted immunodeficiency is reflected in the type of infections which frequently occur. *Pneumocystis carinii*, and herpes group viruses are the main threat. Pneumocystis should be preventable by the prophylactic use of co-trimoxazole for 4–6 months. Cytomegalovirus infections are especially important, particularly as pneumonitis seldom responds to treatment once established. Herpes zoster is quite common, but seldom life threatening. Humoral immunity can remain defective for as long as 2 years. This can result in failure to respond appropriately to encapsulated organisms, such as *Haemophilus influenzae* and pneumococcus.

The time span and nature of the risk of infection is therefore related to the pattern of regeneration of the patients' immune system. This normal pattern can be considerably protracted by GVHD which poses a threat because of direct tissue damage predisposing the patient to infection by delaying the normal pace of immune reconstitution.

PNEUMONITIS

Historically about 25% of patients who went to transplantation developed pneumonitis (Meyers et al 1983). About half these cases were fatal. There are several contributing factors. Of infective causes the most common organism is cytomegalovirus (CMV). In many cases a cause is not found. It is likely that several of these 'idiopathic' cases were attributable to the irradiation schedule then used. Since pulmonary macrophages also become donor type, there is a period of vulnerability to infection of all types. GVHD is the most important risk factor for the development of pneumonitis, indeed there has always been a suspicion that the lung may be a target of the GVHD reaction. The successful prevention of this disease can be expected to reduce the incidence of pneumonitis.

This risk of CMV pneumonitis is substantially dependent on the serological status of the host and donor (Meyers et al 1986). If the patient is seropositive to CMV it is highly likely that the virus will reactivate from the patient who will become culture positive from throat and/or urine. Whether the patient develops pneumonitis may depend on whether there is coexisting GVHD, but may crucially depend on the immune status of the donor to CMV. For example a seropositive patient has an 'educated' immune system, and can mount a response to the virus. On the other hand a seronegative graft is naïve to the virus and cannot cope when confronted by active infection. Such a precise relationship is still debatable, but there is little doubt that it is the seropositive patient that is at higher risk of developing pneumonitis.

By definition the seronegative patient cannot reactivate the virus. In this case it is much more likely that the infection will be derived from the donor, or more probably through the multiple blood transfusions to which they are subjected.

There is little doubt that, although it presents a major logistic problem for the Blood Transfusion Service, if CMV negative donors are exclusively used, the risk of CMV infection in the seronegative recipient can be virtually prevented. Although arguable, it is probably worth giving seronegative blood products to all seronegative recipients, even if the donor is seropositive.

The development of CMV pneumonitis is ominous. Most patients will not survive. There remains, therefore, a considerable incentive to reduce the risk for CMV seropositive patients. There is some evidence to suggest that high dose acyclovir treatment given prophylactically can reduce the risk. The use of high titre CMV immunoglobulin has produced equivocal results.

GRAFT-VERSUS-HOST DISEASE

HLA identity within a family does not exclude the development of GVHD. Identity is also important to engraftment. As will be discussed later, any degree of HLA mismatch will increase the incidence of GVHD and the chances of graft failure. Despite serological matching some manifestation of this disease will occur in about half the patients. The acute or early form is a risk for the first 2 months. In several cases it will comprise an erythematous skin reaction, which if not treated can progress to severe bullous formation. More advanced disease involves the liver or gastrointestinal tract (Gale 1985). Liver failure or severe gastroenteritis with massive fluid loss are the fatal consequences. Once advanced acute GVHD is established it responds poorly to treatment.

A later version of GVHD (chronic GVHD) can occur at any time up to about 15 months post-transplant. The clinical manifestations are more akin to a connective tissue disorder. If it occurs as a continuous process after acute GVHD it is often difficult to treat. If it develops in the absence of any acute disease it is much more responsive to immunosuppressive treatment with prednisolone and/or azathioprine.

Apart from direct tissue injury, GVHD is important because it delays immune reconstitution. There may, however, be an unexpected benefit because there is some statistical data to suggest that in haematological malignancy the more GVHD that is present, the lower the risk of leukaemic relapse (Weiden et al 1979). There is little doubt that acute GVHD is due to T lymphocytes in the donated marrow being stimulated to proliferate in the host by antigen, in, or of, the host. Various methods of prevention have been attempted. Methotrexate or cyclosporin as single agents have not been particularly effective and have significant toxicity. In recent years anti-T lymphocyte monoclonal antibody treatment of the donor marrow before administration, has become available (Prentice et al 1984). There is little doubt that T cell depletion has been highly effective in preventing GVHD, even without any additional immunosuppression. This very powerful technique remains controversial because it has some disadvantages, which have deterred many groups. First it was noted that removal of T cells lead to graft failure in about 15–20% of cases. As previously mentioned graft failure is a rare event in T cell replete transplantation. By implication it is now clear that donor T cells are themselves immunosuppressive of the host, and contribute to the acceptance of the graft. If T cell depletion is in use it is essential to add extra conditioning of the patient. This can most conveniently be done by additional TBI, which can be achieved without much extra toxicity. In transplantation for severe aplastic anaemia, T cell depletion is unwise anyway, because even in T replete allografts rejections occur, and this will probably be compounded by depletion.

The other disadvantage is the potential elimination of the beneficial effects of the putative GVL effect. Since in man a GVL appears to be associated with clinically obvious GVHD, T cell depletion obviously potentially increases the risk of relapse. There are several reports which suggest that the leukaemic relapse rate is increased. But several other factors may be involved, and there are successful T cell depletion series which are not associated with an increase in relapse rate. The risk may be related to the underlying disease, for example the risk of relapse of chronic myeloid leukaemia may be in excess of 50–60% compared with the usual 15–20% in T cell replete allografts. In acute myeloid leukaemia any increase in relapse is less marked. Because of these problems there is at present little overall survival advantage following the introduction of T cell depletion techniques. What has become clear as a result of this experience is that for haematological malignancies an allogeneic or GVL effect may play an important role in the curative potential of allogeneic transplantation.

Strong support for this concept comes from the observation that the relapse rate in twins is nearly twice that seen in sibling allografts with GVHD (Gale & Champlin 1984). The anti-leukaemic effect is associated with GVHD, because the relapse rate in allografts without GVHD is the same as in twins. The GVL effect is therefore not apparent in man in the absence of GVHD.

GVHD remains a serious impediment to successful transplantation. Use of methotrexate in combination with cyclosporin has produced encouraging results, but the toxicity may yet be problematic (Storb et al 1986).

CLINICAL RESULTS OF BONE MARROW TRANSPLANTATION

The vast majority of transplants have been performed for four diseases, namely severe aplastic anaemia, acute and chronic myeloid leukaemia and acute lymphoblastic leukaemia. There is a smaller, but none the less encouraging, body of data accumulating in other disorders such as myelodysplasia, myeloma and non-Hodgkin's lymphoma. Given a more even geographical availability of transplant facilities a major group of potentially curative diseases are the thalassaemia syndromes.

Severe aplastic anaemia

Aplastic anaemia defined as neutrophils $< 200 \times 10^9/l$ and platelets $< 20 \times 10^9/l$ has a poor prognosis and little chance of spontaneous recovery. Responses to antilymphocyte globulin occur, although they are often partial—but nevertheless are probably appropriate to try before resorting to BMT.

Should an HLA matched sibling donor be available, then the first consideration is what is the most appropriate preparation of the host? The marrow does not require to be cleared to create space for the new marrow so total body irradiation has generally not been used. Non-ablative doses of cyclophosphamide (200 mg/kg) over 4 days is the traditional approach and this is probably sufficiently immunosuppressive for patients who have not been sensitized by prior blood transfusions. Since these patients almost by definition require blood product support from diagnosis, the relatively ideal circumstance of transplanting untransfused patients seldom applies. In early series where cyclophosphamide alone was used, rejection was a major problem occurring in about 50% of cases. However, if the recipient had not been previously exposed to transfusion products engraftment and survival was around 90%. Additions to the standard cyclophosphamide therapy have substantially improved the rate of engraftment and survival. The addition of cyclosporin appears to be the simplest and most successful approach, as well as providing a means of post-transplant immunosuppression to prevent GVHD.

The use of unirradiated buffycoat taken from the donor by leucophoresis in the first few days after transplantation is also effective, but does increase the later complication of chronic GVHD. Why donor buffycoat should, as a single modification, dramatically improve engraftment is not clear. The suggestion that it was a source of additional stem cells seems improbable, in the light of subsequent experience of T cell depletion to prevent GVHD; it is more likely that it is a source of T cells which have a sufficient anti-host effect to permit engraftment.

GVHD remains the major risk in aplastic anaemia, and has a major impact on the possibility of cure. To date T cell depletion has been avoided in this disease because of the fragility of engraftment. It is conceivable that it could be safely introduced, provided acceptable additional conditioning of the host was applied—such as nodal irradiation or intravenous anti-T monoclonal antibody.

Young patients have a particularly good result from bone marrow transplant (BMT) and it should probably therefore be offered as early after diagnosis as possible (IBMTR Report 1989). Adult patients still have a better outcome than with alternative treatments, but because of the risk of GVHD and other complications, prior use of antilymphocyte globulin to which some may adequately respond seems justified.

Chronic myeloid leukaemia

Chronic myeloid leukaemia (CML) is a disease of the haemopoietic stem cells characterized by the finding of the Philadelphia chromosome in all cells derived from the leukaemic clone. This cytogeneic abnormality is a result of reciprocal translocation between chromosome 9 and 22 and results in the juxtaposition of the site of the breakpoint in the bcr gene and the abl gene from chromosome 9. This sequence, known as the bcr/abl gene results in the transcription of an abnormal protein product with kinase activity. The molecular-genetic features of this disease have provided sensitive flags with which to identify leukaemic cells, and have been useful in elucidating the effect of transplantation on the disease.

Whether the formation of the Philadelphia (Ph') chromosome is the primary event in this disease is arguable, but it is inevitable for most patients that in due course further genetic changes take place which contribute to disease progression from a relatively stable, haematologically apparently normal, 'chronic' phase which is nevertheless characterized by the presence of the Ph' chromosome in virtually all cells, either to a resistant blastic phase directly, or indirectly via an 'accelerating' phase characterized by lack of responsiveness to previous treatment. The average duration of the chronic phase is 3–4 years, and although there is current enthusiasm about the potential of interferon therapy, this time window has not been altered by any conventional treatment.

Allogeneic BMT is the only potentially curative treatment available and, although there is some variation in individual centre results, should be successful in 50–60% of recipients (Goldman et al 1988). In the context of CML it is necessary to define cure and relapse. While 50–60% of cases will remain haematologically normal, a small proportion will have Ph'-positive cells in the marrow (cytogeneic relapse). The clone may wax and wane for reasons that are not clear. The detection of Ph'-positive cells sometimes, but not always, is a prelude to haematological relapse. More confusing is the recent evaluation using highly sensitive molecular genetic techniques including sequence amplification by polymerase chain reaction technique, that even in cytogenetically negative patients there is evidence of the residual clone. The significance and reliability of this highly sensitive technique is not yet clear. Assuming these observations do not represent an artefact, then perhaps allogeneic BMT does not eradicate the last leukaemic cells, but reduces them to a level that is compatible with cure. It may take several years to unravel the clinical significance of these data.

If a matched donor is available there is no doubt that transplantation is the treatment of choice. Like all transplant candidates there is an upper age limit, beyond which it is probably not in the patient's interest to advocate proceeding, this is usually around 45–50 years. However, since these patients will inevitably die of the disease some centres will attempt patients in the sixth decade. In general, age is a major determinant of outcome in that younger patients (under 30 years) should have a 55–65% chance of cure but in older patients the outlook is 40% or less. Beyond the age split at 30 years there appears to be no further age effect.

Given that a suitable donor exists and that the patient is accepted for transplant, two further issues require to be resolved. First, when in the natural history of the disease, as defined above, should the transplant be done? Second, is it in the patient's interest to reduce the risk of GVHD by manipulating the donor marrow in vitro to remove T lymphocytes? The rationale of this has been described already together with the potential consequences.

There are a number of potential time points in the natural history of CML where BMT could be advocated. For patients who enter blast crisis the prognosis with any other approach is virtually hopeless. BMT at this point may salvage 10%. In accelerating phase about 30% become long term survivors. In both these circumstances the transplant is a last resort, because no other viable option can save the patient. The decision to transplant is therefore easy, but the results not particularly good, largely because the disease has evolved to a more resistant entity. The best result can be expected before this happens, that is, in chronic phase. There is a risk that patients will progress from chronic phase suddenly and unpredictably, but this risk within 12 months from the diagnosis, is only about 10%. Most patients therefore should probably be transplanted at around a year from diagnosis.

Prevention of GVHD with T cell depletion has been a matter of great controversy. In this disease the risk of relapse has been dramatically increased in some series to around 60–70% from the more usual 15–20% when the T cells have not been removed. There remains argument about the details of other treatment given to the patient in these series, for example additional immunosuppression with cyclosporin, and the qualitative type of T depletion used. While the relapse rate has increased, there is not yet any major reduction in survival in T depleted grafts, nevertheless this is likely to emerge in time. It is probably wise in this disease, particularly in younger patients, to use alternative approaches to GVHD prevention.

Acute leukaemia

The early transplant experience in acute leukaemia was adopted only in patients who had relapsed disease refractory to chemotherapy. Many of these patients were unresponsive to blood product support. Although 10% of these very poor risk patients from this initial Seattle series survived this was clearly not the best use of the technique. It was apparent that the survivors tended to be those in the best clinical condition. This led to the current practice of using transplantation in remission of disease. Unlike chronic myeloid leukaemia, patients with acute leukaemia do have therapeutic alternatives which can be curative without resort to transplantation.

Acute lymphoblastic leukaemia (ALL)

As the common leukaemia of childhood with a peak incidence between the age of 2 and 4 years, chemotherapy currently cures about 60–70% of cases. For those who fail treatment, the outlook is largely influenced by the duration of their first remission and whether or not the relapse occurred during or after treatment. For those who relapse early while receiving chemotherapy the prognosis is poor, and once a further remission is achieved, transplantation is fully justified: 30% will survive (IBMTR Report 1989). For those who relapse late the outlook with further conventional therapy is not hopeless. Further durable remissions are possible, but these are seldom longer than the first remission. Proceeding directly to transplant is therefore more debatable, but ultimately BMT is still likely to be the only curative option. There is an argument to permit these patients to enjoy the natural time span of the second remission and delay transplant till the third remission.

In the relatively small number of adults with ALL the curative potential of conventional treatment is probably not more than 30% of those who enter complete remission. This has recently persuaded some groups to offer transplantation in first remission to all adults. Similarly it is possible to identify some subsets of children with ALL who are at high risk of failing conventional treatment and offering BMT instead. These high risk factors are not universally agreed and the clinical data is not sufficiently mature to vindicate such a strategy. At present the projected survival is around 50%, which is probably an improvement but it is probable that some of the high risk factors for chemotherapy will also predict a poor outcome from bone marrow transplant. In the circumstances in which BMT is justified in ALL, a major reason for failure is leukaemic relapse.

Acute myeloid leukaemia (AML)

The majority of patients with AML are over 50 years of age and are not considered for transplantation. There has been considerable progress in the initial treatment of this disease with 75–80% of younger patients entering remission. This is largely attributable to better supportive care during the pancytopenic phase. There is little or no evidence that there has been a corresponding increase in the proportion of those patients who enter remission initially, surviving at 5 years. 70–80% of patients will relapse despite further post-remission chemotherapy: For the last 10 years BMT has been offered to AML patients as consolidation treatment of first remission. The durable survival is 50%, with the risk of leukaemic relapse being 20% (IBMTR Report 1989). Such comparative studies as have been done between chemotherapy and BMT in first remission, have usually favoured transplant but the survival advantage has not always been statistically significant.

Some experience has been gained in transplantation in second remission of AML. About 30% of patients are salvaged at that point, and the main difference from first remission is that about 50% will have a further relapse.

It has recently been pointed out that by the time the patient is admitted to the transplant unit, they have avoided relapse during the waiting time and are already at a lower risk of relapse. The pattern of relapse is around 5% per month in the first 6 months of the remission, so if the patient does not arrive for transplant for 3 months, they are selected and have about a 30% chance of being cured already. An important number of patients who may benefit from transplant will therefore be excluded if there is delay in arranging the transplant. Conversely, some patients (e.g. 30%) are already cured at the time of transplant. This has led to the suggestion that BMT should be reserved for second remission—where 30% can be salvaged which is superior to the 5–10% survival achieved by chemotherapy. When added to the 30% already cured in first remission, this will result in the same overall number of cured patients. The problem is that a substantial proportion of patients who relapse will not achieve a second remission. It also turns out that there is no statistical difference in the overall survival between transplanting patients as the primary treatment of relapse, and transplantation in second remission. This has led to the suggestion that patients should only be transplanted when they relapse from first remission, without any attempt being made to re-induce remission. This is a controversial view, not least because instant access to a transplant unit may not be possible. The prevailing preference is to offer transplant to all suitable patients in first remission. What the upper age limit should be is not well defined. The outcome of transplant beyond the age of 40 is not superior to chemotherapy and the argument to delay BMT is more reasonable. Other factors may come into the decision, such as the CMV status of the transplant.

AML is primarily a disease of the elderly, and only about one-third of patients can be considered on age grounds alone. They have to have been successfully induced into remission, and of those 1 in 3 will have a compatible sibling donor. While BMT is a very important treatment for patients who qualify for it, only about 10–15% of all patients with AML will be candidates. Partly because of unavailability of a donor, BMT will only cure 6–8% of all patients with AML.

AUTOLOGOUS BMT

For the many patients who would benefit from an allograft and are excluded because of age or the unavailability of a matched donor, conventional chemotherapy is a poor option. In recent years autologous BMT has been put forward as an alternative (Linch & Burnett 1986). The strategy is to remove marrow from the patient during a period of disease remission and store it for subsequent use following myeloablative treatment.

This has very widespread potential use because it opens a therapeutic window to permit substantial dose escalation of chemotherapeutic agents, well beyond the limit normally imposed by myelotoxicity. High dose treatment supported by autologous BMT has therefore been explored in a wide range of solid tumours but has so far had limited impact on survival. Although some responses have been seen, these are usually more incomplete or shortlived. In general such a strategy appears to produce hopeful results in responsive malignancies such as acute leukaemias, non-Hodgkin's lymphoma and Hodgkin's disease. These latter disease groups are often cured by conventional first-line treatment, so high dose therapy can only really by justified in those who fail standard regimens. But even in this setting second-line treatment can be curative. There is little doubt that high dose therapy has produced encouraging results, particularly when the disease is still responsive, but it may take some time before its true contribution becomes clear.

The rationale for autograft in acute leukaemia may appear obscure for a number of reasons. It would at first sight seem an illogical approach. Since this is a bone marrow disease, and the justification for applying it is that further relapse in the bone marrow is highly probable, it would appear inevitable that occult disease is being reinfused with the patients' own marrow. It would seem at least necessary to devise methods of cleansing ('purging') the graft of occult leukaemia cells. From previous discussion in relation to the mechanism of cure by allogeneic transplantation, a GVL effect would also be valuable. Since in man this is associated with clinical GVHD, which will not occur in autologous transplantation, it can be anticipated that the relapse rate will be higher. This may, however, be offset by lack of toxicity due to the absence of the immunobiological problems of allograft.

Several transplant groups have nevertheless felt that such an initiative justified using unpurged marrow. If one projected that in clinical remission the residual leukaemic burden was 1×10^8 cells, probably only 1×10^6 would be clonogenic, i.e. are leukaemic stem cells. During harvest probably only 1% of bone marrow cells are removed and perhaps half will not survive the storage procedure. These arguments suggest that 5×10^3 clonogenic leukaemic cells might be in the autograft itself. It is by no means established that such cells will be at all efficient in seeding into the patients. These arguments support the view that purging occult disease may not be a requirement. As it happens syngeneic transplants represent the ideal proto-type of an autograft without contamination, and although the total world experience is small, the relapse rate is about 50%. This is taken as important evidence to support the view that allogeneic transplantation— where the relapse rate is 25%—is associated with an immunologically mediated GVL effect. The general outcome of autologous transplantation AML using unpurged marrow is of a 45–55% longterm survival, i.e. identical to the twin data. This suggests first that any occult leukaemia that is present in the autograft is not clinically important, and second it will be very difficult to evaluate clinically the benefit of purging methods.

A number of approaches to in vitro treatment (purging) of the autograft in both ALL and in AML are potentially useful. In AML no suitably specific monoclonal antibody exists thus excluding immunological approaches. Most effort has been devoted to incubation of the autograft with the active cyclophosphamide metabolite 4-hydroxy-cyclophos-phamide (Yeager et al 1986). This was based on convincing experimental data derived from a rat model. There is, however, little evidence to suggest that human leukaemic stem cells are any more or less sensitive than their normal counterparts. In ALL useful monoclonal antibodies are available to antigens expressed on leukaemic cells but not on haemopoietic stem cells. In vitro such antibodies can be shown to effect up to a 4 log kill of leukaemic cells, while sparing haemopoietic precursors.

Many groups have adopted purging in ALL because it is logical and is supported by in vitro data, but there are no clinical studies which prove its value. This is mainly because even in allogeneic transplantation relapse of disease in the patient remains a major problem. It is not possible to determine whether a relapse has come from the patient or the autograft.

The indications for autologous BMT in acute leukaemia are not different from those for allograft, and appear a viable option for those who lack a donor. Because there is less associated immunosuppression and no mor-

Table 7.2 Comparison of outcome of treatment: conventional treatment versus bone marrow transplantation (% 5-year survival)

Disease	Conventional treatment	Bone marrow transplantation	
		Allogeneic	Autologous
Severe aplastic anaemia	20%	50%	NA
Acute myeloid leukaemia			
(first remission)	25%	50%	45–50%
(second remission)	5–10%	30%	20–30%
Acute lymphoid leukaemia	60–70% (children)	NA	NA
(first remission)	30% (adults)	50–60%	40–60%
(second remission)	15%	30%	20–30%
Chronic myeloid leukaemia	1–2%	50%	NA

NA—not available or not normally offered.

bidity associated with GVHD, older patients can safely be offered this option; it is safe in patients up to the age of 55 years. This approach is therefore potentially available to a much larger proportion of patients with leukaemia than allogeneic BMT.

Somewhat surprisingly the results achieved in AML and ALL in first or second remission are very similar to the allograft results. This suggests that the conceptual disadvantages of a higher relapse rate principally due to lack of a GVL effect has indeed been balanced by the lack of procedural mortality. Most patients who fail do so because of relapse. Procedural deaths usually due to infection or haemorrhage are 5–8%. A number of large national and international trials are now in progress to determine the contribution autograft makes to the overall treatment of AML compared with allogeneic transplantation or modern intensive chemotherapy alone. Two further issues are controversial. Some advocate that the autograft should be reserved only for second remission as has been argued for allograft. It is certainly possible to salvage patients at this stage but the potential difficulties in this approach were highlighted earlier. There must be an age limit where patients might be better off with an autograft, even although a matched donor is available. Where this is, is not known but is probably around 40 years. The overall contribution of transplantation, whether allogeneic or autologous to the major diseases is illustrated in Table 7.2.

TRANSPLANTATION FROM NON-GENOTYPICALLY MATCHED DONORS

Autologous BMT is not an option for patients with immunodeficiency syndromes, aplastic anaemia or chronic myeloid leukaemia. In these diseases there is a considerable incentive to provide a transplant from donors other than fully matched siblings. Two broad choices might be possible, first partially matched members of the extended family or second unrelated donors who are phenotypically but not genotypically matched. It can be anticipated that because of the HLA disparity in these situations securing engraftment and avoiding severe GVHD will be the main technical problems.

Subsequent clinical experience has confirmed that these problems are difficult to overcome and the prospects of success are limited to young patients with a limited degree of mismatch. It has been possible to produce equivalent survival figures to the genotypically matched patients only if minor mismatches are attempted, e.g. a one-locus mismatch. While GVHD tends to be more severe the overall survival is the same. More extensive mismatches are rarely successful. The problems of the mismatch transplant remain very complex.

The use of donors who are serologically matched at the major HLA loci, but who are unrelated to the patient, and therefore not genotypically matched, is now under development. Progress in this area has been inhibited by the logistics of finding a suitable donor within a practical time span. In recent years several national registries have been built up with lists of volunteers of known tissue groups. To have a reasonable chance ($> 50\%$) of finding a donor a registry size of at least 100 000 is required. The possibilities of identifying a suitable donor will depend also on the racial mix within the indigenous population. Even when the considerable administrative difficulties have been overcome, there remains the considerable clinical challenge of achieving engraftment without serious GVHD.

Progress is certainly being made in this direction; such an approach is still in its early development but is likely to be of increasing importance in the future.

FUTURE PROGRESS IN BONE MARROW TRANSPLANTATION

Over the past decade there have been strenuous efforts made to eliminate the procedural complications which accompany allogeneic transplantation and are the major contributors to death in about 30%, and contribute to considerable additional morbidity. The use of CMV negative blood products when the donor and host are CMV seronegative is important. Reliable prevention of CMV disease in CMV seropositive patients remains to be achieved. Newer antiviral agents in combination with high-titre CMV-immunoglobulin shows promise.

There is little doubt that GVHD can be prevented by T depletion techniques. It is possible to overcome reliably the unexpected rejection problems using additional conditioning. The probability of increasing the rate of relapse has yet to be clarified and requires further attention.

Recombinant DNA technology is beginning to provide a number of cytokines for clinical use. Haemopoietic growth factors can accelerate engraftment, and may therefore reduce morbidity in the immediate post-transplant period. It has yet to be shown that this alters survival. Continued careful evaluation is necessary in view of the considerable extra cost these factors are likely to involve. There has been recent speculation that the immunological advantages (GVL) of allograft, and possibly autograft, may be augmented by the cytokine interleukin 2 (IL2). It appears that a population of lymphocytes with cytotoxic potential can be potentiated. The cytotoxic potential against leukaemic cells can be demonstrated in vitro, but so far there is very little clinical data to demonstrate any antileukaemic effect in vivo.

Recurrence of leukaemia remains an important problem, particularly in the autograft setting. More sophisticated delivery of radiotherapy is under development particularly antibody directed radiation. There will be a major effort made to facilitate transplantation between donors who are not sibling matches. It is even possible that, as the safety of the technique improves, a wider spectrum of diseases may become candidates for transplantation—including non-malignant conditions such as connective tissue diseases.

REFERENCES

Gale R P 1985 Graft-versus-host disease. Immunological Reviews 88: 193–214
Gale R P, Champlin R E 1984 How does bone marrow transplantation cure leukaemia? Lancet ii: 28–30
Goldman J M, Gale R P, Horowitz M et al 1988 Bone marrow transplantation for chronic myeloid leukemia in chronic phase. Annals of Internal Medicine 108: 806–814
International Bone Marrow Transplant Registry Report 1989. Bone Marrow Transplantation 4: 221–228
Jacobsen L D, Simmonds E L, Marks E K, Eldredge J H 1952 Recovery from irradiation injury: A review. Cancer Research 112: 315
Linch D C, Burnett A K 1986 Clinical studies of ABMT in acute myeloid leukaemia. Clinics in Haematology 15: 167–186
Lorenz E, Uphoff D, Ried T R, Shelton E 1957 Modification of irradiation injury in mice and guinea pigs by bone marrow injections. Journal of the National Cancer Institute 19:123–130
Meyers J D, Flournoy N, Wade J C et al 1983 Biology of interstitial pneumonia after marrow transplantation. In: Gale R P (ed) Recent advances in bone marrow transplantation. Alan R Liss, New York, pp 405–423
Meyers J D, Flournoy N, Thomas E D 1986 Risk factors for cytomegalovirus infection after human marrow transplantation. Journal of Infectious Diseases 153: 478–488
Prentice H G, Blacklock H A, Janossy G et al 1984 Depletion of T lymphocytes in donor marrow prevents significant graft-versus-host disease in matched allogeneic leukaemia marrow transplant recipients. Lancet i: 472–476
Storb R, Deeg H J, Whitehead J et al 1986 Methotrexate and cyclosporin compared with cyclosporin alone for prophylaxis of acute graft versus host diseases after marrow transplantation. New England Journal of Medicine 314: 729
Thomas E D, Ashley C A, Lochte H L et al 1959 Homografts of bone marrow in dogs after lethal total-body-irradiation. Blood 14: 720–736
Weiden P L, Flournoy N, Thomas E D et al 1979 Anti-leukaemia effect of graft-versus-host disease in recipients of allogeneic marrow grafts. New England Journal of Medicine 300: 1068–1073
Yeager A M, Kaiser H, Santor G W et al 1986 Autologous bone marrow transplantation in patients with acute myelogenous leukaemia using ex vivo marrow treatment with 4-hydroxy-cyclophosphamide. New England Journal of Medicine 315: 141–147

8. Interventional cardiac catheterization in the management of children with heart disease

M. J. Godman

With the introduction of balloon atrioseptostomy for transposition of the great arteries—the commonest cardiac cause of cyanosis in the newborn infant—Rashkind & Miller (1966) demonstrated that the cardiac catheter laboratory could be the setting not just for haemodynamic and anatomical diagnosis but also for therapeutic intervention by the cardiologist. Atrial balloon septostomy rapidly became an established palliative treatment for the newborn infant with transposition of the great arteries and transformed the prognosis for this group of patients, Rashkind and a few others continued throughout the 1960s and 1970s to explore the potential of the cardiac catheter as a tool for treatment as well as diagnosis of congenital heart disease. It was, however, the report from Kan and associates from Baltimore of successful balloon dilatation of pulmonary valve stenosis which accelerated the recognition that interventional cardiac catheter procedures could offer a feasible alternative to surgery in the management of many congenital cardiac defects (Kan et al 1982).

The principal developments have been:

1. the application of balloon dilatation techniques for the relief of pulmonary and aortic valve stenosis, native coarctation and recoarctation of the aorta as well as stenotic lesions elsewhere in the cardiovascular system.
2. the development of devices to occlude the ductus arteriosus and atrial and ventricular septal defects without the need for surgery.
3. the application of techniques developed by radiologists, such as therapeutic embolization of systemic vessels, to treatment of congenital cardiovascular lesions.

As a result of advances in catheter techniques, it is now possible for many of these new techniques to challenge conventional approaches and it seems likely that they will constitute the optimal treatment available for specific lesions in the near future.

113

BALLOON DILATATION

Pulmonary valve stenosis

Pulmonary valve stenosis is characterized by fusion of the valve leaflets with poorly developed or absent commissures. Occasionally the valve may be dysplastic and the pulmonary annulus hypoplastic. Secondary reactive muscular subvalvular obstruction may be associated with severe valve stenosis. Mild pulmonary valve stenosis is well tolerated and the prognosis without treatment is good. Surgical pulmonary valvotomy has been advised when the stenosis is of a moderate or severe degree, defined haemodynamically as a pressure gradient across the pulmonary valve of more than 50 mmHg. Balloon dilatation of the pulmonary valve is now considered as a therapeutic option by most paediatric cardiologists in patients with a gradient of more than 50 mmHg. Continuous wave Doppler ultrasound estimates of the pulmonary valve gradient correlate well with cardiac catheter measurements. Therefore the patient with mild pulmonary valve stenosis can be followed with repeated ultrasound investigations until there is evidence of a degree of obstruction which might merit cardiac catheterization with a view to balloon dilatation.

The technique of balloon dilatation of the pulmonary valve is now well established and many hundreds of successful procedures have been reported since 1982. The dilatation balloons are usually made of transparent polyethylene. Diameters of the inflated balloon range from 2.5 to 25 mm. A balloon diameter is usually chosen with a balloon/pulmonary valve annulus ratio of 1.2–1.4 : 1. Pulmonary valve annular diameter can be assessed either from echocardiography or at the time of angiography. The dilating catheter is usually passed across a long exchange guide wire which is positioned within the left pulmonary artery and the balloon, when in position across the pulmonary valve, is inflated with dilute contrast material to approximately 3–5 atmospheres of pressure. Attempts are made to keep the inflation/deflation cycle to as short as possible—some 5–10 seconds or so—with 3–4 balloon inflations performed several minutes apart. If the pulmonary valve annulus is too large to dilate with a single balloon, two balloons can be simultaneously inflated across the pulmonary valve. Following balloon dilatation the pressure gradient across the pulmonary valve is remeasured and an angiogram performed to demonstrate the adequacy of the relief of obstruction. The technique can be used not only in children but in adults with pulmonary valve stenosis. Although experience with neonates is small it has been used successfully in these patients who often have the most critical form of obstruction (Ali Khan et al 1989). Publication of results from the Valvuloplasty and Angioplasty of Congenital Anomalies (VACA) Registry from the United States indicates that balloon pulmonary valvuloplasty is now the most common interventional procedure performed at cardiac catheterization in children. In the 6-year period of the report (from 1983 to 1989) it accounted for nearly half of all interventional procedures performed (Stanger et al 1990). The results from the Registry confirm earlier reports that balloon pulmonary valvuloplasty is effective in markedly reducing the degree of right ventricular outflow tract obstruction in pulmonary valve stenosis. Although residual obstruction was common immediately after balloon dilatation, it usually consisted of relatively small gradients across the pulmonary valve with higher gradients found at infundibular level. Intermediate follow-up studies have shown subsequent spontaneous reduction of the infundibular pulmonary gradient following balloon pulmonary valvuloplasty.

The overall mortality has been reported as less than 1 in 200 patients with a complication rate of about 5%. Thrombosis of the femoral or iliac vein is the commonest complication particularly in neonates and young infants. Pulmonary incompetence occurs commonly but appears to be of little haemodynamic significance.

There are two subsets of pulmonary valve stenosis in which valvuloplasty may not be so successful. In the patient with a dysplastic pulmonary valve the results may not be as favourable particularly if the stenosis is due to annular hypoplasia rather than abnormal morphology of the valve. Newborn infants may occasionally have critically severe stenosis associated with hypoplastic right ventricles. Although refinements in catheter techniques have extended the application of balloon valve dilatation to this age group, the morbidity and mortality is likely to be higher. Surgical results have, however, been associated with an average mortality of 37% in selected series of newborn babies with critical pulmonary valve stenosis, so the outlook here is not without promise (Stanger et al 1990).

When compared with surgery, balloon dilatation of the pulmonary valve has several apparent advantages:

24-hour hospital admission
No surgical soar
No blood products
Good relief of obstruction
Low morbidity and mortality
Good early to medium term results

The surgical treatment of valvar pulmonary stenosis has been available for over 40 years and it is important not to make comparison between surgical results from an earlier era. Quoted operative mortality varies between 3 and 14% although many major institutions would currently claim results better than these (Nugent et al 1971). None the less, given that mortality following balloon valvuloplasty is low the risks of this technique and the lesser morbidity associated with it, would appear to favour its use over surgical procedures. The recurrence rate of pulmonary valve stenosis is somewhat higher than quoted for surgery but improvements in balloon catheter design and technique, experience already provide evidence that not only the early but the intermediate results from balloon dilatation of the pulmonary valve are likely to be at least as good as those obtained with surgical pulmonary valvuloplasty.

Balloon dilatation of the pulmonary valve can therefore now be regarded as an established treatment for pulmonary valve stenosis and as an effective and safe means of relieving obstruction. Further studies with 5–10 year and longer term follow-up are necessary to confirm unequivocally that it is the treatment of choice rather than surgery.

Aortic valve stenosis

Aortic valve stenosis is frequently a progressive lesion throughout childhood and early adolescence. Severe aortic stenosis may be associated with sudden death in any age group. In the newborn infant severe obstruction can produce heart failure. Balloon dilatation of the aortic valve has not been as widely applied nor become as well established as for the pulmonary valve (Sholler et al 1988). In those centres employing the technique as a treatment, the indications have been essentially similar to those applied in considering patients for surgical aortic valvotomy—a peak systolic pressure gradient in excess of 60–80 mmHg or greater than 50 mmHg in patients with symptoms or electrocardiographic ST-T wave changes (Hsieh et al 1986). The technique is similar to that employed for the pulmonary valve. The balloon catheter is introduced through the femoral artery and advanced over a flexible guide wire which has been positioned within the left ventricle (Fig. 8.1). A balloon is usually chosen with a diameter slightly smaller than that of the aortic valve annulus, thus minimizing the risk of aortic valve rupture and aortic valve regurgitation associated with a larger balloon. Either a single or double balloon may be used and the inflation/deflation time is kept to a minimum. The presence of aortic regurgitation is usually regarded as a contraindication to balloon dilatation because of the anxiety about producing further incompetence. A previous aortic surgical valvotomy, in the absence of regurgitation, is not in itself a contraindication and many good results can be obtained in these patients. In the data from the VACA Registry valvuloplasty was usually successful in reducing the peak systolic left ventricular aortic gradient from 77 ± 2 mmHg to 30 ± 1 mmHg (Rocchini et al 1990). The VACA Registry results report 204 children and infants as having aortic valvuloplasty between 1982 and 1989. The technique was associated with a higher complication rate than that for pulmonary valvuloplasty. As well as death, aortic regurgitation, femoral artery thrombosis or damage, excessive blood loss, life-threatening arrhythmias and damage to other cardiac structures are potential complications. Mild to moderate aortic regurgitation occurred in 10% of the children although both higher and lower incidences have been reported in series from individual institutions. Again, not surprisingly, the risks of the procedure were greatest in infancy. In this group severe valve dysplasia, left ventricular hypoplasia and dysfunction as well as technical difficulties may

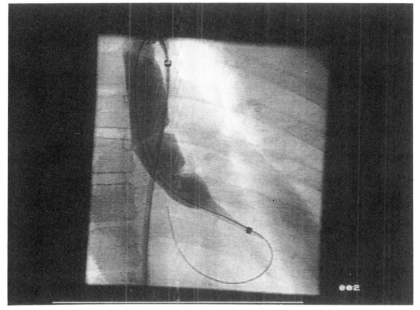

a

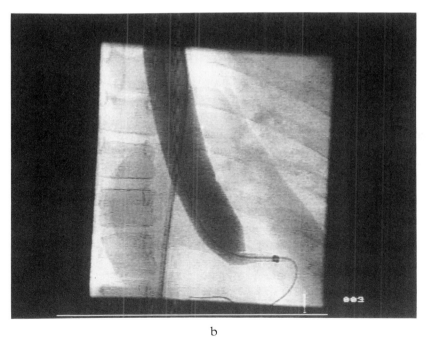

b

Fig. 8.1   (a) and (b) Ciné angiogram recorded during balloon dilatation for congenital aortic valve stenosis. Balloon is inflated unti. indentation is abolished.

militate against a successful result. Improvements in catheter design as well as increasing technical expertise are likely to improve the results in this group.

Whilst it is well documented that the immediate results of aortic valvuloplasty can be acceptable, there is a paucity of data on the intermediate term follow-up, although Sholler and others at 2-year follow-up have reported no re-stenosis or change in aortic valve regurgitation in a series of 80 patients (Sholler et al 1988).

Current data, including that from the VACA Registry, would therefore indicate that whilst balloon valvuloplasty can be a highly effective treatment for the acute relief of valvular aortic stenosis in both infants and children, it has not yet established itself as the treatment of choice for congenital aortic valve stenosis (Choy et al 1987, Wren et al 1987). When the data on surgical results for aortic valve stenosis are reappraised, however, balloon valvuloplasty may be considered as an effective alternative to surgical valvotomy. The surgical mortality for young infants and newborns is 10–15% and in some excellent institutions higher than this. Although the operative mortality of aortic valvotomy beyond the first year of life is less than 2%, re-stenosis of the aortic valve has been reported with a frequency of between 15 and 75% at follow-up with valve regurgitation present in 40–50% of patients. Re-operation has a mortality and the probability of this being required is 19% at 15 years and 35% at 20 years after surgery (Hsieh et al 1986). All these considerations, therefore, continue to make balloon aortic valvuloplasty an attractive, but as yet unproven, alternative to surgical valvotomy.

Coarctation of aorta

Coarctation of the aorta is one of the commonest causes of heart failure in infancy. In this age group, the pathology is most commonly a discrete juxtaductal area of narrowing associated with tubular hypoplasia of the aortic isthmus. The condition is frequently associated with persistence of the ductus arteriosus. In later childhood or adult life, the pathological basis for coarctation is more often only a localized area of juxtaductal narrowing and the clinical presentation is that of arterial hypertension. Surgical repair of coarctation of the aorta has usually been recommended for all infants in heart failure and asymptomatic individuals between the ages of 2 and 4 years or thereafter when recognized.

Experimental work and histological studies on excised segments of human aortic coarctation have demonstrated the feasibility of balloon dilatations but studies have also shown that dilatation is achieved at the expense of damage to the intima and medial walls and tears have been found which have been limited only by the adventitia (Ho et al 1988). There has been widespread concern that a weakened aortic wall may be a precursor for aortic aneurysm formation. Many paediatric cardiologists who have enthusiastically embraced the application of balloon dilatation for the pulmonary and aortic valve have been much more conservative in applying the technique to native coarctation of the aorta.

A balloon catheter diameter is usually chosen to be equal to that of the descending thoracic aorta at the diaphragm from measurement derived from angiography. The catheter is positioned across the coarctation over a guide wire and 3–4 inflations carried out at 4–5 atmospheres of pressure with a total inflation/deflation cycle of 5–10 seconds (Fig. 8.2).

In the VACA Registry there were data on dilatation of 141 native coarctation procedures in 140 patients between 3 days and 29 years (Tynan et al 1990). The immediate results confirmed that native coarctation can be effectively treated in both infants and older children. It was recognized by the VACA Registry Study Group that the results were hampered by incomplete information. None the less, there was a significant decrease in pressure gradient across the aortic coarctation and increase in diameter of the coarctation segment was demonstrated in both infants and older patients although the outcome is often unpredictable for any individual patient. The complication rate in the VACA Study was 17%, the main complication relating to arterial puncture. There were 8 aneurysms reported, 2 early and 6 late. Other papers published recently suggest the incidence of aneurysm is lower than earlier feared and there is increasing recognition that aneurysms may occur with a higher frequency than suspected after surgical repair of coarctation of the aorta both by patch angioplasty and subclavian flap repair (Morrow et al 1988). The factors responsible for aneurysm formation in an individual patient have not yet been fully identified. Balloon size alone does not seem to be of major significance. Variations in technique and the morphology of the coarctation as well as underlying cystic medial necrosis may all be relevant factors. Early re-stenosis can occur especially in young infants and newborns with native coarctations and the technique is probably less applicable to those with a long tubular hypoplastic isthmic segment than in those with a localized discrete narrowing. While some continue to believe that balloon angioplasty will have a place in the management of infants and children with native coarctation of the aorta, the VACA Registry Group continue to sound a cautious note in the application of this form of treatment for coarctation and reiterate the question 'Not can it be done, but should it be done?'

When re-coarctation of the aorta occurs following previous surgery the position may be different and balloon angioplasty is more clearly seen as an alternative and acceptable treatment to surgery than it is for native coarctation. The belief is that perivascular fibrosis after surgery reinforces the outer wall and may increase the safety of subsequent balloon dilatation although there is little firm information to support this. In part though the greater willingness to consider the balloon dilatation technique for re-coarctation of the aorta is a consequence of the perception that re-operation

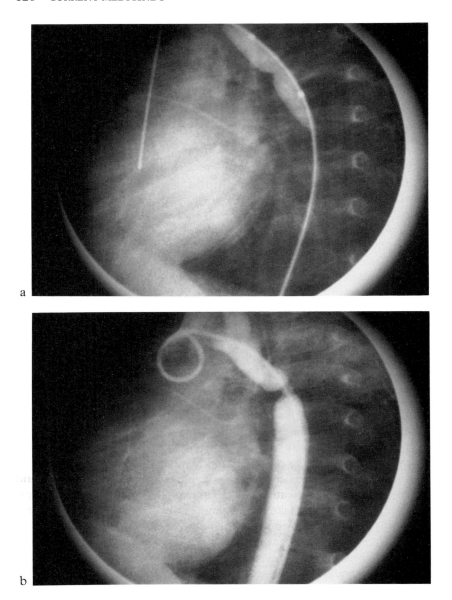

may carry a significantly higher risk than in native coarctation and is associated with mortality rates in various series up to 33% (Hellenbrand et al 1990). In the VACA Study there were 200 patients with re-coarctation of the aorta. An excellent relief of residual or recurrent obstruction was obtained in almost 80% of the total. The Group contrasted this initial success rate with a reported incidence of re-coarctation of 24–30% after second operation for coarctation of the aorta. None the less, some mortality

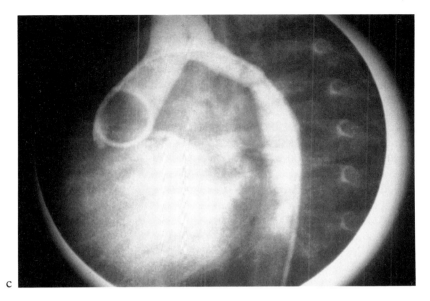

c

Fig. 8.2 (a) Angiogram recorded during dilatation of stenosis following surgically repaired coarctation—indentation is seen. (b) Ciné angiogram pre-dilatation. (c) Ciné angiogram post-dilatation.

was associated with the procedure. In the VACA Study one case of fatal aortic rupture demonstrated that some patients may lack scar tissue and made them vulnerable to fatal aortic rupture. The VACA Registry Group emphasized that as with native coarctation, there is no way of predicting potential success for this technique but it is clear that with further improvements in angioplasty catheters, complications—particularly those associated with femoral artery damage—will be reduced. The advantages of avoiding general anaesthesia, transfusion plus a short hospital stay and results and complication rates which compare favourably with surgical therapy in the long term, make balloon angioplasty a satisfactory alternative to surgery for re-coarctation of the aorta for the majority of paediatric cardiologists. The precise frequency of aneurysm formation and the timing of its appearance still remain to be determined. Magnetic resonance imaging and ultrasound technique will provide the information necessary to determine the medium to long term results of follow-up in these patients. It is likely to be many years before we know conclusively the answers to whether or not this is a preferred treatment to surgery.

Miscellaneous lesions

Balloon dilatation has also been offered widely in a variety of other congenital cardiovascular lesions. Pulmonary arterial branch stenosis may take a variety of forms from a single discrete isolated lesion close to the pulmonary arterial bifurcation to multiple distal stenoses. The Boston Sick Children's Hospital has had the widest experience in the management of the different subsets of the condition and have found that in about 50% of vessels it is possible to increase the angiographic diameter by more than a half with a reduction in pressure gradient and improvement in pulmonary perfusion scans. Follow-up, although limited in duration, suggests that the re-stenosis rate is less than 10%. On the other hand dilatation of pulmonary vein stenosis—a rare and usually fatal lesion—has been unrewarding. In postoperative patients balloon dilatation has been applied successfully to the treatment of stenotic bioprosthetic valves and systemic to pulmonary arterial shunts as well as to the relief of stenosis of intra-atrial baffles after atrial redirection procedures for transposition of the great arteries (Radtke & Lock 1990).

CATHETER CLOSURE OF INTRACARDIAC AND EXTRACARDIAC SHUNTS

Throughout the 1970s Rashkind, who had pioneered catheter creation of atrial septal defects to palliate newborn infants with transposition of the great arteries, continued to work on devices that might be suitable for closure of septal defects or persistent arterial ducts. Many developments from vascular radiology were also increasingly applied to specific problems in congenital heart disease and coils and detachable balloons have been used to close aortopulmonary collateral vessels, arteriovenous malformations and systemic to pulmonary shunts (Fuhrman et al 1984).

Persistent ductus arteriosus

The first surgical closure of a persistent ductus arteriosus (PDA) was by Gross and Hubbard in 1938. In Britain the first non-infected ductus arteriosus was ligated by Sir James Fraser in Edinburgh in 1939. Surgical closure—ligation or division—has become accepted treatment for almost all ductuses and is an operation carried out with very low mortality and morbidity and excellent long term results. Non-surgical closure was pioneered by Porstman in 1967. He used a pre-shaped Ivalon plug introduced via the femoral artery to occlude the ductus. Because of the size of the catheters and plugs the method was not suitable for most children under 5 years of age. In 1979 Rashkind developed a collapsible umbrella device which could also be delivered via either a venous or arterial approach. Mullins introduced an important modification of the technique. He suggested that a long trans-septal sheath be placed transvenously through the duct and the stiff delivery system, to which the device is attached, passed through this to the aortic end of the ductus arteriosus (Rashkind et al 1987). The umbrella device itself has also been substantially modified and the currently commercially produced double umbrellas Rashkind occluder device consists of two opposing spring-loaded discs of polyurethane attached on collapsible spring wires.

The devices come in two sizes, 12 mm in diameter and 17 mm in diameter, and are placed via a long sheath using an 8 or 11 French delivery catheter.

The indications for transcatheter closure of PDA are generally the same as those for surgery. If the duct is too large, however—greater than 9 mm at its pulmonary artery end—it is regarded as unsuitable for catheter closure even with the 17 mm device. It may be difficult also to advance the larger device and in particular the 11 French long sheath through the small vessels of infants weighing less than 9–10 kg and surgery may be the preferred option in these babies if the ductus is assessed as being more than 4 mm in size. The presence of pulmonary vascular disease is regarded as an absolute contraindication.

The technique is usually performed under general anaesthesia or with heavy sedation with ketamine anaesthesia. High quality X-ray and fluoroscopy screening is essential. At the Royal Hospital for Sick Children in Edinburgh the experiences of the team since October 1982 now extends to 89 patients, children and adults: the ages range from 6 months to 78 years with a weight range from 6.6 to 74 kg. Loss of control of the device resulting in embolization occurred in 3 patients, in 2 to the pulmonary artery and 1 to the descending aorta. In 1 of the 2 patients in whom the device had embolized in the right pulmonary artery, it was possible to retrieve it. In the other, surgery was required, at which time the ductus was also ligated. In a frail 68-year-old patient with pulmonary arterial pressure of 110 mmHg in whom the device embolized to the abdominal aorta, it was not retrieved and 6 months later has not been associated with any problems. In the Edinburgh series angiography has usually been performed 15 minutes after implantation and the patient thereafter followed by Doppler colour flow mapping studies to establish whether complete occlusion has been obtained. At 6 months of age there has been a small residual left to right shunt in 8 patients and in 1 of these a second ductus device has been implanted.

The two main problems of the technique therefore are embolization of the device and residual shunt. Refinements in technique and increasing operative experience suggest that embolization should be an uncommon complication and strategies have also evolved which make it more likely that the device can be retrieved with a basket or grabber catheter, thereby avoiding surgical ligation and removal of the device at the same time. In comparison with surgical ligation of the ductus arteriosus, residual leaks are more common with the umbrella closure technique but improvements in operator expertise are likely to reduce this incidence further (Wessel et al 1988). Endocarditis has been reported in one patient and there has also been the report of a patient who had a residual shunt who developed continuing intravascular haemolysis which required its removal. The device is not suitable for use in the premature infant with a ductus arteriosus because of the size and weight of these patients.

For 50 years surgical ligation of the ductus arteriosus has been carried out with a high degree of safety and acceptability but it is likely that catheter closure will become the preferred treatment for almost all cases. The patient usually spends only one day or night in hospital, blood products are avoided, there is no prolonged general anaesthesia or thoracotomy scar and an extended costly hospitalization is avoided.

Atrial septal defect

The first report of successful transcatheter closure of a secundum atrial septal defect with a double umbrella device was in 1976 by King & Mills who reported complete closure in 4 out of 5 patients. Rashkind throughout the 1970s also continued to work in the development of a device but the clinical application of his device has been limited. At the Boston Sick Children's Hospital Lock and colleagues developed a new device which is a modification of the double umbrella Rashkind PDA occlusion system. This has been named the Lock–Clamshell occluder. As the name suggests, the device functions similarly to a clamshell with the hinged arms folding back against themselves.

Lock and his colleagues have recently reported on 34 patients in whom atrial septal defect (ASD) closure was attempted (Rome et al 1990). The size of the defects ranged in diameter from 3 to 22 mm and the size of the occlusion device chosen from 17 to 33 mm. There were two early device embolizations but they were retrieved by catheter without complication. One elderly patient incurred a cerebral embolus before the device placement and died a week later. The follow-up in 31 patients discharged with devices in place has shown no umbrella related complications. Imaging studies have only been obtained in 19 of these patients 6 months or more after device placement but there was no residual shunt in 12 patients: there was a small residual flow through separate previously unrecognized ASDs in 2 and small residual leaks less than 3 mm were present in 5 patients.

This experience therefore is encouraging but Lock's group and others have highlighted existing evidence that the technique will have limitations and will not be applicable to all patients. Those patients who lack a complete rim of septum and in whom placement of the device might compromise important related structures such as the coronary sinus or pulmonary veins, may be poor candidates for transcatheter closures and may constitute 30–50% of all secundum atrial septal defects. It is important therefore that there be accurate assessment of the atrial septal anatomy prior to selection for catheter closure of the atrial septal defect. Biplane transoesophageal echocardiography at present is probably the most useful technique for assessing the atrial septal anatomy in detail.

The technique may have wider application than just in children with isolated secundum atrial septal defects. Some young adults with unexplained embolic stroke may have an elevated incidence of patent foramen ovale. If this apparent relation is causative, i.e. the strokes are due to paradoxical embolus at atrial level, then transcatheter closure of these defects may reduce the incidence. It is likely also that as with other interventional techniques, improvement in experience and modification of design will result in transcatheter closure becoming possible in a larger number of children and adults with isolated secundum atrial septal defects than would appear to be the case at present.

Ventricular septal defect

Catheter closure of ventricular septal defects is still at an early stage. Lock has reported on the use of the Rashkind double umbrella or clamshell occluder in 14 patients (Lock et al 1988). In a further 4 patients in whom catheterization was performed with the intention of closing the defect the attempt was abandoned because the defect was either too small, too close to the aortic valve or too large. In the 14 patients in whom an attempt was made the device abolished or significantly reduced the shunt. Whilst ventricular septal defect closures therefore have been possible with limited morbidity and encouraging success, much further evaluation of its application is required. It seems likely that those defects most suitable will be in the apical or lower third of the muscular part of the septum whilst those closely related to the aortic root or to the septal leaflet of the tricuspid valve such as the common perimembranous ventricular septal defect may prove less amenable to this form of treatment.

NEW DEVELOPMENTS

The application of laser techniques in the management of congenital cardiovascular lesions is still at an early stage. Although the method has been used to preserve ductus patency and treat a variety of obstructive lesions, its role is not yet defined (Radtke et al 1988).

More promising is the use of balloon expandable stents in the treatment of peripheral pulmonary artery stenosis and obstructive venous lesions (Mullins et al 1988).

The advances in interventional catheter techniques have been amongst the most exciting developments in the management of children with heart disease. None the less, many of these procedures offer only palliation and it is sanguine to reflect that it may yet be many years before we know how completely or otherwise they modify the natural history of congenital cardiovascular disease.

REFERENCES

Ali Khan M A, Al-Yousef S, Huhta J C, Bricker J T, Mullins C E, Sawyer W 1989 Critical pulmonary valve stenosis in patients less than 1 year of age: treatment with percutaneous gradational balloon pulmonary valvuloplasty. American Heart Journal 117: 1008–1014

Choy M, Beekman R H, Rocchini A P, Crawley D C 1987 Percutaneous balloon valvuloplasty for valvular aortic stenosis in infants and children. American Journal of Cardiology 58: 608–612

Fuhrman B P, Bass J L, Castaneda-Zuniga W, Amplatz K, Lock J E 1984 Coil embolisation of congenital thoracic vascular anomalies in infants and children. Circulation 70: 285–289

Hellenbrand W E, Allan H D, Golinko R J, Haglet D J, Lutin W, Kan J 1990 Balloon angioplasty for aortic recoarctation: results of valvuloplasty and angioplasty of Congenital Anomalies Registry. American Journal of Cardiology 65: 793–797

Ho J W, Somerville J, Yip W C L, Anderson R H 1988 Transluminal balloon dilatation of resected coarctation segments of the thoracic aorta: histological study and clinical implications. International Journal of Cardiology 19: 99–105

Hsieh K S, Keanes J F, Nadas A S, Bernhard W F, Castaneda A R 1986 Long term follow up up of valvotomy before 1968 for congenital aortic stenosis. American Journal of Cardiology 58: 338–341

Kan J S, White R F Jr, Mitchell S E, Gardner I J 1982 Percutaneous balloon valvuloplasty: A new method for treating congenital pulmonary valve stenosis. New England Journal of Medicine 307: 540–542

King T D, Mills N L 1976 Secundum atrial septal defects: Non operative closure during cardiac catheterisation. Journal of the American Medical Association 235: 2506–2509

Lock J E, Block P C, McKay F G, Baim D S, Keane J F 1988 Transcatheter closure of ventricular septal defects. Circulation 78: 361–368

Morrow W R, Vick G W, Nihill M R, Mullins C E 1988 Balloon dilatation of unoperated coarctation of the aorta: short and intermediate term results. Journal of American College of Cardiology 11: 133–138

Mullins C E, O'Laughlin J, Vick W 1988 Implantation of balloon expandable intravascular grafts by catheterisation in pulmonary arteries and systemic veins. Circulation 77: 188–199

Nugent E W, Freedom R M, Nora J J, Ellison R C, Rowe R D, Nadas A S 1977 Clinical course of pulmonary stenosis. Circulation 56 (suppl 1): I–38–47

Radtke W, Anderson R R, Guerrero L 1988 Laser balloon angioplasty of the ductus arteriosus for palliative shunting (abstract). Circulation 78: II–100

Radtke W, Lock J, 1990 Balloon dilatation. Paediatric Clinics of North America 37: 193–213

Rashkind W J, Miller W W 1966 Creation of an atrial septal defect thoracotomy. Palliative approach to transposition of the great arteries. Journal of the American Medical Association 196: 991–994

Rashkind W J, Mullins C E, Hellenbrand W E 1987 Non surgical closure of patent ductus arteriosus: clinical application of the Rashkind PDA occluder system. Circulation 75: 583–592

Rocchini A P, Beekman R H, Shachar G B, Benson L, Schwartz D, Kan J S 1990 Balloon aortic valvuloplasty: Results of the valvuloplasty and angioplasty of Congenital Anomalies Registry. American Journal of Cardiology 65: 784–789

Rome J J, Keane J F, Perry S B, Spevak P J, Lock J E 1990 Double umbrella closure of atrial defects—Initial clinical applications. Circulation 82: 751–758

Sholler G F, Keane J F, Perry S B, Sanders S P, Lock J E 1988 Balloon dilatation of congenital aortic valve stenosis: results and influence of technical and morphologic features on outcome. Circulation 78: 351–360

Stanger P, Cassidy S C, Girod D, Kan J, Lababidi Z, Shapiro S 1990 Balloon pulmonary valvuloplasty: Results of the valvuloplasty and angioplasty of Congenital Anomalies Registry. American Journal of Cardiology 65: 775–783

Tynan M, Finlay J P, Fontes V, Hess J, Kan J 1990 Balloon angioplasty for the treatment of native coarctation: Results of valvuloplasty and angioplasty of Congenital Anomalies Registry. American Journal of Cardiology 65: 790–792

Wessel D L, Keane J F, Parness I, Lock J E 1988 Outpatient closure of the patent ductus arteriosus. Circulation 77: 1068–1071

Wren C, Sullivan I, Bull C, Deanfield J 1987 Percutaneous balloon dilatation of aortic valve stenosis in neonates and infants. British Heart Journal 58: 608–612

9. Subacute spongiform encephalopathies

R. G. Will

INTRODUCTION

The transmissible spongiform encephalopathies are a group of diseases of the nervous system which affect both animals and man. The most important human form of these disorders, Creutzfeldt–Jakob disease (CJD) was first recognized as a specific clinicopathological entity in 1920, while the disease in sheep, scrapie, has been recognized in the UK for over 250 years. Scrapie was shown to be transmissible in 1899 and the two conditions were linked in 1968 when CJD was transmitted to the chimpanzee by the intracerebral inoculation of brain extract from an affected patient. The transmission of a human CNS disorder with 'degenerative' neuropathology and no evidence of an immune response to the infectious agent was of fundamental importance and prompted extensive research with particular emphasis on the nature of the transmissible agent. Despite major advances in various fields of research, the spongiform encephalopathies were until recently primarily of academic interest, particularly in the human context as CJD is such a rare disease. The status of the transmissible spongiform encephalopathies was transformed in 1986 by the recognition of a novel disease in cattle, bovine spongiform encephalopathy (BSE) (Wilesmith et al 1988). The potential for species to species transmission in the spongiform encephalopathies has led to unprecedented public interest and concern with particular emphasis on the possibility that BSE may represent a risk to the human population. A judgement on the potential risks of transmission from bovine to human is dependent on an assessment of a body of evidence relating to CJD, scrapie and the other spongiform encephalopathies. The intention of this review is to provide an overview of the spongiform encephalopathies with particular reference to the potential public health risk posed by BSE.

DISEASES ASSOCIATED WITH SPONGIFORM ENCEPHALOPATHY

The transmissible spongiform encephalopathies include disorders affecting a range of animal species and three distinct conditions in man (Table 9.1)

Table 9.1   Transmissible spongiform encephalopathies

Host	Disease	Year first described
Man	Kuru	1900
	Creutzfeldt–Jakob disease	1920
	Gerstmann–Straussler syndrome	1926
Sheep	Scrapie	1730
Goat	Scrapie	1872
Mink	Transmissible mink encephalopathy	1947
Mule deer/elk	Chronic wasting disease	1967
Cattle	Bovine spongiform encephalopathy	1986
Nyala/Gemsbok/		1986–1989
Eland/Oryx/Kudu		
Cat	Feline spongiform encephalopathy	1990

Kuru

Kuru is a progressive neurological disorder which affects the people of the Fore linguistic group in the Eastern Highlands of Papua-New Guinea. Clinically, there is progressive ataxia of gait, followed by limb ataxia and dysarthria, but rarely nystagmus. Terminally the patients are unable to stand or walk and, although emotional lability may develop, dementia is unusual. The average duration of illness is 12 months.

Epidemiological evidence suggests that transmission of the agent was effected by the practice of ritual endocannabilism, which was prevalent until 1956. The incubation period ranges from 4.5 years to at least 30 years and the increased incidence in females and children is explained by the differential exposure to brain and internal organs: the adult male population did not consume these tissues. The continuing decline in incidence and the absence of disease in individuals born after 1956 provides further evidence for transmission by ritual cannabalism and confirms that there is no vertical transmission from generation to generation.

Creutzfeldt-Jakob disease (CJD; Fig. 9.1)

This is a rare cause of rapidly progressive dementia with a clinical course which usually extends to only months. Associated clinical features include myoclonic movements of the limbs, ataxia, pyramidal signs and in some cases cortical blindness. Terminally there is a state of akinetic mutism in which the patient lies still and unresponsive. Routine investigations are usually normal including the CT scan which shows cortical atrophy in only a minority of patients but is important in order to exclude other conditions. The electroencephalogram on the other hand is helpful in diagnosis, showing periodic complexes at about 1 per second in the majority of patients, appearances relatively specific to CJD. Diagnostic criteria in these subacute cases have been validated pathologically and by transmission

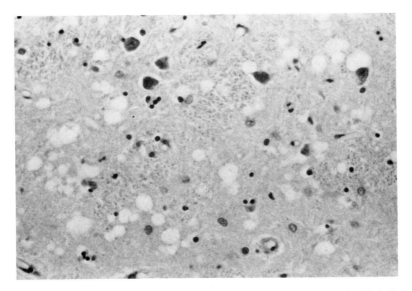

Fig. 9.1   Spongiform change in the basal ganglia of a patient with Creutzfeldt–Jakob disease.
Dark neurons and fibre bundles are interspersed with small vacuoles. (The preparation is
haematoxylin and eosin × 240: This figure is presented courtesy of Dr J. Bell and Dr J.
Ironside, Neuropathology Laboratory, Western General Hospital, Edinburgh.)

studies. In about 10% of cases the course is more protracted and in these
patients the clinical distinction from Alzheimer's disease may be impossible.

Although CJD is associated with a transmissible agent, paradoxically
between 5 and 10% cases are familial with a dominant pattern of inheritance. Modern diagnostic techniques including immunocytochemistry and
molecular genetics have recently suggested that other rare forms of familial
dementia may be related to CJD although these disorders have not yet been
proven to be transmissible.

Gerstmann–Straussler syndrome (GSS)

This is an exceedingly rare disorder, typified by chronic progressive ataxia,
bulbar dysfunction and terminal dementia. The great majority of cases are
familial with a dominant pattern of inheritance and symptoms usually
develop in the third or fourth decade with death ensuing in 3–5 years.

Scrapie

Scrapie is a common disease of adult sheep, affecting up to 30% of flocks in
the UK. The disease develops over months and clinical features include
behavioural change, debilitation, pruritus with rubbing against fixed
objects, grinding of teeth, biting of limbs, and ataxia of gait. Death occurs

from 1 to 8 months after onset of symptoms although rarely the clinical course is more protracted. Scrapie in goats is uncommon and less well characterized.

Transmissible mink encephalopathy (TME)

This is a rare sporadic disease which only affects commercially reared animals and is characterized by behavioural disturbance, ataxia and somnolence. The disease is caused by feeding mink with sheep tissues contaminated with scrapie and outbreaks are devastating with virtually total mortality in adult animals. There is, however, no evidence of lateral or vertical transmission of the agent from mink to mink and the outbreaks are self limiting.

Chronic wasting disease

This is a degenerative neurological disorder affecting mule deer and elk. Only isolated cases have been reported, all originating in North America.

Bovine spongiform encephalopathy (BSE; Fig. 9.2)

BSE was first described in the UK in 1986, although a small number of cases in 1985 were identified retrospectively. Since then cases have been

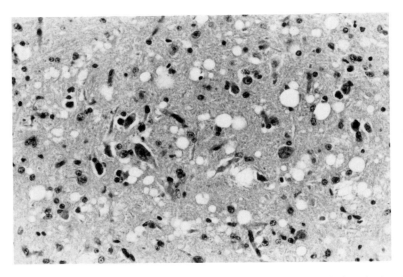

Fig. 9.2   Neuronal and neurophil vacuolation in bovine spongiform encephalopathy (× 240). (This figure is presented courtesy of Crown Copyright 1990: Dr G. Wells, Ministry of Agriculture, Fisheries and Food, Central Veterinary Laboratory, Weybridge, Surrey.)

described in Eire, Northern Ireland, and in cattle exported from the UK to Oman. By mid-1990 over 18 000 cases have been identified in the UK. Clinically there is aggression and other forms of behavioural disturbance (thus the popular term 'mad cow disease') followed by weight loss, ataxia, recumbency, and death 6–8 months from the onset of symptoms. The disease is almost certainly transmitted by cattle feed in the form of commercially produced concentrates which have been contamined by scrapie from sheep carcasses.

BSE was first identified as a spongiform encephalopathy on the basis of the pathological findings and an association with this group of conditions was confirmed recently when the transmission of BSE to mice was reported (Fraser et al 1988).

Isolated cases of spongiform encephalopathy have also been reported recently in captive zoo animals such as the nyala and gemsbok, presumptively due to feeding with commerical concentrates.

Feline spongiform encephalopathy (FSE)

A case of spongiform encephalopathy in a cat was reported from Bristol recently (Wyatt et al 1990). Clinical features including ataxia and somnolence were non-specific and one hypothesis was that the recognition of a spongiform encephalopathy in a cat might have been due to increased surveillance rather than the occurrence of a new disease. Two further cases have subsequently been reported suggesting that FSE is indeed a new disease presumably due to the contamination of pet food with increased titres of agent by inclusion of bovine material contaminated with BSE. Cats have been known to be experimentally susceptible to transmissible encephalopathy for over 10 years and occurrence of FSE does not necessarily imply a change in the species specificity of the scrapie agent but may be due to an increased level of exposure to a transmissible agent.

DEFINITION

These conditions were originally linked by the characteristic neuropathological changes on light microscopy which include vacuolar degeneration of the grey matter of the brain and spinal cord (spongiform change) (Fig. 9.1), astrocytic gliosis and neuronal loss. The distribution of these pathological changes varies between conditions and between individual cases but the presence of spongiform change is pathognomonic. The pathological definition of this group of conditions has been refined using immunocytochemical techniques and by electron microscopy. Scrapie associated fibrils (SAF) are a consistent finding in all these conditions on negative stain electron microscopy and are also pathognomonic.

There is no pathological evidence of an inflammatory response and there is no evidence of an immune response to the transmissible agent, nor interferon production. The pathological changes are progressive and the clinical signs progress in parallel over weeks or months and invariably result in death. Although the clinical course is rapid these conditions are typified by prolonged incubation periods which may range from years to decades. This extended duration between transmission of the agent and the development of clinical signs has complicated the study of the epidemiology of these conditions and the difficulty in establishing the mechanism of natural transmission of the agents is further complicated by the lack of an in vivo marker of infection.

The absence of a test to establish the presence of the infectious agent is of crucial importance. Animals incubating scrapie or BSE cannot be identified before the development of clinical signs. This compromises any programme for eradication of these disorders and has implications for any potential risk to the human population. The limitations in the field study of the spongiform encephalopathies has enhanced the importance of research into the nature of the agent and transmission studies in the laboratory.

THE NATURE OF THE TRANSMISSIBLE AGENT

Much of the evidence on the nature of the causative agent is based on research on the scrapie agent and, although the transmissible agents of the spongiform encephalopathies are remarkably similar, they do exhibit distinct properties, for example differing susceptible species range in laboratory transmission. None the less it is clear that these agents are not conventional viruses on the basis of both biological and physiochemical properties (Gajdusek & Gibbs 1977) (Table 9.2).

Purification techniques have demonstrated that a major component of the infectious agent is a membrane glycoprotein, prion protein (PrP) which is present in many tissues with particularly high concentration in neurones.

Table 9.2 Properties of the transmissible agents distinct from conventional viruses

Biological properties	No inflammatory response
	Chronic progressive pathology
	'Degenerative' histopathology
	No inclusion bodies
	No interferon production of sensitivity
	No virus interference
	No infectious nucleic acid demonstrable
	No antigenicity
Physicochemical properties	Size: filtrable to 25–100 nm pore diameter
	Resistant to: Formaldehyde
	Proteases
	Nucleases
	Heat: incompletely activated at 100°C
	Ultraviolet radiation
	Ionizing radiation

PrP is found as a normal protein in uninfected animals, but in the spongiform encephalopathies PrP is post-translationally modified and may accumulate in the brain as SAF or in the form of extracellular amyloid plaques. The specific change in the structure of the abnormal PrP that allows aggregation has not yet been established but this form of PrP is relatively resistant to degradation by proteinase K. This property has resulted in the development of immunocytochemical techniques that allow the identification of the abnormal protein in brain tissue, although interpretation is complicated by crossreactivity between normal and abnormal forms of PrP.

The persistence of infectivity in highly purified preparations of PrP and the resistance of the agent to treatments likely to denature nucleic acid has led to the proposition that the agent is an infectious protein which controls its own replication. This 'prion' hypothesis invokes a novel biological mechanism of infection and remains unproven, although research currently in progress, for example studies in transgenic rodents, may provide further support to the theory. The alternative view is that the agents of the spongiform encephalopathies contain a specific genome which is likely to be a nucleic acid and that host-coded protein in the form of PrP is a major component, but not infectious in isolation. This is the 'virino' hypothesis and is supported by evidence of virus-like pathogenesis and strain variation in the scrapie agent, provided by transmission studies in the laboratory (Kimberlin 1990). These studies are the only form of bioassay in the spongiform encephalopathies and have provided crucial information on the mechanisms of pathogenesis and factors that influence transmission.

TRANSMISSION STUDIES

Scrapie, TME, CJD, Kuru, GSS and more recently BSE are transmissible in the laboratory to a range of laboratory animals (Prusiner 1987) (Table 9.3).

The susceptible species range varies: for example CJD is transmissible to the chimpanzee while scrapie is not, and there is usually a species barrier to transmission. This barrier may result in prolongation of the incubation period or failure of transmission, but if transmission is achieved to a new

Table 9.3   Host range of spongiform encephalopathies in experimental transmission

Host	Kuru	CJD	Scrapie	TME
Ape	+	+		
Monkey	+	+	+	+
Sheep			+	+
Mink	+		+	+
Cat		+		
Mice		+	+	
Ferret	+			

Table 9.4   Relative efficacy of transmission by route of inoculation

Route	ID 50 (LD 50)
Intracerebral	1
Intraocular	10
Intravenous	10
Intraperitoneal	500–40 000
Subcutaneous	25 000
Oral	40 000

species there may be an alteration in the characteristics of the transmissible agent. This change usually involves a decrease in pathogenicity as judged by the duration of incubation period in the new species, although the incubation period may then shorten on serial passage, suggesting adaption of the agent, perhaps by selection of mutant strains. The concept of differing strains of infectious agents is supported by the identification of at least 15 isolates from scrapie which exhibit distinct properties, both in terms of incubation period and pathogenicity. The possibility of strain selection after cross-species transmission is of importance in assessing the risks of BSE because of the possibility that the agent of BSE may exhibit unpredictible properties following transmission of scrapie to the bovine population. In this context the factors which influence the efficiency of laboratory transmission are of relevance.

Experimental transmission may be effected by a number of routes of inoculation including intracerebral, intraperitoneal, intravenous and oral, but the titre of agent required to achieve transmission varies, with the oral route being least effective (Table 9.4).

In scrapie, after peripheral inoculation, there is a brief 'viraemic' phase and replication is then established in the spleen, lymph nodes and some other tissues in the lymphoreticular system (LRS), including Peyer's patches after oral dosage. Replication plateaus in these tissues and after a delay which may extend to over half the total incubation period infection spreads via the sympathetic nervous system to the thoracic cord and thence to the brain. Study of the spread of the agent after intraocular injection to the contralateral superior colliculus gives an estimate of the intra-axonal spread of scrapie at about 1 mm/day and the delay in clinical expression of infection within the CNS may also relate to limitation of replication within neurones and of spread between neurones.

The implication of the evidence on the pathogenesis of scrapie in mice is that specific tissues may contain high titres of infectivity and that these titres vary in relation to the stage of development of the disease. This is borne out by the evidence of the relative infectivity of tissues in natural scrapie (Table 9.5).

In the early pre-clinical phase the spleen, lymph nodes and other LRS tissues contain high titres of the agent while later in the incubation period

Table 9.5   Classification of tissues by agent titre and duration of incubation in natural scrapie

Titre of infectivity	Preclinical				Clinical	
	< 8	10–14	25	> 25	34–57	38–49
High					Brain Spinal cord	Brain Spinal cord
Medium		LN Spleen Ileum Colon	LN Tonsil Ileum Colon		Tonsil LN Spleen Ileum	Pituitary LN Spleen Colon
Low		Tonsil	Brain (brain stem) Spleen		Pituitary CSF Sciatic nerve Thymus Adrenal Colon	CSF Sciatic nerve Thymus Adrenal Colon
Undetectable	Tonsil Lymph node (LN) Spleen Thymus	Blood clot Serum Faeces Brain	Spinal cord Brain (cortex) Thymus Adrenal	Colostrum	Blood clot Testis Saliva Ovary Thyroid Uterus Heart Fetus Lung Mammary gland Kidney Skeletal muscle	Blood clot Ovary Milk Uterus Faeces Mammary gland Bone marrow Skeletal muscle Kidney

and after the development of clinical signs high titres are found in the CNS. It is of note that sheep muscle contains no detectable titre at any stage and neither does blood or milk. It cannot be concluded that these tissues do not contain any infectious agent but it does suggest that the titre is extremely low. Viraemia has been established in experimental models, for example the transmission of CJD from hamster to hamster by inoculation of buffy coat extract, but this required the inoculation of highly concentrated extracts by the intracerebral route.

The implication from this and other evidence, including the high titres necessary to effect oral transmission of CJD to primates or oral transmission of BSE to mice, is that the dosage of the agent is critical to the efficiency of transmission and may also influence incubation period.

In summary, transmission experiments have established that a number of factors interact to determine whether challenge with a transmissible agent results in disease. These include:

1. The strain of the transmissible agent
2. The route of inoculation
3. The dosage of inoculum

GENETIC FACTORS IN THE SPONGIFORM ENCEPHALOPATHIES

Host factors influence susceptibility, incubation period and the pathological distribution of lesions in some, but not all, of the spongiform encephalopathies. Historically it was recognized that the likelihood of developing scrapie varied between breeds of sheep and the availability of an experimental model of scrapie in mice has enabled the genetic factors which influence susceptibility to be more clearly defined. In mice incubation period is controlled by the Sinc (scrapie incubation period) gene which has two alleles: S7 (short incubation) and P7 (prolonged incubation). When infected with the ME7 strain of scrapie specific breeds of mice homozygous for S7 have a short and predictable incubation period, while P7 homozygotes have a prolonged incubation period and heterozygotes have an incubation period midway between the two. The interaction between the strain of agent and host genotype however varies: with the 22A strain S7 homozygotes have a prolonged incubation period in relation to P7 homozygotes.

A further interesting discovery was that in some models (defined by strain type and genotype) agent replication occurred in the spleen but did not result in clinical disease, the presumption being that the incubation period for replication in the CNS exceeded the life span of the host. A genetic influence of susceptibility has been shown in scrapie in sheep, in which a single gene, the Sip gene (scrapie incubation period), influences incubation period. There is, however, no convincing evidence that host factors influence susceptibility in TME or Kuru (nor as yet in BSE) and in CJD the recent evidence of a genetic component to susceptibility has been dependent on molecular biological techniques rather than transmission studies.

The discovery that PrP was a major component of the infectious agent led to the identification of the PrP gene which is present in all species unrelated to the presence of spongiform encephalopathy. Restriction fragment length polymorphisms (RFLP) associated with PrP in mice were shown to correlate with the Sinc gene and further research confirmed a close linkage between the PrP and Sinc genes (Hunter et al 1987). It has been subsequently established that different amino acid sequences in the PrP gene relate to contrasting Sinc genotype, suggesting that PrP may be the gene product of the Sinc gene. Thus the gene which influences incubation period and/or susceptibility in scrapie may code for a protein which is an essential component of the transmissible agent.

Analysis of the PrP gene in human spongiform encephalopathies has shown that in some familial cases specific anomalies of the PrP gene are associated with disease. For example in a number of pedigrees of GSS a proline/leucine substitution at codon 102 of the PrP gene is present in affected family members but not in unaffected individuals (Hsiao et al 1989). A number of different amino acid substitutions or insertions have been discovered in the PrP gene in familial CJD and more recently in a limited number of cases of sporadic CJD. This raises the possibility that CJD and the other spongiform encephalopathies may be genetic in origin and that the gene product, prion protein, is sufficient in itself to cause disease. One difficulty with this theory is that the property of transmissibility is then necessarily an epiphenomenon, with the implication that spongiform encephalopathies are not in essence infectious diseases. The evidence from basic scientific research must, however, be evaluated in relation to the natural disorders and in particular their epidemiology.

EPIDEMIOLOGY

Although the agents of the spongiform encephalopathies share common properties, the natural diseases have distinct epidemiological characteristics.

Creutzfeldt–Jakob disease

Since the experimental transmission of CJD to primates in 1968, cases of CJD have been reported throughout the world and systematic national surveys are being carried out in a number of countries (Table 9.6).

Despite all this work, the mechanism of natural transmission of CJD remains uncertain, although a number of epidemiological conclusions can be drawn from the evidence (Brown et al 1987).

Table 9.6   Surveys of Creutzfeldt–Jakob disease

Local surveys of CJD		National surveys of CJD	
Slovakia	1977	Italy	1973
Brooklyn & Staten Island	1978	Israel	1974
Burlington, Vermont	1978	England and Wales	1975
Tisza river (Hungary)	1978	Czechoslovakia	1977
Paris	1978	Hungary	1978
Santiago	1980	United States	1979
Southern Italy	1980	Japan	1979
Genoa	1981	France	1979
Parma (Italy)	1983	Chile	1980
Tenerife	1988	Japan	1983
Yamanasi (Japan)	1989	England and Wales	1986
		France	1987
		Finland	1988

CJD has a worldwide distribution and a relatively consistent incidence of 0.5–1 case/million/annum.

The geographical distribution of cases within individual countries largely parallels population density with no convincing evidence of spatio-temporal aggregation of cases. This largely excludes the possibility of transmission from case to case and a history of direct personal contact between individual patients is exceedingly uncommon.

5–10% of cases are familial, but it is not known whether this represents contact transmission, vertical transmission, inherited control of suscepti-bility or genetic integration of the agent.

Accidental transmission of CJD from patient to patient has occurred by a variety of routes including contaminated neurosurgical instruments, corneal transplantation, and administration of human growth hormone. However, these occurrences are exceedingly rare and iatrogenic trans-mission cannot explain the development of CJD in the great majority of patients.

There is no convincing evidence to support zoonotic transmission, and in particular the evidence does not suggest a casual link between scrapie and CJD. There have been reports of CJD in individuals who had consumed sheep brains or sheep eyeballs and there is an extraordinarily high incidence of CJD in Libyan-born Israelis who as a group have a high dietary exposure to sheep tissue. However, an excess of cases in this ethnic group and the recently reported aggregation of cases in Czechos-lovakia may well be related to a high incidence of familial cases rather than increased dietary exposure to scrapie. Furthermore there is no evidence of an increased risk of CJD due to occupational exposure to the scrapie agent and case-control studies have not shown an increased exposure to sheep meat in affected patients in relation to controls. CJD has been described in a life-long vegetarian and the incidence of CJD in Iceland is relatively low despite endemic scrapie and the historical practice of consuming scrapie affected animals. Most significantly CJD occurs with the expected incidence in countries such as New Zealand and Australia which are free of scrapie, and also in Japan where scrapie has only recently been reported in imported stock from Canada despite high levels of veterinary surveillance.

In conclusion, scrapie has not been shown to present any demonstrable risk to the human population, although the cause of CJD in individual sporadic cases is not known. No mechanism of natural transmission in CJD has been identified and case to case transmission cannot explain the rarity and spatial dispersion of cases. The possibility of a carrier state or infection with recovery cannot be excluded without a diagnostic test for the presence of the agent and it is also possible that the infectious agent is widespread in the environment with disease only developing in those with a rare genetic predisposition.

Scrapie

Although genetic factors influence susceptibility, scrapie is undoubtedly an infectious disease. Scrapie can spread from flock to flock by the importation of infected but apparently normal sheep and also spreads from dam to offspring. The exact mechanism of lateral transmission is uncertain but cross-contamination by the oral route is almost certainly involved: for example uninfected sheep may develop scrapie after grazing on contaminated pastures. The mechanism of transmission from dam to offspring is also uncertain but intrauterine infection is unproven and postpartum oral contamination by placenta, which contains high titres of the scrapie agent, may be important. Eradication of scrapie has proved exceedingly difficult because of the occurrence of both lateral and vertical transmission and because infected but clinically normal animals cannot be identified.

Bovine spongiform encephalopathy

Since the recognition of BSE in 1986 detailed epidemiological information has been obtained in all new cases and by mid-1990 the total number of confirmed cases exceeded 18 000. Careful collection and analysis of data at the Central Veterinary Laboratory suggested early in the course of the epidemic that this was an extended common source epidemic and the likely source of infection was scrapie-contaminated feed in the form of commercially produced concentrates. Study of the production methods of this material revealed a change in production methods in the early 1980s, including continuous rather than batch processing and the abandonment of solvent extraction, which may have allowed a higher titre of scrapie agent in the final product. An alternative hypothesis, that the change in production methods allowed recycling of contaminated bovine material from a previously rare and unrecognized spongiform encephalopathy in cattle cannot be excluded, but the possibility of a change in the scrapie agent itself is unlikely because of the widespread geographic distribution of cases throughout the UK within a relatively short period.

The government responded to the occurrence of BSE by setting up a group of experts, the Southwood Committee, who concluded that the risk of transmission of BSE to the human population was remote (Southwood Committee Report 1989). None the less a number of specific actions were recommended, resulting in statutory measures which have subsequently been extended. These have included the destruction of all clinically affected animals, a ban on the feeding of ruminant-derived protein to ruminants, and a ban on the use of specified bovine offals (including all tissues with a potentially high titre of agent such as brain, spinal cord, etc.) in human food.

The ban on feeding of potentially infected material to cattle in July 1988 was designed to prevent further cases of BSE by oral transmission of the agent. However, it is not known whether vertical or lateral transmission will occur within the cattle population, although it is possible, by analogy with TME, that cattle will be a dead end host. The future course of the epidemic is therefore uncertain: if there is no cross-infection the epidemic should decline after 1992 and disappear in the early years of the next century; if there is maternal transmission from dam to calf the epidemic will none the less decline over a similar period because only a minority of calves reach adulthood and are able to breed; if there is lateral transmission the condition may become endemic. A difficult problem in deciding on specific action to accelerate the decline in the epidemic is the absence of an in vivo marker for infection. All cattle exposed to potentially infected material before July 1988 are potentially incubating the disease, although the within herd incidence does not suggest that a high proportion of cattle are actually infected. Transmission from dam to calf, although this is still hypothetical, could occur in affected animals and also in clinically normal animals incubating the disease. Control measures are therefore likely to be exceedingly difficult and an important measure may be to ensure that careful records are kept of breeding and cattle movement so that if research in progress suggests, for example, vertical transmission appropriate action can be taken.

Does BSE represent a risk to the human population?

This question has prompted a volume of informed and ill-informed comment in the media relating to a matter of understandable public concern. A judgement on the possibility of transmission of BSE to the human population depends on an assessment of the scientific evidence relating to the spongiform encephalopathies which I have attempted to summarize, rather than intuitive assertions.

The epidemiological evidence does not suggest that scrapie is a significant pathogen to man and it is reasonable to assume that scrapie in cattle will not therefore pose a risk to the human population. Humans have been exposed to scrapie for over 250 years without demonstrable harm despite the probability that there has been significant dietary and occupational exposure to the scrapie agent. The possibility that the characteristics of the scrapie agent may have been altered by transmission across the species barrier must however be considered, although previous experiment does not suggest that this is likely to result in an increased pathogenicity to man. Transmission experiments currently in progress provide support for this view: primates inoculated with BSE remain healthy well after they would have been expected to develop clinical disease if inoculated with CJD or GSS. However, it will take many years to establish the properties of the BSE agent because of the necessarily protracted nature of transmission experiments and it is clearly prudent to minimize any potential human exposure to the agent.

Transmission of the spongiform encephalopathies is dependent on a number of factors including dosage of inoculum, route of inoculation and interaction with host genetic factors. One approach to an assessment of the risk of BSE is to examine these factors as they apply to the human population. The pathogenesis of the spongiform encephalopathies is similar in natural and laboratory induced disease and the titre of the agent is highest in specific tissues such as brain, spinal cord and components of the LRS. Although cattle exhibiting signs of clinical disease are destroyed, it is possible that such tissues as spleen and lymph nodes from cattle incubating the disease may contain high titres of the agent.

The ban on the human consumption of specified bovine offals is therefore of great importance as it excludes the possibility of dietary exposure to organs from apparently healthy animals which potentially contain high titres of the agent. Consumption of other tissues, including muscle, from healthy animals is not restricted but the evidence from transmission studies suggest that such tissues are exceedingly unlikely to represent a risk because they do not contain detectable titres of agent. Furthermore, the oral route is by far the least efficient route of transmission and meat for human consumption is usually obtained from animals which are slaughtered at an age when significant titres of the agents are unlikely to be detectable even in the LRS. Animals currently reared for meat production are no longer exposed to potentially contaminated feed and cannot be infected unless there is vertical or horizontal transmission. In conclusion, the evidence provides powerful support to the view that the consumption of beef is exceedingly unlikely to represent a risk to the human population.

Of greater concern is the possibility that inoculation of the agent may pose a higher risk and in particular that those occupationally exposed to high risk tissue such as brain, for example abbatoir workers or butchers, may be at risk through accidental inoculation in cuts or lacerations of the skin. Guidelines have been issued to relevant professions but it is important to remember that occupational exposure to the scrapie agent has not been demonstrated to be associated with an increased risk of developing CJD. The tragic occurrence of CJD in human growth hormone recipients suggests that extreme caution should be taken with any medicinal products or implants potentially contamined with the BSE agent. This has prompted action by the Committee for the Safety of Medicines and all medicinal products of bovine origin are now sourced from countries which are known to be free of BSE, for example Australia and New Zealand. Although this action is clearly essential, iatrogenic transmission of CJD and the transmission of kuru have both involved passage of an agent adapted to humans either by inoculation in the CNS or by the oral consumption of large quantities of high risk tissue. Transmission by human growth hormone has similarly required the transmission of an adapted agent following repeated injection of potentially contaminated material over a period of years.

In conclusion, experimental and epidemiological evidence provides strong support for the view that the risks of BSE to the human population are likely to be remote. It is, however, clearly incorrect to suggest that there is no risk and a judgement as to whether the current legislative measures are sufficient will inevitably vary according to personal experience, circumstance and attitude to risk. Decisions, however, have to be taken by the authorities in response to BSE and, although based on the scientific evidence, these decisions may have major economic and political implications. Continuing research in the spongiform encephalopathies is essential and in the future may suggest that an extension of current legislative controls is necessary. One part of this research is the continuing study of the epidemiology of CJD and this may allow a future judgement on whether the Government response to the development of BSE has been effective in preventing any potential risk to the human population.

REFERENCES

Brown P, Cathala F, Raubertas R F, Gajdusek D C, Castaigne P 1987 The epidemiology of Creutzfeldt–Jakob disease: Conclusion of a 15-year investigation in France and review of the world literature. Neurology 37: 895–904
Fraser H, McConnell I, Wells G A H, Dawson M 1988 Transmission of bovine spongiform encephalopathy to mice. Veterinary Record 123 p 472
Gajdusek D C, Gibbs C J Jr 1977 Unconventional viruses causing the spongiform virus encephalopathies. A fruitless search for the coat and core. In: Viruses and environment (Proceedings of the Third International Conference on Comparative Virology, Mont Gabrial, PQ Canada). Chapter 5: pp 79–98
Hsiao K, Baker H F, Crow T J et al 1989 Linkage of a prion protein missense variant to Gerstmann–Straussler syndrome. Nature 338: 342–344
Hunter N, Hope J, McConnell I, Dickinson A G 1987 Linkage of the scrapie-associated fibril protein (PrP) gene and Sinc using cogenic mice and restriction fragment length polymorphism analysis. Journal of General Virology 68: 2711–2716
Kimberlin R H 1990 Transmissible encephalopathies in animals. Canadian Journal of Veterinary Research 54: 30–37

Prusiner S B 1987 An introduction to scrapie and Creutzfeldt–Jakob disease research. In: Prusiner S B, McKinley M P (eds) Prions: novel infectious pathogens causing scrapie and Creutzfeldt–Jakob disease. Chapter 1: pp 1–15

Southwood Committee Report 1989 Report of the Working Party on Bovine Spongiform Encephalopathy. Department of Health and Ministry of Agriculture Fisheries and Food. ISBN 185197 405 9

Wilesmith J W, Wells G A H, Cranwell M P, Ryan J B M 1988 Bovine spongiform encephalopathy: Epidemiological studies. Veterinary Record 123: pp 638–644

Wyatt J M, Pearson G R, Smerdon T, Gruffydd-Jones T J, Wells G A H 1990 Spongiform encephalopathy in a cat. Veterinary Record 126: 513

FURTHER READING

Agriculture Committee (Fifth Report): Bovine Spongiform Encephalopathy (BSE). House of Commons 10 July 1990. Report and Proceedings of the Committee together with Minutes of Evidence and Appendices.

Brown P 1980 An epidemiologic critique of Creutzfeldt–Jakob disease. American Journal of Epidemiology 2: 113–135

Brown P 1988 The clinical neurology and epidemiology of Creutzfeldt–Jakob disease, with special reference to iatrogenic cases. In: Novel infectious agents and the central nervous system. Ciba Foundation Symposium pp 3–23

Prusiner S B, Hadlow W J (eds) 1979 Slow transmissible diseases of the nervous system. Volumes 1&2. Academic Press, New York

Prusiner S B, McKinley M P (eds) 1987 Prions: novel infectious pathogens causing scrapie and Creutzfeldt–Jakob disease. Academic Press, New York

ter Meulen V, Katz M (eds) 1977 Slow virus infections of the central nervous system. Springer-Verlag, New York

10. Malaria

H. M. Gilles

INTRODUCTION

Malaria remains the most important parasitic infection in the world with an estimated 1 billion persons at risk (Fig. 10.1). The situation is most serious in sub-Saharan Africa, where transmission of *Plasmodium falciparum* malaria is very high, basic health services are often rudimentary and uncontrolled migration to the cities with their conglomerates of 'shanty towns' has created new or extended transmission sites. Most of the estimated 2.5 million people who die from malaria every year are children under 5 years.

The relentless spread of chloroquine resistant *P. falciparum* malaria (Fig. 10.2) has been an ominous development of the past 20 years. In some parts of the world e.g. Thailand and Vietnam, multidrug resistance is widespread and diminished susceptibility of the parasite to quinine is increasingly reported.

There are four species of malarial parasites, *Plasmodium falciparum, P. vivax, P. ovale* and *P. malariae*. In this review, I shall deliberately highlight *P. falciparum* infection, since this is the species that is responsible for virtually all the global mortality associated with malaria and for a substantial portion of its morbidity.

Transmission

All types of malaria are predominantly transmitted by female anopheline mosquitoes. Transmission can however occur by blood transfusion, syringe passage among drug addicts, and transplacental transfer of parasites.

Imported malaria

The exponential increase in long distance travel for leisure, business or other purposes has resulted in a rise in the importation of malaria into non-endemic areas.

In Great Britain in 1989, almost 2000 cases were reported to the Malaria

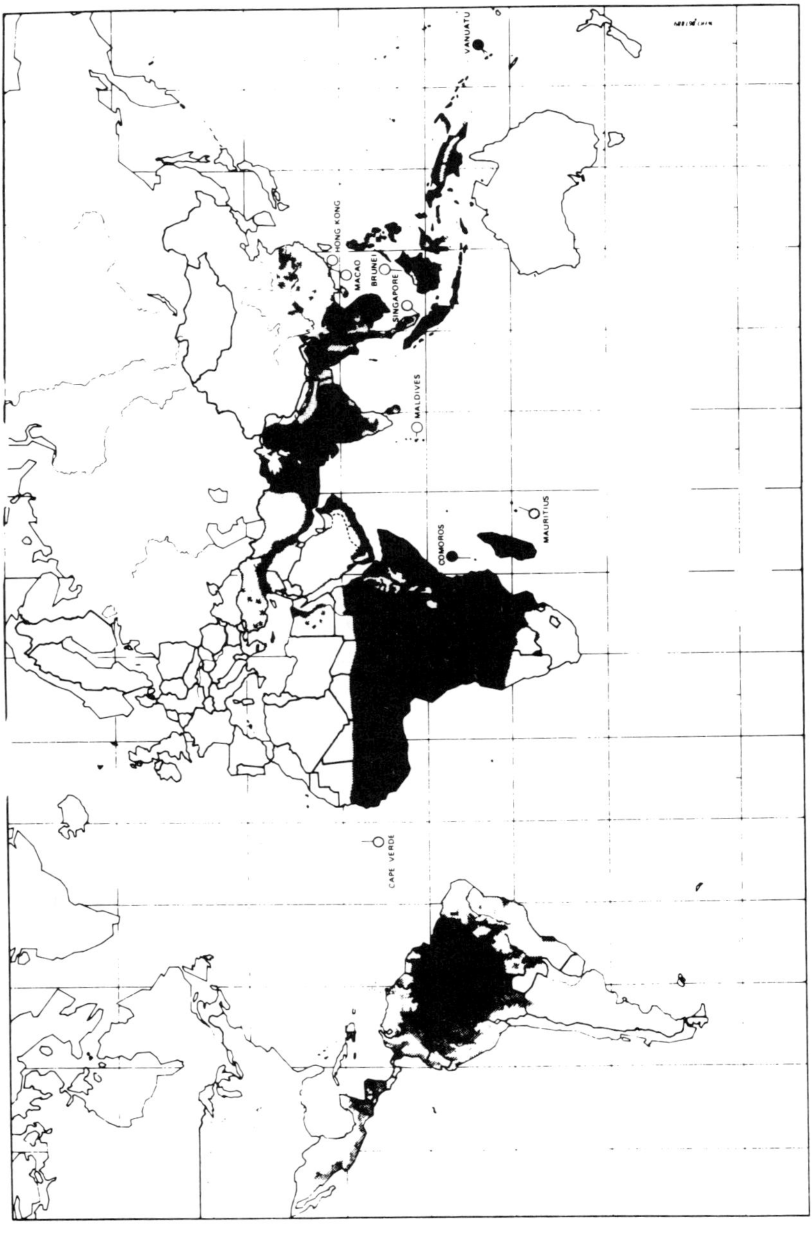

Fig. 10.1 Global status of malaria, 1990.

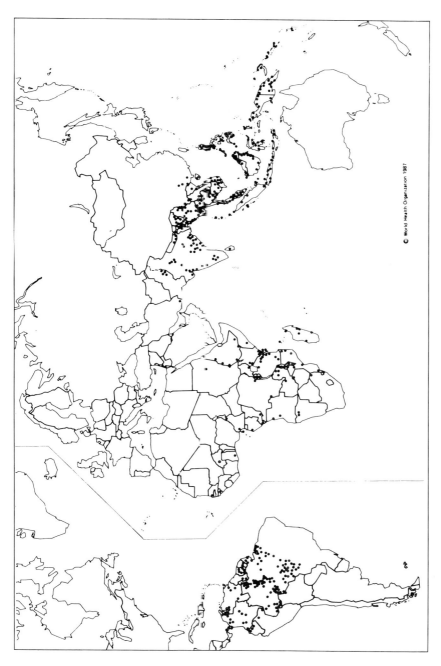

Fig. 10.2   Global status of chloroquine–resistant *P .falciparum*, 1990.

Reference Laboratory of the London School of Hygiene and Tropical Medicine. The distribution of the various species was:

P. falciparum   : 1072
P. vivax   : 734
P. ovale   : 101
P. malariae   :   33
Mixed infections   :   47

When the time interval was reported, the majority of cases occurred within one month of returning from an endemic area; 202 cases occurred in children under the age of 10 years, not infrequently such children having visited their parents living overseas during school holidays.

For the second year in succession the number of *P. falciparum* has exceeded those of *P. vivax;* whereas in the past the reverse was the case. This is an ominous trend since *P. falciparum* is a killer whereas *P. vivax* is usually not. Most of the cases of falciparum were contracted in West Africa (645); East Africa (150) and Central Africa (45): these being the great danger areas for *P. falciparum* transmission. Between January and September 1990, 1688 cases of malaria have been reported of which 836 were due to *P. falciparum*.

In the USA in 1988, 1023 cases of malaria were reported with 6 deaths, all due to *P. falciparum*; while in Canada in 1989 5 deaths occurred from falciparum malaria.

In the past 20 years, 34 cases have been reported in Europe of **'airport malaria'**, acquired by people living near or working in airports, who had not travelled overseas. These patients were bitten by infected mosquitoes arriving in aircraft from the tropics—one study of 27 aircraft from Nairobi yielded 150 adult mosquitoes. Six air cargo handlers working on an aircraft from Zaire were infected in Brussels airport of whom 1 died.

One of the weirdest examples of malaria transmission outside the endemic area occurred when 2 passengers who boarded an Ethiopian Airline plane at Heathrow Airport and alighted in Rome, developed malaria on their return to the UK having obviously been infected on board the aircraft—**'commuter malaria'**.

CLINICAL FEATURES

Malaria is usually an acute febrile illness characterized by episodic fever due to asexual reproduction of plasmodium within red corpuscles (schizogony).

A.   Plasmodium falciparum malaria: malignant tertian malaria

The presentation of uncomplicated malignant tertian malaria is very variable and can mimic many other diseases. Fever is a very common, though

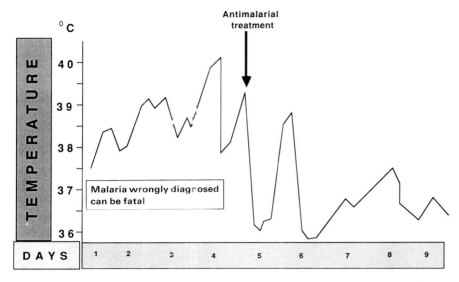

Fig. 10.3 Temperature chart characteristic of falciparum malaria. Note: continuous daily (not tertian) fever.

not an invariable presenting symptom; it is initially persistent rather than tertian and may or may not be accompanied by rigors (Fig. 10.3). The patient sometimes complains of aches and pains all over the body. Jaundice may be present as well as anaemia and on physical examination the liver and spleen may be palpable. This mundane presentation is frequently mis-diagnosed as influenza or viral hepatitis. Abdominal pain and diarrhoea are inconsistent features. Unless diagnosed and promptly treated, the clinical picture deteriorates at an alarming speed and severe manifestations and complications appear (Looareesuwan et al 1990) (Table 10.1).

Particularly severe manifestations can occur in non-immune travellers, migrant workers and in all age groups in areas where the endemicity of

Table 10.1 Complications of acute falciparum malaria

Brain	Altered consciousness → coma, convulsions and psychiatric manifestations
Kidney	Oliguria and acute renal failure, acute tabular necrosis
Liver	Hepatosplenomegaly Jaundice and acute hepatocellular necrosis
Lung	Acute pulmonary oedema
Haemolysis	Acute intravascular haemolysis, anaemia, haemoglobinuria, disseminated intravascular coagulation
Circulatory collapse	Gram-negative septicaemia
Blood	Gram-negative septicaemia
Hypoglycaemia	Drug-induced, liver glycogen depletion, inhibition of gluconeogenesis

malaria is low. By contrast, in parts of the world where falciparum malaria is holo- or hyperendemic, severe malaria is most likely to occur among young children over the age of 6 months, primigravidae, persons who have lived away from the area for several years, splenectomized persons and patients receiving immunosuppressive therapy. Older children and adults in these areas acquire a partial immunity to malaria. Paradoxically, AIDS does not seem to enhance the severity of malaria.

Apart from jaundice, clinical signs of hepatic dysfunction are unusual, although biochemical disturbances, e.g. elevation of serum enzymes, are common and the serum albumin is low. Muscle damage (rhabdomyolysis) with general myalgia and myoglobinuria has been reported.

Cerebral malaria

By definition the patient is comatose using the Glasgow Coma scale of Teasdale & Jennett (1974); other encephalopathies locally prevalent, e.g. bacterial meningitis and viral encephalitides, have been excluded and malaria parasites are demonstrable on a peripheral blood smear. In young children, the depth of coma may be assessed by observing the response to standard painful or vocal stimuli (Molyneux et al 1989). Convulsions are common in both adults and children. Retinal haemorrhages are very variable; exudates are unusual and papilloedema is rare. A variety of transient eye movement abnormalities, e.g. divergent eyes, conjugate deviation, have been noted. Fixed jaw closure and tooth grinding are common. Neck stiffness is not uncommon but overt signs of meningeal irritation are absent. The commonest neurological picture is one of a symmetrical upper motor neurone lesion. Motor abnormalities such as hypertonicity, posturing or opisthotonos occur. The opening pressure at lumbar puncture is usually normal in adults; the CSF is clear, there are less than 10 cells/μl, the protein is raised as is the CSF lactate. A variety of non-specific EEG abnormalities have been described while computerized tomography (CT) scans of the brain are usually normal. Hepatosplenomegaly is a common accompaniment of cerebral malaria and the abdominal reflexes are invariably absent.

In 10% of African children, especially when the disease is complicated by hypoglycaemia, lasting neurological sequelae occur (Taylor et al 1988). In some young children the opening pressure at lumbar puncture may be raised.

Hypoglycaemia

This is increasingly being recognized as a complication of severe malaria. The diagnosis can easily be overlooked because several of its clinical features are also typical of severe malaria. It has been described in three settings: (1) patients who are treated with quinine or quinidine, (2) pregnancy, and (3) patients, especially young children, with severe disease (White et al 1987, Taylor et al 1988). Possible causes of hypoglycaemia—apart from quinine/quinidine-induced hyperinsulinaemia—include: (a) increased glucose consumption by the host and the parasites, (b) hepatic glycogen depletion, and (c) inhibition of hepatic gluconeogenesis.

Renal dysfunction and failure

Renal impairement is virtually confined to adults. There is a rise in serum creatinine and urea, oliguria and eventually anuria due to acute tubular necrosis. Renal failure is usually oliguric but may occasionally be polyuric. The mechanism of acute tubular necrosis in malaria is not fully understood. Studies of renal blood flow have shown cortical ischaemia and medullary congestion as in other forms of acute tubular necrosis.

Acidosis

Acid-base disturbances and other metabolic abnormalities as well as hypovolaemia and hyponatraemia are relatively common in falciparum malaria. Concentrations of lactate in the blood and cerebrospinal fluid are high.

Malarial haemoglobinuria

The classical description of 'blackwater fever' occurring in a non-immune Caucasian patient taking quinine irregularly for prophylaxis or presumptive treatment, accompanied by mild or absent fever and scanty or absent parasitaemia, is now extinct.

Malarial haemoglobinuria, however, still occurs; it is uncommon and is usually associated with hyperparasitaemia and/or severe disease.

When haemoglobinuria occurs in 'partially immune' persons, it is likely to be due to glucose-6-phosphate dehydrogenase (G-6-PD) deficiency (Gilles & Ikeme 1960) or some other erythrocyte enzyme abnormality.

Anaemia

Anaemia is a common finding in severe malaria. Its degree, in general, correlates with parasitaemia, schizontaemia, serum total bilirubin and creatinine concentration. The mechanisms are multifactorial and complex (Weatherall & Abdalla 1982) involving haemolysis, dyserythropoiesis, immune factors, iron sequestration and abnormal splenic activity. In African children it is a common presenting feature (McGregor et al 1956); parasitaemia is often low but there is abundant malarial pigment in the cells of the reticuloendothelial system reflecting recent or resolving infection.

Spontaneous bleeding/disseminated intravascular coagulation (DIC)

Bleeding gums, epistaxis, petechiae and subconjunctival haemorrhages occur. DIC, complicated by clinically significant bleeding (e.g. haematemesis, melaena) occurs in less than 10% of patients and is more frequent in non-immune patients with imported severe malaria.

Hyperpyrexia

This is particularly common in children and is associated with convulsions, delirium or coma. It must be differentiated from heat stroke in unacclimatized visitors to the tropics or if there is a history of excessive exercise.

Circulatory collapse ('algid malaria')

Some patients are admitted in a state of collapse with a systolic BP less than 80 mmHg in the supine position; a cold, clammy cyanotic skin; constricted peripheral veins; rapid feeble pulse etc. In Thailand and elsewhere, this clinical picture was often associated with a Gram-negative septicaemia.

Idiopathic pulmonary oedema

This is one of the most dreaded complications of severe malaria carrying with it a very high mortality (over 50%). It usually appears several days after chemotherapy has been started and at a time when the patient's general condition is improving and the peripheral parasitaemia is diminishing. It must be differentiated from the iatrogenically produced pulmonary oedema resulting from fluid overload.

The first indication of impending pulmonary oedema is an increase in the respiratory rate preceding the development of other chest signs.

The mechanisms involved in the idiopathic malarial pulmonary oedema—which resembles the adult acute respiratory distress syndrome—are unknown.

Hyperparasitaemia

Although in general and especially in non-immunes, high parasite densities e.g. 5–10% or over are associated with severe disease; in holo-hyper-endemic areas of malaria partially immune children can tolerate surprisingly high levels (20–30%) often without clinical symptoms.

It is important to realize that multi-organ failure frequently occurs in severe malaria and several of the above listed complications may occur simultaneously in any one individual.

Important differences in the history and clinical presentation of severe malaria between adults and children are given in Table 10.2.

Table 10.2   Differences between severe malaria in adults and children

History, signs or symptoms	Adults	Children
1. Cough	Uncommon	Common
2. Convulsions	Common	More common
3. Antecedent history	5–7 days	1–2 days
4. Resolution of coma	2–4 days	1–2 days
5. Neurological sequelae	Rare	Occur in about 10%
6. Jaundice	Common	Uncommon
7. Pretreatment hypoglycaemia	Uncommon	Common
8. Pulmonary oedema	Common	Rare
9. Renal failure	Common	Rare

Pathophysiology of cerebral malaria

Studies carried out recently have attempted to elucidate a longstanding controversy: the pathophysiology of cerebral malaria. Hypotheses include cellular 'sludging', increased vascular permeability, an immunologically mediated reaction, and cellular 'sequestration'. Some of these hypotheses were based exclusively on animal models. Unfortunately, the natural history and clinical features of malaria in monkeys and rodents bears little relation to that in man and extrapolations have proved largely unjustified.

The 'sludging' hypothesis considered that the pathological events in cerebral malaria were the result of obstructed microcirculatory flow or the local release of unidentified toxic materials from the malaria parasites. This early theory (put forward nearly 50 years ago) has been considerably refined in recent years and the molecular mechanisms involved are being elucidated. The evidence that immune factors are involved in the pathogenesis of acute cerebral malaria are generally considered unconvincing.

Currently the mechanical 'sequestration' hypothesis seems to be the most generally acceptable.

Two principal mechanisms have been proposed to explain the phenomenon of sequestration. Decreased deformability of the parasitized red cells may be a contributory factor—but this cannot be the sole explanation for a variety of reasons e.g. selective sequestration in different vascular beds; *P. vivax* enlarges the erythrocyte but does not sequester.

Infected erythrocytes may adhere to vascular endothelium due to a specific molecular interaction. This is currently referred to as 'cytoadherence'. In vitro models of cytoadherence are providing information about both potential parasite adhesives and host receptors. Several candidate molecules have been identified and this area bears careful scrutiny in the coming years.

Recent studies also suggest that anaerobic cerebral glycolysis takes place in cerebral malaria.

Tumour necrosis factor (TNF, cachectin) contains several properties that suggest that this cytokine may have a role in the pathophysiology of cerebral malaria. In Malawian children plasma TNF levels are significantly associated with severity of disease and mortality. TNF is known to increase the adhesive properties of endothelial cells and leucocytes, and it is feasible that TNF may moderate or accelerate the cytoadherence of parasitized red cells to cerebral venular endothelium resulting in sequestration. The role of TNF could be proven if a beneficial effect of anti-TNF antibody can be demonstrated in patients with severe cerebral malaria. Other cytokines e.g. interleukins 1, 2 and 6, and interferon also require investigation.

B.   Plasmodium vivax/P. ovale malaria: Benign tertian

The classical descriptions of the malaria paroxysm stage are more commonly seen in *P. vivax* and *P. ovale* infections than in falciparum malaria. The fever is of the tertian type especially if the infection has been initially misdiagnosed for some other febrile illness, or is relapsing after inadequate treatment. Hepatosplenomegaly occurs frequently. In addition to jaundice, patients may have mild abnormalities of liver function and transient bilirubinuria. The disease is rarely directly fatal, although death from a ruptured enlarged spleen and chronic anaemia occasionally occurs. Thrombocytopenia is common in both vivax and falciparum malaria. Possible causes include intravascular lysis, enhanced splenic uptake or sequestration, and decreased platelet production. For all pratical purposes, it can be assumed that *P. vivax* and *P. ovale* infections wherever they have been acquired will respond satisfactorily to treatment with a combination of chloroquine and primaquine (see later); even though a recent report of a *P. vivax* infection acquired in Papua-New Guinea resistant to chloroquine has appeared in the literature.

In both *P. vivax* and *P. ovale*, 'hypnozoites' (dormant stage of the parasite) persist in the liver. These may develop months or even years after the initial infection and are also responsible for the characteristic relapses that occur unless radical treatment is given.

C.   Plasmodium malariae: Quartan malaria

The most important clinical feature of this infection is its ability to produce an immune-complex nephropathy, especially in children living in endemic areas. It is now generally accepted that unlike *P. vivax* and *P. ovale*, *P. malariae* does not have a 'hypnozoite' (dormant state) in its life-cycle. A radical cure is therefore achieved with chloroquine alone, since to date no cases resistant to the drug have been reported.

D.   Malaria in pregnancy and neonates

The impact of malaria on 'non-immune' and 'partially immune' pregnant women is different; moreover, even among the 'partially immune', important differences occur between primiparae and multiparae for reasons that have yet to be satisfactorily explained.

Pregnancy malaria in 'non-immune'

Maternal death, abortion, stillbirth, premature delivery and low birth weight have all been reported.

Hypoglycaemia is common, may be asymptomatic or manifest itself by abnormal behaviour, sweating and sudden loss of consciousness which can easily be misdiagnosed as cerebral malaria.

Acute pulmonary oedema may be present on admission, develop while in hospital or occur immediately after delivery.

Pregnancy malaria in 'partially immunes'

The florid manifestations of severe falciparum malaria are rarely seen in 'partially immune' pregnant women whether primigravidae or multigravidae.

Placental parasitaemia is common and in primigravidae (but not in multigravidae) has been shown to be associated with low birthweight and increased neonatal mortality (McGregor et al 1983). In holo-hyperendemic areas, the association between maternal malaria and abortion, premature labour and stillbirth is far from convincing.

Acute falciparum malaria can cause a sudden and catastrophic fall in haemoglobin concentration in primiparae during the second trimester of pregnancy. The correlation between the severe anaemia and peripheral parasitaemia is very poor. It is known, however, that the placenta is a site of preferential sequestration and development of the parasite.

Congenital malaria

Congenital malaria is a well-documented phenomenon. It seems to be commoner in areas of low than of high transmission. Infants born to 'non-immune' mothers who develop parasitaemia manifest clinical illness while those born to 'partially immune' mothers are usually asymptomatic.

E.   Inherited red cells factors and malaria

Over the years, epidemiological, clinical, in vitro culture and autopsy evidence has accumulated to demonstrate that some of the inherited red cell disorders protect against the lethal effects of falciparum malaria. The wealth of evidence indicates that the heterozygous sickle trait, heterozygous alpha- and beta-thalassaemia, female heterozygous G-6-PD deficiency and hereditary ovalocytosis, significantly protect carriers against death from malignant tertian malaria. The evidence of heterozygous HbE individuals is at present inconclusive while that for haemoglobin C is negative.

DIAGNOSIS

A. Clinical

The most important element in the clinical diagnosis of malaria is to have a high index of suspicion irrespective of whether one is practising in endemic or non-endemic areas.

Because the distribution of malaria is variable even in countries where it is known to be prevalent, the geographical and travel history is as important here as in temperate countries.

Malaria can mimic many other diseases which are also common in malarious countries. The most important of these are all types of meningitides, typhoid fever and septicaemia. Other differential diagnoses include hepatitis, leptospirosis, the relapsing fevers, haemorrhagic fevers, all types of viral encephalitides and, in Africa, trypanosomiasis.

In pregnant women, malaria must be distinguished from sepsis arising in the uterus, urinary tract or breast. In children, convulsions due to malaria must be differentiated from febrile convulsions (where coma unusually lasts for longer than half an hour after the ictal phase).

B. Parasitological

In the majority of cases, examination of the peripheral blood will reveal malaria parasites in thick and thin blood films.

Thick films are more useful than thin films in the detection of a low parasitaemia. Although occasional reports have described individuals dying from proven cerebral malaria in whom there was no detectable peripheral parasitaemia, in the majority of patients with severe malaria high parasite counts are seen unless previous treatment has been given (this is becoming increasingly common in the tropics) or a highly synchronous infection occurs. The geometric mean parasitaemia in 131 Malawian children with cerebral malaria was $410\,000/mm^3$ (Molyneux et al 1989). In holo-hyperendemic areas (where at any time 60–70% of children may have parasitaemia), parasitaemias below $10\,000/mm^3$ may be incidental and a careful search for an alternative aetiology should be made before the symptoms are attributed to malaria. None the less, there is no harm in treating the patient for malaria providing the above precaution has been taken.

While high parasite densities can usually be equated with severity of disease, the reverse is not always true. White and Krishna (1989) have pointed out there may be wide differences between the number of parasitized cells in the peripheral blood and the number sequestered, and that rapid changes may be expected in synchronous infections. Frequent (every 4–6 hours) monitoring of the parasitaemia is very important.

The microscopic diagnosis of malaria parasites is not easy and is often found wanting in laboratories both in the tropics and in temperate countries.

Parasites and malarial pigment have also been found by fine needle aspiration of the bone marrow and the dermis. The presence of malaria pigment in monocytes is a useful indication of the diagnosis of malaria especially in anaemic children. Probes labelled with radioisotopes and synthetic oligonucleotide probes labelled with alkaline phosphatase are being evaluated, while a variety of other tests are being developed. Sooner or later all of them will have to be adapted to be useful in a clinical setting.

C.   Laboratory

Thrombocytopenia is almost invariable and peripheral leucocytosis is found in most patients with severe disease.

Elevations of plasma urea, creatinine, bilirubin and serum enzymes e.g. aminotransferases and 5-nucleotidase may be found. The severely ill patients are acidotic, with low capillary plasma pH and bicarbonate concentrations. Fluid and electrolyte disturbances—sodium, potassium, chloride, calcium, phosphate—are variable.

Concentrations of lactate in the blood and cerebrospinal fluid are high in both adults and children.

Blood glucose should be frequently monitored for the early detection of hypoglycaemia; in hypoglycaemic children, the cerebrospinal fluid has a correspondingly low glucose concentration.

PROGNOSIS

The clinical and laboratory parameters which indicate a poor prognosis are summarized in Table 10.3 (White et al 1985, Molyneux et al 1989). The number of these risk factors (clinical and laboratory) exhibited by each patient can be counted, the total providing a 'bedside prognostic index'. In a Malawian study, children with a prognostic index of 4 or greater were 8 times as likely to die or suffer sequelae as those with an index below 4 (Molyneux et al 1989).

TREATMENT

Drugs used to treat malaria

Quinine

At present, quinine remains the drug of choice for the treatment of severe and complicated malaria in chloroquine-resistant areas and wherever the sensitivity is unknown. It should always be given by rate-controlled in-

Table 10.3   Prognostic indicators of severe malaria in children and adults

Clinical
1.   Age <3 years
2.   Deep coma (score o/5)
3.   Witnessed convulsions
4.   Absent corneal reflexes
5.   Organ dysfunction (e.g. renal failure; pulmonary oedema)
6.   Retinal haemorrhages (in some areas only)

Laboratory
1.   Hyperparasitaemia (250 000–1 000 000/μl)
2.   Peripheral schizontaemia   (>5->20%)
3.   Peripheral leucocytosis   (>12 000/μl)
4.   Packed cell volume less than 20%
5.   Haemoglobin less than 4.4 mmol/l   (<7.1 g/dl)
6.   Blood glucose less than 2.2 mmol/l   (<40 mg/dl)
7.   Blood urea nitrogen more than 21.4 mmol/l   (>60 mg/dl)
8.   Low CSF glucose
9.   Creatinine more than 265 μmol/l   (>3.0 mg/dl)
10. High CSF lactate   (>4 mmol/l)
11. Raised venous lactate > 6 mmol/l
12. Elevation of serum enzymes (amino transferases) over 3-fold
13. Elevated plasma alanine
14. Increased plasma 5-nucleotidase
15. Low antithrombin III levels
16. Tissue necrosis factor levels > 500 pg/ml

fusion, never by bolus intravenous injection. It can be administered by deep intramuscular injection in the anterior thigh ideally using more dilute solutions of quinine dihydrochloride (e.g. 60 mg/ml rather than 300 mg/ml) adjusted to neutral pH to reduce the pain. Quinine appears to be safe for use in pregnancy (Looareesuwan et al 1985). The pharmacokinetics of quinine have been subject to considerable study and are by no means straightforward. For a detailed review of the subject see White (1990).

Mild adverse effects are common—'cinchonism' (tinnitus, hearing loss, nausea, uneasiness, dysphoria and blurring of vision); while serious cardiovascular and neurological toxicity is rare. Hypoglycaemia is the most serious common adverse effect. In suspected quinine posioning, activated charcoal orally or nasogastrically accelerates elimination. Quinine interacts with several other drugs, including some of the other antimalarials, digoxin, phenytoin and rifampicin. Quinidine is not a substitute for quinine and should only be used if quinine is not available, since it is more cardiotoxic than quinine.

Chloroquine

This is still the most widely prescribed antimalarial in the tropics. Chloroquine is a 4-aminoquinoline derivative which is effective against the asexual erthrocyte forms of *P. falciparum* and *P. vivax* together with the sexual forms of *P. vivax*. It is virtually inactive against sporozoites or the exo-erythrocytic tissue stages of plasmodial infection even when given in large doses. Its mechanism of action is not completely understood. However, it is known that the parasitized erythrocyte concentrates chloroquine at least 100-fold more than the unparasitized erythrocyte.

Chloroquine is rapidly and completely absorbed following oral adminis-tration. It is about 50% bound in the plasma and extensive tissue binding takes place with high concentrations in the erythrocytes, liver and ocular tissues, 50–70% is eliminated as parent compound with smaller amounts present as monodesethylchloroquine. The elimination half-life of chloro-quine is dose-dependent being around 70–100 hours after usual doses. Because of the extensive tissue binding of this drug, a loading dose is essential if effective plasma concentrations are to be obtained. Other antimalarials interfere with hepatic metabolism of chloroquine by enzyme inhibition; these include amodiaquine and primaquine. Despite resistance, it still provides symptomatic relief and reduces morbidity and mortality in many endemic areas. Like quinine, it should always be given by slow rate-controlled intravenous infusion and never by bolus injection. It can also be given intramuscularly and subcutaneously at a reduced dosage from that recommended for intravenous infusion. Oral therapy should be substituted as soon as possible. Where injection is not available, it can be given by nasogastric tube. Side effects include nausea, vomiting, headache, uneasi-ness, dysphoria, blurred vision, hypotension and pruritus. Chloroquine poisoning is manifested by coma, convulsions, dysrhythmias and hypo-tension. Myopathy and retinopathy only occur after long-term prophy-lactic use: usually when more than 100 g have been taken over five years or more.

Proguanil

This drug is the safest antimalarial and has been used as a prophylactic for very many years either alone or lately in combination with chloroquine. Proguanil is a biguanide drug which is well absorbed orally and is meta-bolized to the active triazine compound, cycloguanil. Proguanil is concen-trated in erythrocytes and is also found in high concentrations in liver and kidney. Mild and transient gastrointestinal effects occur after treatment. It can safely be given to pregnant women. A high prevalence of mouth ulceration has been reported in recent years.

Amodiaquine

Amodiaquine is another 4-aminoquinoline derivative generally considered to be a useful substitute for chloroquine when oral treatment is required. As far as is known, its pharmacokinetics are similar to those of chloroquine. A related compound, amopyroquine, is available in some Francophone countries in Africa and this may be given by intramuscular injection using the same precautions and dosages as chloroquine.

Mefloquine

This is effective against all malaria species, including multidrug resistant *P. falciparum*. Structurally it resembles quinine, being a quinoline methanol compound available as the hydrochloride salt. Naturally resistant parasite populations have been reported from various parts of the tropics. It is only available in tablet form and it may be given in severe malaria (15 mg/kg to a maximum of 1 g) following a parenteral course of quinine, but not earlier than 12 hours after the last quinine course in order to avoid cardiovascular toxicity. Mefloquine is rapidly absorbed, has a large volume of distribution and a long half-life of 14–40 days. Mefloquine is highly bound to plasma proteins and does not appear to have significant drug interactions, although the potential for serious interactions with quinine require further investigations. The pharmacokinetics of mefloquine in children are not well elucidated (Karbwang & White 1990). Toxic effects include nausea, abdominal discomfort, vertigo, sinus arrhythmia, bradycardia and hypotension. Acute psychosis or a transient encephalopathy with convulsions are serious though relatively rare and transient side effects.

Sulfadoxine-pyrimethamine (S 500 mg + P 25 mg)

This combination has been widely used both as an adjunct to quinine therapy in severe malaria, in the treatment of uncomplicated malaria in partially immune subjects and as a prophylactic. Pyrimethamine is a dihydrofolate reductase inhibitor which is readily absorbed from the gastrointestinal tract and is active against the erythrocytic forms of malarial parasites, but does not have any effect on the exoerythrocytic tissue forms. Because of resistance of falciparum malaria to pyrimethamine, it has been used in combination with long-acting sulphonamides, such as sulfadoxine. Both drugs have long half-lives, that of pyrimethamine being of the order of 100 hours and sulfadoxine being of the order of 200 hours. It is now no longer recommended for prophylaxis because of an unacceptable mortality estimated to be between 1:11 000 and 1:25 000 recipients. It should not be given in late pregnancy or to the neonate because of the theoretical risk of provoking kernicterus. An intramuscular preparation exists, but is painful and is used only for treatment of severe malaria where chloroquine or quinine are not available. No severe reactions have been reported when the oral preparation has been used as a single dose treatment.

Halofantrine

This is a phenanthrene-methanol recently introduced into clinical practice. It is active against multidrug resistant falciparum malaria. There is, however, no parenteral preparation and oral absorption of the drug is poor, although it can be increased if taken with a fatty meal. Like all effective antimalarials, halofantrine has a large volume of distribution. Its elimination half-life lies between 1.3 and 6.6 days. Reported adverse effects are few—abdominal pain, diarrhoea and pruritus being the most frequent.

Quinghaosu

To date, clinical trials of artemesinine and related compounds—the amino-ether: artemether (intramuscular); and the hemisuccinate: artesunate (oral and intravenous)—indicate that these compounds are superior to the quinoline antimalarials for the treatment of both uncomplicated and complicated malaria. These drugs are sesquiterpinelactones extracted from plants of the artemesian family. Recrudescence rates have, however, been high. The clinical pharmacology of these compounds is poorly understood and there is still no agreement on which compound should be developed for general use. Their rapidity of action, novel molecular structure and mode of action augurs well for the future and they deserve detailed and careful study as they may have a major role to play in the future treatment of severe malaria.

Regimes in use

The treatment of malaria is both antiparasitic (chemotherapy) and supportive (management of complications). Both are of equal importance.

A.   Plasmodium falciparum malaria

Malignant tertian malaria is a medical emergency. It progresses rapidly from a relatively mild infection to a catastrophic illness. Because of this, in cases of doubt or if parasitological diagnosis is likely to be delayed, presumptive treatment is justified.

Chemotherapy for uncomplicated attacks is relatively straightforward and is summarized in Table 10.4. For areas where chloroquine-resistant *P. falciparum* occurs, several alternatives are feasible, their choice usually depending upon availability of drug.

The treatment of severe falciparum malaria is complex. Before dealing with specific chemotherapy certain points of a general nature must be made. Ideally, the patients should be admitted to an intensive care unit as both good nursing care and careful attention to fluid balance is vital. Daily or more frequent monitoring for hypoglycaemia should be carried out.

Table 10.4   Treatment of uncomplicated falciparum malaria

Areas where parasites sensitive to chloroquine
Chloroquine
    Day 1   10 mg Base/kg followed by 5 mg Base/kg after 6 hours
    Days 2 and 3   5 mg Base/kg

Areas where parasites resistant to chloroquine*
                 either
1. Quinine
      10 mg Salt/kg 3 times per day for 3–7 days
             plus
    Sulfadoxine (500 mg)-Pyrimethamine (25 mg)-Fansidar®
      3 tabs in single dose
             or
    Tetracycline
      250 mg 4 times per day for 7 days
             or
2. Mefloquine
      7.5 mg Base/kg twice in one day (maximum 1 g)
             or
3. Halofantrine
      8 mg Base/kg 6-hourly × 3 doses (repeated 15 days later in non-immunes)
             or
4. Sulfadoxine (500 mg)-pyrimethamine (25 mg)-Fansidar®
      3 tabs in single dose (for partially immunes)

---

* Choice of regimen depends on location and drug availability
Note: If quinine *not* available, quinidine in similar dosage can be used.
       Tetracycline not to be given to pregnant women and children under 10 years old.
       Mefloquine not recommended (at present) for pregnant women.

Comatose patients should always have their cerebrospinal fluid examined especially if the diagnosis is in doubt. The antimalarial therapy should be initiated parenterally, oral treatment being commenced as soon as the patient can take the drugs reliably by mouth. Doses should be calculated on a mg/kg basis. It is important not to confuse the doses of salt and base: quinine is usually prescribed as salt, whereas chloroquine is prescribed as the base. Harmful and unproven adjuvant treatments should be avoided.

The chemotherapy of severe falciparum malaria is summarized in Table 10.5. Response should be monitored by frequent clinical examination, including recording of fluid balance, temperature, pulse, blood pressure, venous jugular pressure etc. and blood films every 4–6 hours.

The management of the complications of falciparum malaria is given in Table 10.6. Exchange transfusion has become fashionable in certain locations. However, it should be appreciated that only successful cases are reported in the literature giving a biased view of its effectiveness. Moreover, the equipment and amounts of compatible blood required for total exchange are rarely available in areas endemic for malaria and the risks of the procedure in the tropics are high, involving, for example, transfusion-related viral infections and increased risk of bacterial infection. Partial

Table 10.5   Treatment of complicated or severe falciparum malaria

Chloroquine-sensitive falciparum malaria
Chloroquine constant rate i.v. infusion
10 mg Base/kg over 8 hours → 15 mg Base/kg over next 24 hours
or
Chloroquine i.m. or subcutaneous injection
3.5 mg Base/kg every 6 hours

Chloroquine-resistant falciparum infection or where sensitivity unknown
1.   Quinine dihydrochloride
7 mg/kg i.v. infusion by pump over 30 minutes
↓
10 mg/kg diluted in 10 ml/kg isotonic fluid i.v. infusion over 4 hours
repeated every 8 hours until swallowing achieved then change to oral
therapy with
↓
Quinine salt
10 mg/kg 8-hourly for 7 days
or
2.   Quinine dihydrochloride
20 mg/kg i.v. infusion over 4 hours
↓
10 mg/kg infusion over 4 hours as above
repeated 8-hourly until swallowing achieved then oral regime as above
or
3.   Quinidine gluconate base
10 mg/kg i.v. infusion over 1–2 hours
↓
0.02 mg/kg/min by infusion pump for 72 hours until swallowing established
then quinine tablets orally for 7 days as above
or
4.   Quinidine gluconate base
15 mg/kg i.v. infusion over 4 hours
↓
7.5 mg/kg infusion over 4 hours repeated 8-hourly until swallowing
established then quinine tablets orally for 7 days as above.

Where significant degree of quinine resistance (e.g. Thailand)
add to quinine/quinidine regime—
Tetracycline 250 mg 4 times daily for 7 days (except pregnant women and
children below 10 years)

Note: 1.   Loading dose of quinine/quinidine omitted if patient has received either drug or
mefloquine in preceding 24 hours.
2.   In patients requiring more than 48 hours parenteral therapy reduce
quinine/quinidine dosage by one half to one third (i.e. 5–7 mg/kg 8-hourly).

exchange transfusion may be a promising and more practical alternative.

Ancillary treatments which have been recommended for cerebral malaria from time to time, but which are all of unproven value or are positively detrimental to the patient include corticosteroids, other anti-inflammatory agents, other agents used to treat cerebral oedema (e.g. urea), low molecular weight dextran, adrenaline, heparin, prostacyclin, oxpentifylline, hyperbaric oxygen, and cyclosporin A.

Table 10.6   The management of the severe complications of falciparum malaria (Warrell et al 1990)

	Manifestation/complication	Immediate management*
1.	Coma (cerebral malaria)	Maintain airway, nurse on side, exclude other treatable causes of coma (e.g. hypoglycaemia, bacterial meningitis). Give prophylactic anticonvulsant (10 mg/kg of barbiturate). *Avoid harmful adjuvant treatments such as corticosteroids, heparin and adrenaline*
2.	Hyperpyrexia	Tepid sponging, fanning, cooling blanket antipyretic (paracetamol 15 mg/kg)
3.	Convulsions	(Prevent with intramuscular phenobarbital). Maintain airway, treat with intravenous or rectal diazepam (adults 10 mg, children 0.15 mg/kg) or intramuscular paraldehyde injection (0.1 ml/kg in glass syringe)
4.	Hypoglycaemia	Measure blood glucose, give 50% dextrose injection followed by 5% or 10% dextrose infusion
5.	Severe anaemia (packed cell volume > 15%)	Transfuse fresh whole blood or packed cells if pathogen screening is available
6.	Acute pulmonary oedema	(Prevent by avoiding excessive rehydration). Prop up at 45°, give oxygen, venesect 250 ml of blood into donor bag, give diuretic (frusemide iv), stop intravenous fluids
7.	Acute renal failure	Exclude dehydration: strict fluid balance, peritoneal dialysis (haemodialysis if available)
8.	Spontaneous bleeding and coagulopathy	Transfuse fresh whole blood, Vitamin K injection 10 mg intravenously, if the prothrombin or partial thromboplastin times are prolonged
9.	Metabolic acidosis	Exclude or treat hypoglycaemia, hypovolaemia and Gram-negative septicaemia. Give oxygen. Correct arterial pH to 7.2 or above
10.	Shock, 'algid malaria'	Suspect Gram-negative septicaemia. Take blood cultures. Give parenteral antimicrobials, correct haemodynamic disturbances
11.	Aspiration pneumonia	Give parenteral antimicrobials, change position, physiotherapy, give oxygen

* It is assumed that quinine or chloroquine infusion will have been started in all cases.

B.   Plasmodium vivax/ovale malaria

The treatment of benign tertian malaria is straightforward and is summarized in Table 10.7.

C.   Plasmodium malariae

The treatment of quartan malaria is summarized in Table 10.7. Quartan malaria is usually sensitive to chloroquine therapy.

Table 10.7   Treatment of *P. vivax, P. ovale* and quartan malaria (*P. malariae*)

P. vivax and P. ovale malaria
Chloroquine
    Day 1   10 mg/Base/kg followed by 5 mg Base/kg after 6 hours
    Days 2 and 3   5 mg Base/kg
                         plus
Primaquine
    Days 4–17   15 mg/day*†

Quartan malaria (*P. malariae*)
Chloroquine
    Day 1   10 mg Base/kg followed by 5 mg Base/kg after 6 hours
    Days 2 and 3   5 mg Base/kg

---

* Double in Chesson-type strain areas (e.g. Solomons, Philippines, Thailand, New Guinea).
† For G-6-PD positive patients 45 mg/week for 8 weeks.

Emergency self-treatment

Self-treatment is only justified if medical services are not available and if a person feels unwell 7 days after the first exposure to malaria. It is assumed in this context that such a person would have taken the first dose of prophylactic drug one week prior to departure, as is usually recommended. The only three drugs worthy of serious consideration for emergency treatment are:
(1)   sulfadoxine-pyrimethamine (a single oral dose of 3 tablets)—with the obvious well-recognized reservation of sulphonamide sensitivity;
(2)   halofantrine 8 mg/kg at 6-hourly intervals × 3 doses in 1 day, and
(3)   mefloquine 15 mg/kg in a single oral dose (maximum 1000 mg).
    A 7-day course of quinine, though effective, is not a realistic option since most persons will not persist with self-treatment for that long.

PREVENTION

The prevention of malaria must be considered separately for travellers and indigenous people born and living in endemic malarious areas of the world. Neither themes are simple nor straightforward and differing views are held by various authorities. An important factor to consider in all people is the adoption of measures of self-protection both by long-established and by recently adopted methods.

A.   Self protection: general measures

The well-known measures of self-protection such as wearing long sleeves, using insect repellants and net screening during sleep are now more important than ever. Bed net protection may be enhanced by regular impregnation of material with permethrin at a concentration of 0.2 g/m^2 every 6 months. Attention should also be paid to the possible use of impregnated curtains to cover eaves, windows and doors when the house construction is appropriate.

B.   Travellers

It is important to bear in mind that the risks for malaria in any country or situation must be balanced against the hazards of chemoprophylaxis (Phillips-Howard & West 1990). For neither set of risks are there sufficiently detailed data for unequivocal choice. Advice must therefore be kept simple and clear to encourage good compliance. It must provide reasonable (if not absolute) protection against malaria, must minimize the risks of adverse effects and should be applicable to most travellers involved. For most areas the combination of daily proguanil and weekly chloroquine meets the above requirements. Both proguanil and chloroquine are safe to use in pregnancy.

Experience with mefloquine as a prophylactic drug is still comparatively small. Its use should be restricted to short visits of 3 weeks or less to areas of high transmission and multidrug resistance. Careful monitoring is required particularly in relation to its most alarming side effect—psychotic disturbances. Its main use is in rural areas of South-East Asia; however, it can also be justified in parts of Kenya and Tanzania (Table 10.8).

Encouraging results have been reported with new combinations such as proguanil + gantrisin. Doxycycline has also been shown to be effective in certain circumstances, but considerably more experience of these combinations in non-immunes is required before they can be generally recommended.

Table 10.8   Chemoprophylaxis of malaria

A. Most parts of the world	
	Proguanil (200 mg) daily
	plus
	Chloroquine (300 mg) weekly
B. Rural areas of South-East Asia, Coastal Kenya and Tanzania	
either	Proguanil (200 mg) daily
	plus
	Chloroquine (300 mg Base) weekly
or	Mefloquine (250 mg) weekly
C. Papua-New Guinea and South Pacific Islands	
Some authorities recommend	
	Chloroquine (300 mg Base) weekly
	plus
	Dapsone (100 mg) + Pyrimethamine (12.5 mg)—*Maloprim*® weekly

Note: 1. *None of the recommended drugs give 100% protection.*
       2. Start 1 week before departure, continue throughout stay and for 4 weeks after return.
       3. Mefloquine prophylaxis should continue only 2 weeks after return. This drug is *not* recommended for persons requiring fine coordination and special performance, e.g airline crews, persons using heavy or dangerous equipment, or pregnant females.

C.   Indigenous populations

The only groups of indigenates for whom chemoprophylaxis is currently justified are pregnant women, children under 5 years of age and certain special 'risk' groups.

Pregnancy

It is my personal view that primiparae should be protected against malaria with an appropriate safe drug throughout their pregnancy. In the Third World, attendance at antenatal clinics rarely occurs before the first 2 months thus minimizing considerably the risk of teratogenic effects. For many areas a curative dose of chloroquine (25 mg/kg given over 3 days when first seen) followed by chloroquine prophylaxis (300 mg base weekly) throughout the rest of the pregnancy and the first month of the puerperium still gives adequate protection. Regrettably, in areas of extensive chloroquine- and multi-drug resistance, careful monitoring of the primiparae and early treatment of attacks may be the only option at present.

Children under five

Despite the excellent results obtained in the Gambia, I do not believe that regular chemoprophylaxis for the first 5 years of life is a feasible strategy in most malarious areas of the world, either logistically or in face of the major compliance difficulties of the regime. There could be a place for this strategy in countries where the transmission season is short, the population is relatively small and primary health care attitudes are well developed.

Special 'risk' groups

Patients who are receiving long-term corticosteroid therapy, or are immunosuppressed, and individuals homozygous for the abnormal haemoglobins (e.g. SS, thalassaemia/HbE) should be protected against malaria if possible.

D.   Prophylaxis in special circumstances

Labour forces and military personnel, a proportion of whom even when indigenous, may not be immune—should be protected against malaria during their period of exposure.

CONCLUSION

Malaria still constitutes one of the major problems of public health in the world. Although promising new antimalarial drugs continue to be developed, resistance to existing drugs is spreading due to the greater populations in affected countries; the widespread habit of inadequate and/or improper self-treatment and to increasing mobility of representatives of these populations.

It seems likely that the final solution to malaria lies not in better treatment of this potentially devastating parasitic infection, but rather in vaccination procedures to avoid colonization by the parasite in the first place. Regrettably, we seem to be some way from this desirable situation even at the close of the 20th century.

In the meantime our prime goal must be to reduce the morbidity and mortality from the disease.

ACKNOWLEDGEMENT

Liberal use has been made in this article of the information contained in the publication entitled 'Severe and complicated malaria' (Warrell et al 1990). This publication was based on the deliberations of two informal WHO sponsored meetings held in 1985 and 1988 of which I was chairman.

REFERENCES

Gilles H M, Ikeme A C 1960 Haemoglobinuria among adult Nigerians due to glucose-6-phophate dehydrogenase deficiency with drug sensitivity. Lancet ii: 889–891

Looareesuwan S, Phillips R E, White N J et al 1985 Quinine and severe falciparum malaria in late pregnancy. Lancet ii: 4–8

Looareesuwan S, Phillips R E, Kaetswang J, White N J, Flegg D A 1990 *Plasmodium falciparum* hyperparasitaemia: use of exchange transfusion in seven patients and a review of the literature. Quarterly Journal of Medicine 277: 471–481

McGregor I A, Gilles H M, Walters J H, Davies A H, Pearson F A 1956 Effects of heavy and repeated malaria infections on Gambian infants and children. British Medical Journal ii: 686–692

McGregor I A, Wilson M E, Billewicz W Z 1983 Malaria infection of the placenta in the Gambia, West Africa; its incidence and relationship to stillbirth, birthweight and placental weight. Transactions of the Royal Society of Tropical Medicine and Hygiene 77: 232–244

Molyneux M E, Taylor T E, Wirima J J, Borgstein J 1989 Clinical features and prognostic indicators in paediatric cerebral malaria: a study of 131 comatose Malawian children. Quarterly Journal of Medicine 71: 441–459

Phillips-Howard P A, West L J 1990 Serious adverse drug reactions to pyrimethamine-sulphadoxine, pyrimethamine-dapsone and to amodiaquine in Britain. Journal of Royal Society of Medicine 83: 82–85

Taylor T E, Molyneux M E, Wirima J J, Fletcher K A, Morris K 1988 Blood glucose levels in Malawian children before and during the administration of intravenous quinine for severe falciparum malaria. New England Journal of Medicine 319: 1040–1047

Teasdale G, Jennett B 1974 Assessment of coma and impaired consciousness: a practical scale. Lancet ii: 81–84

Weatherall D J, Abdalla S 1982 The anaemia of *Plasmodium falciparum* malaria. British Medical Bulletin 38: 147–151

White N J, Krishna S 1989 Treatment of malaria: some considerations and limitations of the current methods of assessment. Transactions of the Royal Society of Tropical Medicine and Hygiene 83: 767–777

White N J, Warrell D A, Looareesuwan S, Chanthavanich S, Phillips R E, Pongpaew P 1985 Pathophysiological and prognostic significance of cerebrospinal-fluid lactate in cerebral malaria. Lancet i: 776–778

White N J, Miller K D, Marsh K et al 1987 Hypoglycaemia in African children with severe malaria. Lancet i 708–711

FURTHER READING

Karbwang J, White N J 1990 Clinical pharmacokinetics of mefloquine. Clinical Pharmacokinetics 19: 264–279

Gilles H M, Warrell D A 1992 Bruce-Chwatt's essential malariology. 3rd edn. Heinemann, London, p 104

Warrell D A, Molyneux M E, Beales P F 1990 Severe and complicated malaria. Transactions of Royal Society of Tropical Medicine and Hygiene 84(2): 1–65

White N J 1990 Clinical pharmacokinetics of antimalarial drugs. Clinical Pharmacokinetics 10: 187–215

WHO 1990 Practical chemotherapy of malaria. Technical Report Series 805. Geneva

11. Gastrointestinal bleeding and non-steroidal anti-inflammatory drugs

D. A. Henry

INTRODUCTION

The possibility that upper gastrointestinal haemorrhage (UGIH) can complicate therapy with non-steroidal anti-inflammatory drugs (NSAIDs) should be familiar to everyone who prescribes these drugs. However, until the last few years there was surprisingly little systematic research into the topic. Since 1985 the relevant literature has expanded rapidly. Despite this, uncertainty remains as to the actual level of risk posed by these drugs, and the extent to which this risk may vary from individual to individual depending on their underlying susceptibilities. Estimates of the number of deaths from ulcer complications which are attributable to NSAIDs have varied from 200 to over 3000 annually in the UK (Blower & Armstrong 1986, Somerville et al 1986). Even if only the lower figure is correct, ulcer complications due to NSAIDs are still one of the most important adverse reactions from modern drugs If the higher figure is correct, we are faced with a substantial public health problem and corrective action is indicated.

In reviewing this major topic, I have chosen to highlight some areas of recent development. These are: mechanisms of damage; the growing evidence of damage to multiple sites in the gastrointestinal tract; the epidemiological evidence of risk of UGIH to the individual and to the community; the importance of the levels of exposure to NSAIDs within communities; and the quality of evidence supporting different strategies for the prevention of UGIH.

MECHANISMS OF DAMAGE

NSAIDs exert most of their beneficial effects through inhibition of prostaglandin synthesis. Prostaglandins have a number of functions in the stomach. They are antisecretory; they influence bicarbonate secretion, mucus production and cellular renewal, and increase mucosal blood flow. Drugs which inhibit prostaglandin synthesis might be expected to cause mucosal damage through interference with any of these actions.

However, the mechanisms of damage which currently are proposed are complex and do not completely explain the clinical manifestations (Szabo et al 1989). It is naïve to assume that one mechanism, for instance inhibition of prostaglandin synthesis, will produce the variety of manifestations of injury observed. An example is aspirin which can acetylate proteins and, during absorption, hydrolysis of the molecule may yield hydrogen ions which back diffuse into the mucosa (Rainsford et al 1983; Szabo et al 1989). These are properties which are not shared by the more modern drugs and which may lead directly to damage without inhibition of prostaglandin synthesis. The NSAIDs in common use today probably vary in their actions on the mucosa. In general there is poor correlation between the degree of prostaglandin inhibition produced by the drugs and the extent and severity of the resulting mucosal lesions. However, despite the heterogeneity of their effects, there appears to be some correlation between the degree of vascular injury, the inhibition of mucus biosynthesis and the degree of ulcerogenicity in experimental models (Szabo et al 1989).

Recent work has highlighted a crucial role for microvascular injury in the pathogenesis of mucosal damage from NSAIDs. A possible sequence of events as outlined by Szabo et al (1989) is reproduced in Fig. 11.1. The initial step may be vasoconstriction due to the loss of vasodilator prostaglandins or an increased production of leukotrienes, which are vasoconstrictor. Production of leukotrienes increases when the enzyme cyclooxygenase is inhibited by NSAIDs, resulting in more arachidonate being processed by the lipoxygenase pathway (Rainsford 1987).

Attention has shifted recently from mechanisms of direct damage to those of mucosal adaptation and repair. Adaptation is the process by which chronic exposure of the mucosa leads to a lessening of the extent and severity of the mucosal injury seen after a single dose of a NSAID. The explanation of adaptation is uncertain but Graham et al (1988a) consider that it probably involves increased cellular regeneration. Repair of mucosal defects may proceed by a process of cellular restitution if the injury is superficial (Fig. 11.1). Restitution involves the migration of cells from underlying layers without cellular division (Graham et al 1988a). It has been suggested that this process may depend on the preservation of mucosal blood supply (Morris 1986). Deeper ulcers heal by a process of cellular regeneration starting in gastric glands at the ulcer edge. Recent work in patients with gastric ulcers has shown that epithelial regeneration is

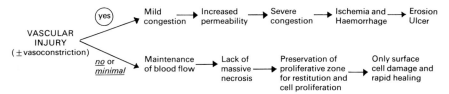

Fig. 11.1   The central role of vascular injury in the pathogenesis of drug-induced gastric erosions and ulcers (after Szabo et al 1989). Reproduced by permission of ADIS Press Ltd and the author.

inhibited by NSAIDs (Levi et al 1990a). This action may contribute to the initial formation of an ulcer and to its failure to heal.

Continuing research into the underlying mechanisms of NSAID damage may permit production of safer drugs (Szabo et al 1989). However, as will become apparent, deriving epidemiological estimates of the risk of serious upper gastrointestinal damage from this class of drugs has proved difficult, so demonstrating that a theoretical advantage of a particular drug in the laboratory translates into a substantial benefit in practice will not be easy.

DAMAGE TO MULTIPLE SITES IN THE GASTROINTESTINAL TRACT

NSAIDs appear capable of damaging the entire gastrointestinal tract. Other than the familiar problems in the stomach and duodenum, the manifestations include oral ulceration, oesophageal injury and haemorrhage, and haemorrhage and perforation of the intestine.

Ulceration of the oral mucosa is unlikely to be a major source of gastrointestinal bleeding, but is a fairly common adverse reaction to NSAIDs, although the role of the drugs is often overlooked. Recently a series of cases of oral reactions to NSAIDs was reported to the Australian Drug Regulation Authority. While damage to the oral mucosa can be part of a systemic reaction to a drug, this series included many cases of ulceration where there were no other general features of an adverse reaction and in which a NSAID was the sole suspected cause.

Oesophagitis and oesophageal ulceration are also complications of NSAIDs and the latter can lead to bleeding and to stricture formation. Two case control studies have indicated that the relative risk of benign oesophageal stricture with NSAIDs lies between 3 and 7 (Heller et al 1982, Wilkins et al 1984).

Recently, research has been directed at the pathogenesis, histology and clinical manifestations of diffuse injury to the small intestine. Work using radiolabelled markers and leucocytes has demonstrated a link between the use of NSAIDs and diffuse intestinal inflammation resulting in increased intestinal permeability and protein loss (Bjarnason et al 1986, Bjarnason et al 1987). Multiple discrete strictures, some of which were narrow diaphragm-like structures, markedly narrowing the lumen, have been demonstrated radiologically in patients receiving long-term therapy with NSAIDs (Levi et al 1990b). Several cases of intestinal obstruction have been reported (reviewed by Aabakken & Osnes 1989), and diffuse intestinal damage may cause loss of blood and protein, contributing to the anaemia and hypoalbuminemia which is evident in some elderly patients who take NSAIDs for long periods. Crohn's disease-like distal ileitis has been demonstrated (Bjarnason et al 1984) which is of interest in view of the reports of patients whose inflammatory bowel disease has been shown to relapse with use of NSAIDs (reviewed by Aabakken & Osnes 1989). The overall importance of these recent findings is unclear. While there is no denying that NSAIDs are capable of inducing changes in the small intestinal mucosa, most of the reports of clinical consequences are anecdotal and in this area further well controlled epidemiological studies are needed. Gastroduodenal haemorrhage and perforation remain the most important adverse effects of NSAIDs on the gastrointestinal tract.

In contrast, there has been little experimental study of large bowel damage from NSAIDs. There have been case reports of rectal ulcers and haemorrhage in patients using suppository formulations, which are persuasive because of the site of the lesions. Also there are instances of relapse of ulcerative colitis in patients taking NSAIDs which could be chance associations (reviewed by Aabakken & Osnes 1989). There has been only one published controlled study of intestinal haemorrhage, conducted by Langman et al (1985). This was a large case control study of 161 cases of intestinal haemorrhage and the same number of age and sex-matched controls. There was no association between intestinal haemorrhage and cardiovascular drugs, but use of NSAIDs was associated with a relative risk for bleeding of 2.6 (95% CI 1.4–4.9). The authors estimated a minimum incidence of intestinal haemorrhage of around 10/100 000/year for the whole population. From their figures it can be estimated that the proportion of cases in the community which are attributable to NSAIDs lies between 10 and 15%. The annual incidence in non-users, therefore, would be 8–9/100 000 and the risk for users in the range of 20–25/100 000. This is lower than the estimates for upper gastrointestinal haemorrhage, which remains a much more important cause of morbidity and mortality.

Studies of the association between NSAIDs and upper gastrointestinal haemorrhage

Most information on the beneficial and adverse effects of modern drugs comes from two sources—clinical trials conducted before and after marketing and voluntary adverse reaction reports submitted by health professionals to reporting agencies once a new drug is in widespread use. Neither of these sources is optimal in defining the risks of UGIH for those who take NSAIDs. Generally, clinical trials are not large enough to detect infrequent events such as bleeding. They are usually of short duration and the participants tend to be healthier than those who receive the drugs after they are released for general use. However, clinical trials continue after marketing and eventually a large body of information accumulates. Chalmers and his colleagues (1988) have shown how the technique of meta-analysis can be used to define the risk of haemorrhage from clinical trials of NSAIDs.

Meta-analysis is a technique for reviewing, combining and synthesizing information from clinical studies, and it has the considerable advantage of increasing statistical power to detect the association between use of

NSAIDs and infrequent but serious complications. In their meta-analysis of 100 clinical trials involving over 12 000 patients, Chalmers et al (1988) recorded an incidence of UGIH of 373/100 000 in subjects randomized to NSAIDs, which was 3 times higher (relative risk 3.0) than the incidence in the control group. Interestingly, this estimate of the relative risk agrees well with that derived from formal epidemiological studies (see below). The difficulty in interpreting the results of this meta-analysis is that the trials were not set up to measure gastrointestinal haemorrhage, so there was no consistent definition of this outcome. It is difficult to tell how serious the gastrointestinal bleeding was. It should be noted that although the individual trials included in the meta-analysis involved 1 or 2 drugs, the results of the statistical pooling can only be applied to the *class* of drug and it is not possible to infer that one particular agent is more or less likely to cause problems than the others. The general disadvantages of clinical trials remain, in that the duration of therapy tends to be short and the patients included in the trials are a rather select group. Nevertheless, this exercise is an important example of the use of meta-analysis in detecting infrequent adverse drug reactions.

Analysis of voluntary adverse reaction reports (e.g. the Committee on Safety of Medicines 'yellow card' scheme) has contributed only modestly to our knowledge of risks of UGIH with NSAIDs. Voluntary reporting by health professionals to journals, national agencies and manufacturers is a very important information source. In fact, it is the usual means by which uncommon adverse effects are first detected. However, when an association is well known, as is the case with UGIH and NSAIDs, one of the incentives to reporting, the novelty of a new association, is not present and reporting rates tend to be low. Australian experience suggests that 3% or less of cases of UGIH in patients taking NSAIDs are reported to the national centre by health professionals. With such a small sample, the incidence cannot be estimated and a temporary enthusiasm for reporting such events with a new drug can distort the reporting patterns giving the impression of a disproportionate risk with that agent.

EPIDEMIOLOGICAL STUDIES

Most of the important epidemiological studies of UGIH and NSAIDs have been published since 1985. These investigations have taken two general forms—case control studies and cohort studies. In case control studies, cases of the disease, usually subjects hospitalized with upper gastrointestinal haemorrhage, have their prior use of NSAIDs compared with that of controls who are usually selected from a community sample or from hospital admissions who have diseases believed to be unassociated with NSAIDs. The underlying principle is that controls should be similar to cases except that they do not have the disease of interest. Controls should represent the 'background' use of NSAIDs in the community. Controls are essential in studies of this type because NSAIDs are very widely used in most communities, increasing the likelihood of a chance association between use of NSAIDs and occurrence of upper gastrointestinal haemorrhage. The fact that a patient with UGIH has taken NSAIDs does not mean that the drug was the cause of the problem. In case control studies, the measure of association is the ratio of the odds of NSAID use in subjects with bleeding compared with that of controls, which is an approximation of the relative risk of bleeding in users compared with non-users.

By contrast in cohort studies, subjects are defined initially by their exposure to NSAIDs and are then followed to determine their rate of upper gastrointestinal haemorrhage, which is compared with that of a control group who are similar to the exposed group except that they have not received the drugs. The measure of association is the ratio of the incidence of bleeding in NSAID users to that in non-users, which is the relative risk. The conduct of cohort studies has been facilitated by the development, in some countries, of large computerized data bases which hold information on prescriptions dispensed to defined populations and subsequent diagnoses made on an outpatient or inpatient basis. Electronic linkage of these data bases has led to a number of studies of the relationship between NSAIDs and upper gastrointestinal haemorrhage.

Sources of bias in epidemiological studies

All epidemiological studies are subject to a range of errors which may bias their results. A full discussion of this topic is beyond the scope of this review. However, it is possible to summarize the main sources of bias which will affect the results of epidemiological studies of NSAIDs. With case control studies it is important to determine how cases have been defined; how similar cases and controls are with respect to factors which will determine their use of NSAIDs; and how prior use of NSAIDs by cases and controls has been ascertained. With cohort studies the key factors are the representativeness of the study population, the comparability of controls, and the methods used for ascertainment of exposure and outcome.

Review of published epidemiological studies

In a traditional narrative review each study is considered independently on its merits and apparent conflict in the results of different studies tends to be highlighted. However, it is possible to regard the available literature as a population of studies which, if broadly compatible, will generate a range of estimates of risk within which the 'typical' value will lie. It is also possible to analyse the results of different studies to obtain a pooled estimate of the overall effect and to determine whether their results are homogeneous. In other words, are the apparent differences in the study outcomes simply due to the play of chance? This approach was used by Hawkey (1990) in a recent statistical overview of the epidemiological studies. Of course it can always be argued that studies can never be regarded as truly homogeneous, as they are drawn from different populations at different points in time using different methods of variable quality.

One approach to the problem of analysing disparate sets of data is called 'sequential meta-analysis'. In this method, studies are sorted by some characteristic, for instance, year of publication, country of origin, or quality, and their results are then pooled *in sequence* so that the impact of each additional study, with its different characteristic, on the overall estimate of effect and measure of homogeneity can be assessed. In this article I have used the technique of sequential meta-analysis in order to provide a concise review of all of the epidemiological studies of the association between NSAIDs and upper gastrointestinal haemorrhage.

Literature review and methods

An attempt was made to identify all studies published in English language journals using Medline and the bibliographies of original papers and previously published reviews. Each study was classified as a case control or a cohort study and quality assessed on a simple unweighted scale in which each of the important characteristics capable of introducing bias (see section above) was scored. The raw data from each study were then extracted and re-analysed. Studies were ranked on their total score and pooling was carried out using the logarithm of the odds ratio for each study weighted by its standard error (Fleiss 1981). This method means that the larger studies have a bigger effect on the final measure of association than the smaller studies.

Case control studies of upper gastrointestinal haemorrhage and NSAIDs

The results of 10 case control studies are given in Table 11.1. The individual studies generated quite a wide range of odds ratios for UGIH with recent or current use of NSAIDs—from 2.7 to 15.7. From the table it can be seen that the poorer quality case control studies (towards the bottom of the table) generally gave higher odds ratios. There are two main reasons for this. Patients suffering upper gastrointestinal haemorrhage tend to be elderly. The elderly tend to be high users of NSAIDs and age is therefore an important confounder of the relationships between drug use and disease. In addition, patients with a recent bleed tend to be questioned closely about their prior consumption of NSAIDs, while control patients are not. Unless investigators pay particularly close attention to the need to control for age, and use a uniform method for determining prior use of NSAIDs, they (predictably) will obtain an inflated estimate of the relative risk.

Sequential meta-analysis is of some help in deciding where the 'typical'

Table 11.1   Case control studies of upper gastrointestinal haemorrhage and use of non-steroidal anti-inflammatory drugs

Authors	Ranking	Odds ratio**	95% Confidence interval for odds ratio	Pooled odds ratio††	95% confidence interval for pooled odds ratio	P (Homogeneity)‡
Griffin et al (1988)*	1	4.1	2.8–6.0			
Somerville et al (1986)	2 =	3.2	2.0–5.0			
Quader & Logan (1988)*	2 =	2.9	1.3–6.3			
Henry et al (1990)	2 =	2.7	1.8–4.1	3.3	2.6–4.1	$P > 0.50$
Bartle et al (in press)	5	3.5	1.3–9.8	3.3	2.6–4.1	$P > 0.70$
Levy et al (1988)	6	9.1	3.4–25.0	3.4	2.8–4.3	$P > 0.20$
Armstrong & Blower (1987)†	7 =	15.7	10.0–24.7			
Clinch et al (1983)	7 =	8.1	2.6–25.0	4.6	3.8–5.6	$P < 0.0005$
Caradoc-Davies (1984)	9 =	15.5	7.2–33.4			
Smedley et al (1988)	9 =	3.9	1.6–9.4	4.9	4.1–5.9	$P < 0.0005$

* Included only patients who had died of ulcer complications.

† Included patients who had died or required emergency surgery for ulcer complications.

** Ratio of the odds of NSAID use in patients with bleeding compared with controls. This is an approximation of the relative risk of bleeding in NSAID users compared with non-users.

†† All studies were pooled in a sequence determined by their quality score. Each figure in this column refers to the pooled odds ratio for all studies to that point, including the study on that line.

‡ Refers to the probability of the variation in study outcomes occurring by chance.

Note: These analyses were carried out using the raw data provided in the authors' tables of results and the calculated odds ratios may differ somewhat from those given in the published papers.

value lies in this series of studies. The inclusion of the four poorest quality studies increases the pooled odds ratio and introduces marked heterogeneity (last column of Table 11.1). In the end, the exercise is subjective, but it appears that the better quality studies are homogenous in their outcomes and pooling gives a typical odds ratio of 3.3–3.4 with a confidence interval between 2.6 and 4.1. This is in close agreement with the results of the first meta-analysis of this topic published recently by Hawkey (1990).

But what does an odds ratio (relative risk) of 3.3 mean? For an individual it means that the use of NSAIDs triples the risk of UGIH which he or she would otherwise have had. The actual level of risk cannot be estimated directly from case control studies which do not usually measure incidence. Incidence can, however, be estimated from cohort studies (see below). However, from the case control studies it is possible to speculate on the public health impact of these drugs. NSAIDs are extremely widely used— from 15% to over 20% of elderly subjects in some countries (Henry 1988). This level of use and a relative risk of 3.3 leads to a prediction that 20–30% of all cases of upper gastrointestinal haemorrhage in these communities are directly attributable to the use of NSAIDs. In the UK alone this is around 2000–3000 cases annually in subjects over the age of 60 years.

In Table 11.1 it is worth noting that two of the better quality case control studies, those of Griffin et al (1988) and Quader & Logan (1988), included fatal cases of ulcer complications. Despite this, their odds ratios fall in the range of values from the other studies, suggesting that although NSAIDs increase the risk of developing ulcer complications they do not necessarily increase the case fatality rate. This was confirmed by a separate case control study which compared drug use by cases who died of ulcer complications with controls who had survived an episode of ulcer haemorrhage or perforation (Henry et al 1987). If there is no increase in the case fatality rate from UGIH in patients who have been taking NSAIDs, it can be assumed that around 1 in 10 elderly patients whose bleeding has been precipitated by the drugs will die. In the UK this is equivalent to 200–300 deaths annually, far short of some of the extreme estimates which have been made (Blower & Armstrong 1986).

Cohort studies

The results of the cohort studies require careful interpretation. The range of relative risks is wide, from almost no elevation in risk (Beard et al 1987, Jick et al 1985), to a relative risk of around nine (Fries et al 1989) (Table 11.2). The high value is probably not representative of most users of NSAIDs as it came from a study of a fairly select group of patients with rheumatoid arthritis. The remaining studies, which should more accurately reflect community use of NSAIDs in the United States, Canada and Scotland, appear somewhat heterogenous, according to the analysis, but have yielded a narrow range of relative risks with a pooled estimate of

Table 11.2   Cohort studies of upper gastrointestinal haemorrhage and NSAIDS

Authors	Ranking	Relative risk**	95% confidence interval for odds ratio relative risk	Pooled relative risk††	95% confidence interval for pooled relative risk	P (homogeneity)‡
Beard et al (1987)*	1	1.4	0.9–2.10			
Guess et al (1988)	2 =	3.4	2.1–5.6			
Beardon et al (1989)	2 =	2.1	1.8–2.5	2.1	1.8–2.4	P < 0.025
Jick et al (1985)*	4	1.0	0.9–1.8	2.0	1.7–2.3	P < 0.005
Carson et al (1987)	5 =	1.5	1.2–2.0			
Bloom (1989)	5 =	3.3	1.4–7.7	1.9	1.7–2.2	P < 0.005
Fries et al (1989)†	6	9.3	2.9–29.7	1.9	1.7–2.2	P < 0.025

* Excluded patients with duodenal ulcer.
† Patients with rheumatoid arthritis only.
** Ratio of the incidence of bleeding in patients taking NSAID compared with controls.
†† All studies were pooled in sequence determined by their quality score. Each figure in this column refers to the pooled relative risk for all studies to that point, including the study on that line.
‡ Refers to the probability of the variation in study outcomes occurring by chance.

Note: These analyses were carried out using the raw data provided in the authors' tables of results and the calculated values may differ somewhat from those given by the authors.

around two. This is lower than the pooled relative risk estimate from the case control studies and the respective confidence intervals of the pooled estimates from the two study types do not overlap, indicating that the difference is unlikely to be due to chance. The reasons for the discrepancy between these groups of studies is not clear, but it may be that even the best case control studies are still subject to biases which tend to inflate the estimates of relative risk.

Although, intuitively, our preference may be for the prospective study design, it is necessary to ask whether cohort studies should be regarded as the gold standard in this instance. Of particular note is the marked variation in the figures for *incidence* of ulcer complications in users of NSAIDs. Table 11.3 provides estimates of incidence which vary by more than an order of magnitude, even in the non-exposed subjects. Some of this variation can be explained. For instance, the low rate quoted by Jick et al (1985) refers to a relatively young population. The incidence of ulcer complications is known to increase sharply with age. The high incidence in patients with rheumatoid arthritis receiving NSAIDs may indicate a particular susceptibility to adverse reactions amongst this group who have a severe systemic disease. The high incidence in the study of Carson et al (1987) no doubt reflects the fact that they measured all cases of UGIH, not just those who were admitted to hospital. Nevertheless, the cases were not validated and the rate is unusually high. Likewise, the incidence estimated from the study of Beardon et al (1989) in Scotland, which relates to hospitalizations, is surprisingly high and difficult to reconcile with a much lower estimate from the same region which was made previously by Johnston et al (1973) using more traditional methods. Johnston et al (1973) suggested that the overall rate of hospitalization with UGIH is 116/100 000 which accords well with the results of a wide range of studies from the UK, Sweden, US, Germany and Hong Kong (full list of references available from the author).

I have laboured the point about the unexpectedly high estimates of incidence of UGIH from some recent record linkage studies but it is important, as these results (superficially) seem to support claims that use of NSAIDs results in a rate of ulcer complications of 1 to 2% or more (1000–2000/100 000/year) (Fries et al 1989, Knill-Jones et al 1990). While such high rates may apply to selected patients with a previous history of peptic ulcer or those who have rheumatoid arthritis, they certainly do not apply to the average user of NSAIDs in the community. The only group who are likely to benefit from promoting such inflated figures are the manufacturers of anti-ulcer drugs who make claims about the value of their products as prophylactic therapy to unselected users of NSAIDs.

Characteristics of patients and their ulcers

Much has been made of an entity called 'NSAID gastropathy' (Roth 1986).

Table 11.3   Incidence of upper gastrointestinal haemorrhage in users and non-users of NSAIDs derived from recent cohort studies

Authors	Study population	No. of users of NSAIDs	Outcome studies	Validation of diagnosis	Estimated incidence of UGIH*	
					Exposed $\times 10^{-5}$	Non-exposed $\times 10^{-5}$
Beard et al (1987)	Members of health maintenance organization United States	34 509 aged > 64 y	Hospitalization with gastrointestinal haemorrhage excluding bleeding duodenal ulcer	Yes	174	158
Jick et al (1985)	Members of health maintenance organization United States	100 000 aged < 65 y	Hospitalization with gastrointestinal haemorrhage excluding bleeding duodenal ulcer	Yes	21	20
Beardon et al (1989)	Residents of a defined region: United Kingdom	25 959 All ages	Hospitalization with ulcer haemorrhage or perforation	No	922	441
Carson et al (1987)	Medicaid population United States	47 136 All ages	All upper gastrointestinal haemorrhage	No	1525	996
Fries et al (1989)	Cohort of patients with rheumatoid arthritis	1684 All ages	Hospitalization with upper gastrointestinal diseases	Yes	1232	132

* Estimate incidence of UGIH in patients who were exposed to NSAIDs compared with the incidence in controls.

Note: These analyses were carried out using the raw data provided in the authors' tables of results and the calculated values may differ somewhat from those given by the authors.

Amongst its claimed characteristics are a preponderance of acute mucosal lesions, particularly in the stomach, the tendency of patients with frank ulcers to be elderly and female, a lack of warning symptoms of ulceration and localization of lesions in the stomach rather than the duodenum. It is important to recognize that some of these features are as likely to be related to the age of the patients who use NSAIDs as the drugs themselves. An exception is the high incidence of 'silent' ulceration in patients taking NSAIDs, which does not seem to be due to confounding by age (Hawkey 1990).

The extent to which age increases the risk of serious ulcer complications with NSAIDs is not entirely clear. Few well controlled studies have stratified relative risk by age. An exception is the study of Griffin et al (1988) which showed no increase in relative risk in age bands from 60 up to 80+ years. There is evidence, however, from a rather poorly controlled study that relative risk is higher in subjects over 60 than those under 60 years (Armstrong & Blower 1987). Griffin et al (1988) showed no further increase in relative risk with rising age beyond 60 years. It is important to interpret these data correctly. Although relative risk may not rise further in the very elderly the absolute risk associated with NSAIDs certainly does. This is because the very elderly have a much higher background risk of ulcer complications in the absence of NSAID therapy. This means that for a given relative risk, the risk difference which is attributable to the drugs in the elderly will be greater than in younger subjects.

Regarding the site of ulcer complications with NSAIDs, recent data have clarified some issues. Well controlled studies have demonstrated that there are increased rates of bleeding from both gastric and duodenal ulcers (Somerville et al 1986, Griffin et al 1988). In contrast, there is controversy regarding the evidence for an increased risk of *uncomplicated* duodenal ulcer with use of NSAIDs. An experimental study detected a high rate of acute mucosal ulceration in the duodenum in subjects studied endoscopically before and after a course of NSAIDs (Ehsanullah et al 1988). However, a well controlled epidemiological study found no association between symptomatic duodenal ulcer and use of NSAIDs (Duggan et al 1986).

LEVELS OF USE OF NON-STEROIDAL ANTI-INFLAMMATORY DRUGS

If NSAIDs were used only for serious disorders, the levels of risk for major gastrointestinal complications which have been defined by epidemiological studies would be quite acceptable. Problems arise largely because of the very wide extent of their use. For a range of common painful musculo-skeletal conditions, NSAIDs have replaced simple analgesics, particularly in elderly subjects. An appreciation of the extent of their use can be obtained from three sources: total prescriptions, sales figures and prevalence studies.

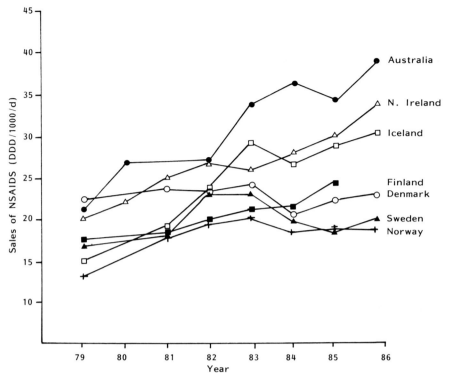

Fig. 11.2   This shows the growth in total sales of NSAIDs (excluding hospital sales) for a number of countries during the 1980s.

The number of prescriptions written for NSAIDs always sound impressive: US (population 240 million) 99 million prescriptions (Edelson et al 1990); UK (population 56 million) 24 million prescriptions (Knill-Jones et al 1990); Australia (population 17 million) 11 million prescriptions (Henry unpublished data). However, these figures on their own mean relatively little. Without knowing the year of study, the average duration of therapy, the average number of courses in a year or the age of the recipients, conclusions cannot be drawn about the number and types of subjects who have been exposed.

Annual sales data for NSAIDs are no better than prescription numbers, but because they are published regularly it is possible to determine usage trends. In Fig. 11.2 I have summarized sales data for NSAIDs from a number of countries (full list of references available from author). The data refer to non-hospital sales and have been converted to an internationally accepted measure of 'exposure'—the number of Defined Daily Doses (DDD) per 1000 individuals/day. In most countries the 1980s were a period of rapid growth in sales of NSAIDs but there were marked international differences in the volumes of sales. It is not possible to conclude with certainty that higher total sales indicate a larger number of users. They could also be explained by a smaller number of users consuming a larger average daily dose. The DDD is an arbitary unit and may differ from the prescribed daily dose. However, Australia which leads the field in Fig. 11.2 has traditionally been a high user of analgesics and can probably lay claim to the dubious distinction of having the highest consumption of NSAIDs.

Prevalence data are hard to come by. The best source is the usage levels reported for controls in carefully conducted case control studies. These data should be representative of the communities from which they were drawn. In general, use by controls has been higher in Australia and the UK than in the US. Somerville et al (1985) recorded use of NSAIDs in around 15% of controls aged 60 years and over in the UK. In Australia, we have found that over 20% of controls (aged 50 years and over) had taken NSAIDs in the previous week. In the US, Griffin et al recorded use of NSAIDs in 11% of controls aged over 60 years. The ranking of these data corresponds roughly to that of the sales levels discussed earlier.

The importance of these very high levels of consumption lies in the resulting population risk. Although the risk of serious gastrointestinal problems for an individual is usually low, the drugs assume responsibility for a high proportion of the cases of the disease, and the resulting deaths. This proportion (aetiologic fraction) varies from around 20% in the US to over 30% in Australia. Because individual risk is modest but the population risk is high the strategies we adopt for reducing or preventing risk should reflect this.

PREVENTION OF UPPER GASTROINTESTINAL DAMAGE

Damage to the upper gastrointestinal mucosa from NSAIDs has come to be regarded as a market by manufacturers who would like to promote co-prescription of their anti-ulcer drugs. If this practice became widespread the potential market would be enormous. Given that the problem was created by other drugs it is tempting, although perhaps overly simplistic, to suggest that limiting exposure of the population is the best approach to the problem. This approach has been criticized on the grounds that it is rarely feasible to discontinue NSAIDs in patients with serious inflammatory diseases (Szabo et al 1989). However, the wide international variation in the use of NSAIDs (Fig. 11.2) is unlikely to be explained by differing disease prevalence and probably reflects variation in practice style. This fact alone suggests that in some countries (e.g. Australia) prescribing of NSAIDs is excessive.

It is not simply the decision to start the drug which leads to problems, but also forgetting to stop it. It is not unusual to ask an elderly patient with a recent severe ulcer haemorrhage why she has been taking NSAIDs to find that she is unaware of the true nature of the drug or the original indication. Subsequent withdrawal can often be carried out without a significant flare up of any underlying inflammatory disorder.

However, it has to be acknowledged that some patients depend heavily on NSAIDs and are better off taking them despite the risks of major gastro-intestinal complications. Individuals at particular risk are the very elderly and those who have had previous ulceration, particularly if this has been complicated. The question arises as to which compounds afford the greatest protection from serious ulcer complications. Although there has been a great deal of research in this area it has done little to answer this important question. This is because the trials of anti-ulcer drugs have used as their endpoints short-term acute changes in the upper gastrointestinal mucosa seen at endoscopy. They have not tested the effects of co-prescription on symptomatic ulceration or ulcer complications. Clearly such trials would need to be large and as such, expensive, but given the implications of such widespread therapy and the size of the potential market, it is not an unreasonable requirement.

Despite the limitation of the available trials some conclusions can be drawn about the short-term effects of different anti-ulcer drugs in amelior-ating or preventing acute mucosal damage from NSAIDs. The histamine H_2 antagonist, sucralfate, and a prostaglandin analogue, misoprostol, have been tested in randomized controlled trials, co-prescribed with a wide range of NSAIDs. The results of these trials can be summarized as follows. Several studies have demonstrated a poor or absent effect of H_2 receptor antagonists in preventing gastric lesions (Roth et al 1987, Ehsanullah et al 1988, Robinson et al 1989). However, in two of these studies H_2 receptor antagonists were effective in preventing duodenal damage (Ehsanullah et al 1988, Robinson et al 1989). The performance of sucralfate in preventing gastric mucosal injury has been variable (Stern et al 1989). In a relatively large trial, misoprostol was effective in preventing acute gastric ulcers (Graham et al 1988b). In comparative trials, misoprostol has been shown to be superior to both H_2 receptor antagonists and sucralfate in preventing gastric mucosal lesions, and equivalent to H_2 receptor antagonists in preventing duodenal lesions (Lanza et al 1988a, b, Agrawal et al 1990).

However, all of these trials relate to short-term mucosal damage, not symptomatic or complicated peptic ulcer. The true benefits of therapy are still a matter of speculation and it cannot be assumed that such benefits necessarily exceed the risks of continued therapy with NSAIDs with the superimposed side effects of the co-prescribed anti-ulcer drug. In the case of misoprostol, the most promising agent, the main side effect is diarrhoea, which affected 39% of recipients using the higher of two doses in the largest trial, leading to discontinuation of therapy in 6% (Graham et al 1988b). The diarrhoea can be severe and the resulting hypovolaemia could be a serious complication in elderly subjects receiving diuretics or angiotensin converting enzyme inhibitors.

CONCLUSIONS

The last few years have yielded research which has increased our knowledge of the mechanisms of UGIH damage resulting from the use of NSAIDs. Research and clinical reports have indicated that the damage may extend beyond the traditional boundaries, particularly to the small intestine. Epidemiological studies have indicated that users of NSAIDs have 2 to 3 times the risk of serious ulcer complications as non-users. However, the absolute level of risk to the 'typical' user of these drugs is still controversial, but probably not very large. Some recent very high estimates of risk probably do not apply to the majority of subjects and should not be used as a justification for blanket co-prescription of prophylactic anti-ulcer drugs. In view of the extremely widespread use of NSAIDs the population risk is probably more important than the individual risk and this is best managed by limiting the exposure of the population.

ACKNOWLEDGEMENTS

My grateful thanks go to Jane Robertson who did much of the background research for this article and to Margaret Bond who did the word processing.

I am also indebted to Ciba-Geigy Australia Ltd who provided drug usage data which are not generally available in Australia.

REFERENCES

Aabakken L, Osnes M 1989 Non-steroidal anti-inflammatory drug-induced disease in the distal ileum and large bowel. Scandinavian Journal of Gastroenterology 24 (Suppl 163): 48–55

Agrawal N, Stromatt S, Brown J 1990 Comparative study of misoprostol and sucralfate in the prevention of NSAID-induced gastric ulcers. Clinical and Experimental Rheumatology 8 (Suppl 4): 107

Armstrong C P, Blower A L 1987 Non-steroidal anti-inflammatory drugs and life-threatening complications of peptic ulceration. Gut 28: 527–532

Bartle W R, Gupta A K, Lazor J 1986 Nonsteroidal anti-inflammatory drugs and gastrointestinal bleeding. Archives of Internal Medicine 146: 2365–2367

Beard K, Walker A M, Perera D R, Jick H 1987 Non-steroidal anti-inflammatory drugs and hospitalization for gastroesophageal bleeding in the elderly. Archives of Internal Medicine 147: 1621–1623

Beardon P H G, Brown S V, McDevitt D G 1989 Gastrointestinal events in patients prescribed non-steroidal anti-inflammatory drugs: a controlled study using record linkage in Tayside. Quarterly Journal of Medicine 71: 497–505

Bjarnason I, Williams P, So A et al 1984 Intestinal permeability and inflammation in rheumatoid arthritis. Effects of non-steroidal anti-inflammatory drugs. Lancet ii: 1171–1174

Bjarnason I, Williams P, Smethurst P et al 1986 Effect of non-steroidal anti-inflammatory drugs and prostaglandins on the permeability of the human small intestine. Gut 27: 1292–1297

Bjarnason I, Zanelli, G, Prouse P et al 1987 Blood and protein loss via small-intestinal inflammation induced by non-steroidal anti-inflammatory drugs. Lancet 2: 711–714

Bloom B S 1989 Risk and cost of gastrointestinal side effects associated with nonsteroidal anti-inflammatory drugs. Archives of Internal Medicine 149: 1019–1022

Blower A L, Armstrong C P 1986 Ulcer perforation in the elderly and non-steroidal anti-inflammatory drugs. Lancet 1: 971

Caradoc-Davies T H 1984 Nonsteroidal anti-inflammatory drugs, arthritis, and gastrointestinal bleeding in elderly in-patients. Age and Ageing 13: 295–298

Carson J L, Strom B L, Soper K A et al 1987 The association of nonsteroidal anti-inflammatory drugs with upper gastrointestinal tract bleeding. Archives of Internal Medicine 147: 85–88

Clinch D, Banerjee A K, Ostick G, Levy D W 1983 Non-steroidal anti-inflammatory drugs and gastrointestinal adverse effects. Journal of the Royal College of Physicians of London 17(4): 228–230

Chalmers T C, Berrier J, Hewitt P et al 1988 Meta-analysis of randomised controlled trials as a method of estimating rare complications of non-steroidal anti-inflammatory drug therapy. Alimentary Pharmacology and Therapeutics 2S: 9–26

Duggan J M, Dobson A J, Johnson H, Fahey P 1986 Peptic ulcer and non-steroidal anti-inflammatory agents. Gut 27: 929–933

Edelson J T, Tosteson A N A, Sax P 1990 Cost-effectiveness of misoprostol for prophylaxis against nonsteroidal anti-inflammatory drug-induced gastrointestinal tract bleeding. Journal of the American Medical Association 264: 41–47

Ehsanullah R S B, Page M C, Tildesley G, Wood J R 1988 Prevention of gastroduodenal damage induced by non-steroidal anti-inflammatory drugs: controlled trial of ranitidine. British Medical Journal 297: 1017–1021

Fleiss J L 1981 Statistical methods for rates and proportions. John Wiley, New York, pp 165–168

Fries J F, Miller S R, Spitz P W et al 1989 Toward an epidemiology of gastropathy associated with nonsteroidal antiinflammatory drug use. Gastroenterology 96: 647–655

Graham D Y, Smith J L, Spjut H J, Torres E 1988a Gastric adaptation. Gastroenterology 95: 327–333

Graham D Y, Agrawal N M, Roth S H 1988b Prevention of NSAID-induced gastric ulcer with misoprostol: multicentre, double-blind, placebo-controlled trial. Lancet 2: 1277–1280

Griffin M R, Ray W A, Schaffner W 1988 Nonsteroidal anti-inflammatory drug use and death from peptic ulcer in elderly persons. Annals of Internal Medicine 109: 359–363

Guess H A, West R, Strand L M et al 1988 Fatal upper gastrointestinal haemorrhage or perforation amongst users and non-users of non-steroidal anti-inflammatory drugs in Saskatchewan, Canada 1983. Journal of Clinical Epidemiology 41: 35–45

Hawkey C J 1990 Non-steroidal anti-inflammatory drugs and peptic ulcers. British Medical Journal 300: 278–284

Heller S R, Fellows I W, Ogilvie A L, Atkinson M 1982 Non-steroidal anti-inflammatory drugs and benign oesophageal stricture. British Medical Journal 285: 167–168

Henry D A, Johnson A, Dobson A, Duggan J 1987 Fatal peptic ulcer complications and the use of non-steroidal anti-inflammatory drugs, aspirin, and corticosteroids. British Medical Journal 295: 1227–1229

Henry D A 1988 Side-effects of non-steroidal anti-inflammatory drugs. Baillière's Clinical Rheumatology 2(2): 425–454

Jick H, Feld A D, Perera D R 1985 Certain nonsteroidal antiinflammatory drugs and hospitalization for upper gastrointestinal bleeding. Pharmacotherapy 5: 280–284

Johnston S J, Jones P F, Kyle J, Needham C D 1973 Epidemiology and course of gastrointestinal haemorrhage in north-east Scotland. British Medical Journal 3: 655–660

Knill-Jones R, Drummond M, Kohli H, Davies L 1990 Economic evaluation of gastric ulcer prophylaxis in patients with arthritis receiving non-steroidal anti-inflammatory drugs. Postgraduate Medical Journal 66: 639–646

Langman M J S, Morgan L, Worrall A 1985 Use of anti-inflammatory drugs by patients admitted with small or large bowel perforation and haemorrhage. British Medical Journal 290: 347–349

Lanza F L, Aspinall R L, Swabb E A et al 1988a Double-blind, placebo-controlled endoscopic comparison of the mucosal protective effects of misoprostol versus cimetidine on tolmetin-induced mucosal injury to the stomach and duodenum. Gastroenterology 95: 289–294

Lanza F, Peace K, Gustitus L et al 1988b A blinded endoscopic comparative study of misoprostol versus sucralfate and placebo in the prevention of aspirin-induced gastric and duodenal ulceration. American Journal of Gastroenterology 83: 143–146

Levi S, Goodlad R A, Lee C Y et al 1990a Inhibitory effect of non-steroidal anti-inflammatory drugs on mucosal cell proliferation associated with gastric ulcer healing. Lancet 336: 840–843

Levi S, de Lacey G, Price A B et al 1990b 'Diaphragm-like' strictures of the small bowel in patients treated with non-steroidal anti-inflammatory drugs. British Journal of Radiology 63: 186–189

Levy M, Miller D R, Kaufman D W et al 1988 Major upper gastrointestinal tract bleeding. Archives of Internal Medicine 148: 231–285

Morris G P 1986 Prostaglandins and cellular restitution in the gastric mucosa. In: Thomson A B R (ed) Protective and therapeutic effects of gastrointestinal prostaglandins. American Journal of Medicine 81(2A): 23–29

Quader K, Logan R F A 1988 Peptic ulcer deaths: How many occur at home or after non-steroidal anti-inflammatory drug prescribing? Gut 29: A1443

Rainsford K D 1987 Effects of lipoxygenase inhibitors and leukotriene agonists on the development of gastric mucosal lesions induced by non-steroidal anti-inflammatory drugs. Agents & Actions 21: 316–319

Rainsford K D, Schweitzer A, Brune K 1983 Distribution of the acetyl compared with the salicyl moeity of acetyl salicylic acid: acetylation of macromolecules in organs wherein side-effects are manifest. Biochemical Pharmacology 32: 1301–1308

Robinson M G, Griffin J W, Bowers J et al 1989 Effect of ranitidine gastroduodenal mucosal damage induced by nonsteroidal anti-inflammatory drugs. Digestive Diseases and Sciences 34: 424–428

Roth S H 1986 Nonsteroidal anti-inflammatory drug gastropathy. We started it—can we stop it? (editorial). Archives of Internal Medicine 146(6): 1075–1076

Roth S H, Bennett R E, Mitchell C S. Hartman R J 1987 Cimetidine therapy in nonsteroidal anti-inflammatory drug gastropathy. Archives of Internal Medicine 147: 1798–1801

Smedley F H, Taube M, Leach R, Westell C 1988 Non steroidal anti-inflammatory drugs: retrospective study of bleeding and perforated peptic ulcers. Gut 29: A1443

Somerville K, Faulkner G, Langman M 1986 Non-steroidal anti-inflammatory drugs and bleeding peptic ulcer. Lancet 1: 462–464

Stern A I, Ward F, Sievert W 1989 Lack of gastric mucosal protection by sucralfate during long-term aspirin ingestion in humans. American Journal of Medicine 86(6A): 66–69

Szabo S, Spill W F, Rainsford K D 1989 Non-steroidal anti-inflammatory drug-induced gastropathy. Medical Toxicology and Adverse Drug Experience 4: 77–94

Wilkins W E, Ridley M G, Pozniak A L 1984 Benign stricture of the oesophagus: role of non-steroidal anti-inflammatory drugs. Gut 25: 478–480

FURTHER READING

Hawkey C J 1990 Non-steroidal anti-inflammatory drugs and peptic ulcers. British Medical Journal 300: 278–284

Henry D A 1988 Side-effects of non-steroidal anti-inflammatory drugs. Baillière's Clinical Rheumatology 2(2): 425–454

Langman M J S 1989 Epidemiologic evidence on the association between peptic ulceration and antiinflammatory drug use. Gastroenterology 96: 640–646

Rainsford K D 1989 Mechanisms of gastrointestinal toxicity of non-steroidal anti-inflammatory drugs. Scandinavian Journal of Gastroenterology 24 (Suppl 163): 9–16

Szabo S, Spill W F, Rainsford K D 1989 Non-steroidal anti-inflammatory drug-induced gastropathy. Medical Toxicology and Adverse Drug Experience 4: 77–94

Best management

12. A 13-year-old newly diagnosed diabetic patient

S. A. Greene, A. C. MacCuish

INTRODUCTION

Insulin-dependent diabetes mellitus (IDDM, type 1 diabetes) is the commonest metabolic disorder in childhood and adolescence but remains comparatively rare. It is reported most frequently in Northern European countries: WHO figures (1988) give an incidence in Scotland of around 20 new cases per 100 000 population per annum, probably twice that in the South of England and exceeded only by Sweden and Finland. The catchment area of an average district general hospital will include no more than 10–20 new cases annually. Virtually all new patients are aged under 40 years at diagnosis, the majority presenting in childhood or adolescence, with distinct 'peaks' at ages 5–7 and 12–14 years. Adolescence is one of the most difficult times for a young person to cope with the onset of a chronic disease. It presents special problems which may not be encountered in younger children or adults and forms a common ground where the responsibilities of paediatricians and adult diabetologists overlap.

DIAGNOSIS

IDDM does not usually present clinically until at least 85% of pancreatic beta cell mass is lost and the establishment of consistent hyperglycaemia, with the inevitable osmotic diuresis, includes thirst, polyuria and weight loss. Apart from a few rare diseases, no other condition will enter the differential diagnosis, which is confirmed by the detection of glycosuria (Diastix strips) and the presence of hyperglycaemia. A persistently raised blood glucose level (fasting $>8\,mmol/l$ or random $>11\,mmol/l$) is diagnostic. Recourse to oral glucose tolerance testing should never be necessary at this age. Ketonuria is common on presentation, confirming severe insulin deficiency, but frank ketoacidosis should be rare provided that the practitioner refers the child to hospital that day, by telephone, rather than seeking a formal appointment in writing. The diagnosis of IDDM is always a potential emergency and there is no place for the leisurely referral letter.

ARRANGEMENT OF DIABETIC CARE

Much debate has surrounded the choice of referral to a paediatric or an adult diabetic clinic and local arrangements vary. In some areas, paediatricians routinely transfer their patients to an adult clinic at the age of 13 years; in others, the paediatric clinic may retain responsibility (perhaps in a special adolescent clinic) until the school leaving age or the late teens. The latter system has the particular advantage for child and family of supervision in a peer-group clinic which is able to expend much time in education, explanation, reassurance and practical support. The spectre of a young child in a large, impersonal adult clinic predominantly of elderly patients, some disabled by blindness or amputation, is not to be encouraged. Adult diabetologists have become increasingly convinced of the merits of a specialist adolescent clinic and usually possess the essential infrastructure (e.g. regular clinic services of a diabetes nurse specialist and dietitian), frequently lacking in the paediatric hospital. Unfortunately, more than a quarter of health boards in the UK still have no designated paediatric diabetic clinic, although the situation is improving steadily under the impetus of the British Diabetic Association (BDA) (British Paediatric Association Working Party 1990).

Therefore, the referring doctor must make a choice which is informed by knowledge of the local facilities available for both childhood and adult diabetic patients. The clinic should offer services of a consultant physician with special interest in diabetes, a diabetes nurse specialist and a diabetic dietitian, with open family access by informal self-referral. Supporting hospital services should include assays for blood glucose, haemoglobin A1 or other glycated protein and microalbuminuria. Ready availability of ophthalmology, chiropody and social work services together with easy access to a psychologist or psychiatrist and special provision for ethnic minority groups, especially Asian patients, is desirable.

In an ideal world, the patient will attend a combined clinic, under the joint care of a paediatrician and adult physician, to cover the difficult adolescent years when so many young persons are lost to follow-up.

SHOULD 'CURE' BE ATTEMPTED?

Type 1 diabetes is an autoimmune disease. Much is now known about its pathogenesis and immune-related markers have been identified which accurately predict its development in susceptible individuals. Even although the bulk of beta cell mass is destroyed before the development of clinical disease, it is tempting to consider intervention at this late stage with immunomodulation therapy, in the hope of reversing the process and restoring carbohydrate tolerance to normal.

Numerous clinical trials, often uncontrolled or poorly-designed, have addressed this possibility over the last 7 years. There is now a broad consensus that cyclosporin A is the immunosuppressant of choice and, if the drug is exhibited within 6 weeks of first diagnosis of childhood diabetes, biphasic insulin secretion and a return to normal carbohydrate tolerance will be observed in perhaps 20% of subjects. It has also become equally clear that immunotherapy is required permanently and that clinical diabetes reappears almost immediately if the drug is withdrawn.

This approach would be a formidable and potentially dangerous prospect for a child aged 13 years. Enthusiasts have suggested that it is justified, based upon the poor prognosis of young people growing up with diabetes and the knowledge that the youngest patients are most at risk from death or disablement by diabetic vascular complications in early adult life (Deckert et al 1978). However, there is an equally compelling body of evidence which indicates that these complications may be delayed, mitigated or possibly prevented by good longterm diabetic control (Green et al 1985). Moreover, cyclosporin A is both non-specific and toxic: it frequently induces nephrotoxicity in children and renal damage may persist when the drug is withdrawn. At present, routine use of cyclosporin A (or other immuno-suppressant) seems unjustified and unethical (American Diabetes Association 1990).

OUTPATIENT OR INPATIENT CARE?

If the child is moderately dehydrated, nauseated, vomiting or in frank ketoacidosis, hospital admission is essential. Uncomplicated cases, i.e. around 80% of children presenting with diabetes, can be managed on an outpatient basis. The first consultation is usually fraught with difficulty: parents are devastated by the diagnosis and the child is frightened or tearful. When the diagnosis is confirmed, the essential needs are firstly, a clear and simple explanation of diabetes for the patient and family; secondly, an introduction to the diabetes team who will be involved in education and continuing care; and thirdly, the exhibition of insulin therapy. The parents will wish an environment and staff from whom they can find comfort, reassurance and expert advice and are entitled to expect that their fears and questions, often unframed at the first visit, can be answered immediately by telephone.

The first visit will involve a venepuncture (urea and electrolytes, haemoglobin A1, etc.). It is unwise to introduce the notion of capillary blood sampling by fingerprick at this stage. Baseline measurements of height and weight are obtained and physical examination, which should be essentially normal but must include measurement of blood pressure, is the prelude to insulin treatment.

THERAPY

Insulin

The choice of insulin formulation is a seemingly daunting prospect but is

Table 12.1 Suitable human insulins (all U100, i.e. 100 units/ml)

Type	Proprietary Name
Soluble (short-acting)	*Actrapid (pyr) Human Velosulin (emp) Humulin S (prb)

Isophane (NPH)
  (intermediate-
  acting)
	*Protaphane (pyr)
	Human Insulatard (emp)
	Humulin I (prb)

Pre-mixed
  suspensions
  (soluble: NPH)
	*PenMix 30:70 (pyr)
	Actraphane 30:30 (pyr)
	Human Mixtard 30:70 (emp)
	Human Initard 50:50 (emp)
	Humulin M1, M2, M3, M4 (prb)
	(range for 10:90 to 40:60 ratio)

* Available in Penfill cartridges (150 u) for NovoPen delivery system.

comparatively simple. In the young adolescent, treatment by twice-daily injections of intermediate-acting insulins (NPH or isophane) will almost invariably be used. If the patient is well grown (>40 kg), markedly hyperglycaemic and possessed of the normal appetite of a teenager, a pre-mixed suspension of soluble (regular) and isophane insulin, injected before breakfast and before the evening meal, is preferable. Numerous formulations are available but a 30:70 or 20:80 mixture of soluble isophane will cover virtually all requirements. Human formulations of insulin are used in preference to others. These are prepared by semisynthesis from pork insulin or by recombinant DNA technology, using bacteria or yeasts as host cells, and have the merit of minimal antigenicity when given subcutaneously (MacPherson & Feely, 1990). A short list of suitable preparations is given in Table 12.1.

Human insulins differ from their predecessors of animal origin (beef and pork insulin) by rather more rapid absorption from the subcutaneous space and generally shorter duration of effective hypoglycaemic action. These properties probably explain some of the concerns that have surfaced in the past two years and in particular, the belief that their use renders the patient more prone to sudden, unexpected or severe hypoglycaemia with an absence of warning symptoms. To date, there is no convincing evidence to suggest that human insulins are more dangerous for the patient than their well-established animal counterparts. Many of the difficulties with hypoglycaemia observed in modern diabetic practice, reflect an over-zealous approach to achieving normoglycaemia, resulting in occasional episodes of dangerously low glucose levels. Diabetics, particularly diabetic children, should not be coerced into maintaining a blood glucose concentration consistently in the 'normal' range (i.e. $\leqslant 5.5$ mmol/l in our 13-year-old): figures of 6–11 mmol/l—and often a good deal higher—are ideal levels if normal family life is not to be disrupted by recurring hypoglycaemia.

Insulin dose will be determined by trial and error and varies according to the patient's weight, the occurrence of growth spurts and the effects of exercise or infection. A starting dose of around 0.5 units/kg is usual with about two-thirds of the total dose given in the morning. Thus a teenager weighing 43 kg will receive approximately 22 units per day, 14 units before breakfast and 8 units before the evening meal. These doses may fall rapidly and substantially within a few days of starting therapy, reflecting the so-called 'honeymoon phase' of partial remission as hyperglycaemia is corrected: almost all patients still produce some endogenous insulin at this time and indeed, 6–10% may actually not require further exogenous insulin for some weeks or even months.

Insulin delivery systems

Insulin is self-administered only subcutaneously by presterilized disposable plastic syringes with integral needle. The syringe can safely be re-used to give repeated injections—up to 5 times is recommended by the BDA—with no risk to the patient and obvious cost benefits.

The large majority of young diabetics still use presterilized syringes but the availability of other injection devices has risen dramatically in the past 5 years. Chief amongst these are the various pen injection devices, which hold a prefilled insulin cartridge (usually 150 units) and have some mechanism for precise dispensing of the required dose by twisting the barrel or pressing a plunger. Insulin pens were originally developed to permit intensified therapy; however, this approach to good control is inappropriate for a 13-year-old and may alienate the patient. Insulin cartridges of isophane and premixed insulin suspensions are now available and are possibly the simplest means of injecting insulin in a twice-daily regimen. A teenager will feel more comfortable with a pen which can be carried in the pocket, schoolbag or blazer and is ready for use with minimum fuss, rather than submit to the ritual of drawing up insulin from a bottle stored in a refrigerator. Available cartridges are listed in Table 12.1.

By contrast, insulin pumps, i.e. portable electromechanical devices for continuous subcutaneous insulin infusion (CSII) have no place in the treatment of adolescent diabetes. Quite apart from cost (£500–£1000 each), they are clumsy and uncomfortable for a teenager to wear, confer no metabolic advantages over conventional regimens, cannot be used to inject isophane insulins and carry unacceptable added risks of hypoglycaemia or ketoacidosis.

Diet

Recent years have witnessed the welcome recognition that young persons with diabetes have the same nutritional requirements as all other teenagers. Insulin therapy should reflect a child's lifestyle and preferred eating habits

Table 12.2   Carbohydrate exchanges in diabetes mellitus

Definition	One exchange is any food portion containing 10 g carbohydrate (whether in mixed, unrefined or highly-refined form)
Measurement	Exchanges are not weighed, but expressed as simple domestic measures of common foods e.g. one small/½ large slice of bread one small potato/6 chips one apple, orange, pear, banana ⎫ each contains 10 g one carton yoghurt/⅓ pint milk ⎬ carbohydrate one ice-cream/packet of crisps etc. etc.
Distribution	Exchanges are distributed throughout the daily eating pattern. The nature of each exchange reflects individual dietary preferences

e.g.		Breakfast		Mid-am		Lunch		Mid-pm		Tea		Bedtime
27 exchanges	=	6	+	2	+	6	+	3	+	8	+	2
270 g CHO	=	60 g	+	20 g	+	60 g	+	30 g	+	80 g	+	20 g

rather than being used as an excuse to coerce the patient and family into adopting a diet that is rigid, complex and often low in carbohydrate content.

A careful, detailed diet history is essential and should be obtained by the dietitian within a few days of diagnosis. Some compromises with pre-diabetic eating habits are inevitable: for example, a more regular distribution of carbohydrate throughout the day may be the most important way to avoid extremes of hypo- and hyperglycaemia. The family will also need to become familiar with the carbohydrate content of common foodstuffs, based upon the exchange system (1 exchange = 10 g carbohydrate); despite its drawbacks, this system remains the simplest means of equating carbohydrate values between different foods (Table 12.2).

The modern diabetic diet should provide about half the daily energy intake as carbohydrate, not more than 40–42% as fat and the balance as protein. These suggested proportions do not deviate greatly from the normal diet of most schoolchildren in the UK but do require some changes in the traditional Western high-fat, low-carbohydrate diet. It is neither necessary nor desirable to alter the protein intake and in a child at age 13 years no vitamin supplementation should be necessary.

Carbohydrate consumption from unrefined, fibre-rich sources (such as fruit) should be encouraged but there is no evidence that simple sugars (sucrose) or disrupted polysaccharides (crisps, mashed potatoes) are harmful in diabetes. Most children have a great liking for crisps, confectionery, sweet biscuits, etc. and it is perfectly safe for some part of the day's carbohydrate to include those foods. A balance between desirable and acceptable is the key to success. It is difficult to equate a medical emphasis on savoury rather than sweet foods with the desire to limit dietary sodium intake in diabetes because of its relationship to blood pressure.

Energy intakes are often formidably high in teenage boys, and may rise further with growth spurts. Absolute energy expenditure increases up to 15 years in girls and 18 years in boys. The clinic records of growth velocity (i.e. height and weight charts) must be monitored in relation to the dietary intake. Our 13-year-old will probably have a total energy intake of around 2500 calories, split as 48–50% carbohydrate, 40% fat, 12–13% protein. This implies a daily intake of about 270 g carbohydrate, i.e. 27 'exchanges' distributed throughout the main meals and snacks of the day.

Binge eating is frequent in young adults with diabetes and should be considered at times of unstable blood glucose control. Similarly anorexia is seen in some young diabetic girls.

Dropping unnecessary snacks is usually helpful in establishing a regular meal plan.

Obesity is a problem particularly in pubertal girls. This appears to be related to their daily insulin dose. Care must be taken not to 'chase' abnormal glycaemic control by continually increasing the dose. A reduction in calories is usually only successful with a concomitant reduction in insulin dose.

There is virtually no place for the special 'diabetic' foods of an earlier era. Such foods are distinguished by high cost and high energy content but are largely harmless. On the other hand, low-calorie sweeteners (saccharin or aspartame) are valuable, particularly when added to the fizzy drinks, e.g. diet Coke, so beloved by teenagers. The Nutrition Sub-Committee of the BDA has lately published a comprehensive paper which reviews the dietary recommendations for children and adolescents with diabetes and is recommended for further reading (Kinmonth et al 1989).

Education

Diabetic life can be marred if the initial education of the patient and family is unsatisfactory. This task is best done by the diabetes nurse. Successful educators teach with clarity and simplicity, demonstrating techniques by practical example (injections, fingerprick blood sampling, etc.). The learning curve for each new patient is different and education is a continuous process at home and in the clinic. Audiovisual aids are widely available but never supplant the individual tutor. The commonest mistake of inexperience is to teach too much, too soon, and to assume rather than confirm that the message is received and understood. An audit of success or failure—a simple checklist—is invaluable and summarized in Table 12.3.

Capillary blood glucose testing should be initiated within the first 7–10 days. Most children accept this but find it more unpleasant than self-injection of insulin; a balance must be struck between the need for information, and repeated trauma to small fingertips. In the early stages, it is sufficient with a twice-daily insulin regimen to aim for the '2-point' profile on 2–3 days per week, i.e. blood glucose estimation just before the morning and evening insulin injections. A little later the '4-point' profile can be

Table 12.3   Education checklist

1. Simple understanding of diabetes
2. Sites of insulin injection
   Giving injections (syringe or pen)
   Drawing up insulin (syringe)
   Setting dose/changing cartridge (pen)
3. Urine tests (ketones/glucose)
   Fingerprick blood sampling
   Blood glucose strips/reflectance meter
4. Self-adjusting insulin dose
   (relation to blood glucose)
5. Diet prescribed and explained
6. Hypoglycaemia—symptoms, treatment,
   prevention
   Use of glucagon
7. Visits to home and school (nurse specialist)

introduced (blood glucose pre-breakfast, pre-lunch, pre-tea, pre-bed) and these measurements will tell whether the short-acting insulin component of the mixture is necessary or adequate. Most children dislike home blood glucose monitoring whereas parents welcome it. Parental oversampling should be discouraged, although parents derive great comfort and reassurance in the ability to make instant measurement of their child's blood glucose, especially at night or if hypoglycaemia is feared.

The occasional child and family will refuse to undertake home blood glucose monitoring and in such cases there is still a place for urinary glucose testing. All adolescents and their families should know how to test for ketonuria, the early herald of metabolic decompensation and should know how to act upon a positive test. All families need a basic inventory of equipment to be kept at home (Table 12.4), the items supplied initially by the clinic and subsequently renewed by prescription from the general practitioner.

Table 12.4   Basic inventory of home equipment

Insulin	2 × 10 ml bottles of each type (syringe users)
	2 × 5-cartridge packs (pen users)
Injection equipment	3 × 10 pkts disposable syringes with needles (syringe users)
	1 × 10 pkt disposable syringes (pen users: for emergency)
	2 pen delivery systems (pen users)
	40 × 27 G disposable needles (pen users)
Monitoring equipment	Disposable lancets plus device for fingerprick
	1 × 50 pk blood glucose reagent strips
	1 × 25 pk urine glucose test strips
	1 × 25 pk urine ketone test strips
Information	Individual dietary prescription
	Other educational literature
	Clinic/staff telephone numbers
	BDA information

A positive attitude is the most important key to successful management of diabetes. Unfortunately, insulin therapy is a 'blunt instrument' in comparison to the complex homeostatic feedback controlled endogenous insulin system and, therefore, overall daily amounts of insulin are very similar in most patients. Frequent adjustments of insulin dose are usually unnecessary, and if taking place require investigation of other aspects of management: diet, emotion, physical development.

Lifestyle considerations

A child aged 13 years spends more than half of his life at school. This causes concern to the parents and to the school. Therefore the school should be visited by the diabetes nurse or community liaison sister, to instruct the teaching staff in the rudiments of diabetes. The school must know what to do in an emergency (the commonest being hypoglycaemia) and must have a clear line of communication to the diabetic clinic if help is needed.

Formal periods of aerobic exercise are a natural part of school life and often the first occasion when a risk of hypoglycaemia is encountered. Prevention is better than cure. The simplest, best prophylaxis is to take additional refined carbohydrate (the ubiquitous Mars Bar) before the sports period.

Insulin dose will almost inevitably rise after the honeymoon phase. Fluctuations in dose will be compounded by growth spurts, the preferred activity pattern, the progression through puberty, compliance or otherwise with diet and intercurrent infection. The last influence is a particularly potent precipitant of ketoacidosis and thus demands early medical help and particularly close metabolic monitoring of the patient. Most of the common infectious diseases of adolescence can be managed without recourse to hospital admission but any cause of repeated vomiting and/or diarrhoea, e.g. acute gastroenteritis, will require intravenous provision of fluids and carbohydrate.

Delivery of continuing care

Diabetes is a chronic disorder requiring self-management by the patient. Whilst accepting that practical advice regarding insulin injections, monitoring techniques and dietary therapy may be given at the standard clinic attendance, routine clinic appointments are an inefficient system for maintaining enthusiasm in teenagers, who often vote with their feet and fail to come to clinics particularly when left to their own devices. Special format clinics for the older teenager, with evening sessions and a younger atmosphere, with group participation from other teenagers can alleviate anxieties, making the adolescent more receptive to advice, instruction or encouragement.

Non-clinic activities play as prominent a role in the delivery of care to this age group. Camps, either nationally organized by the BDA or locally by the diabetes team, give many teenagers the confidence to progress with the management of their diabetes and are often helpful in allaying their fears. UK national initiatives such as the 'Young Diabetics Project' have proved valuable not only delivering care and advice, but obtaining information for services for young people with diabetes, as well as acting as a self-care support group either on a national or local basis.

PROBLEMS

Hypoglycaemia

Symptomatic hypoglycaemia always occurs if blood glucose is <2 mmol/l and frequently at rather higher levels if blood glucose is declining rapidly. The phenomenon is probably the most dreaded aspect of diabetes by patient and parents. If hypoglycaemia occurs frequently it will disrupt domestic life, fragment education and demoralize the family. Severe and prolonged episodes carry the threat that permanent intellectual impairment will ensue.

Most hypoglycaemic episodes are rapid in onset following abnormal bouts of exercise or after a forgotten or delayed meal. Prompt action results in a full and complete recovery. Prolonged episodes, especially those occurring at night, result in persistent symptoms even after the blood glucose has been corrected; these include nausea, headache and a general washed-out feeling. Thus it is particularly important that the causes, indicators and recognition of hypoglycaemia are explained with particular care. At one time, it was commonplace to deliberately induce hypo-glycaemia as part of the education process. Although the practice has now been generally abandoned, it did provide the individual with an experience of his or her particular symptom complex under entirely safe conditions.

The treatment of choice is simple sugar in easily assimilable form. Glucose tablets (Dextrosol) are readily available from pharmacies, highly soluble, quickly effective but rather expensive. Many teenagers find them nauseating and almost any form of favoured confectionery—preferably one that can be stored or carried without melting—is equally acceptable. Carbohydrate in liquid form is very useful, especially if the patient is becoming distant and must be cajoled to swallow: close friends should be given advice on hypoglycaemic episodes and may be encouraged to attend the clinic with the patient.

The safest preparation to treat established hypoglycaemia, where the capacity to swallow is dubious or has been lost, is glucagon. The family should be familiar with the use of this drug which can be stored indefinitely in lyophilized form, reconstituted in seconds with distilled water and injected via one of the patient's own syringes. The therapeutic dose is 1 mg and is equally effective whether injected subcutaneously, intramuscularly

or (involuntarily) intravenously. Glucagon will restore normal consciousness within 10 minutes in all but the most severe cases and must be followed
by the ingestion of carbohydrate to prevent relapse into coma.

If a single dose of glucagon fails to correct the hypoglycaemia, a doctor
must be called to administer dextrose (50 ml of 50% solution intravenously). This is no easy task if peripheral veins are small and the child is
struggling. It is not a treatment of first choice since it demands the presence
of a doctor and is inevitably followed by painful phlebitis. It is, however,
dramatically effective.

Failure to restore full consciousness by the above measures implies
hypoglycaemia has been severe and prolonged, although a postictal phase
must be suspected if a seizure has occurred. If the patient remains uncon-
scious despite a capillary blood glucose of 17 mmol/l, hospital admission is
indicated. The presence of cerebral oedema should be considered, often
with supporting clinical signs other than continuing coma, and treated in
the same manner as cerebral oedema during ketoacidosis (see below).

Not infrequently, hypoglycaemia causes nocturnal seizures and may be
confused with idiopathic epilepsy. It is wise to base all advice on the
presumption of hypoglycaemia. In particularly difficult cases, with real
uncertainty, it may be necessary to admit the child to hospital for hourly
nocturnal blood glucose estimations withdrawn through a suitable peripheral venous line. In a long clinical practice, we have only identified four
diabetic teenagers who were unlucky enough to have coexistent idiopathic
epilepsy. Finally, the symptoms of hypoglycaemia are readily mimicked by
the diabetic teenager who is disenchanted with life in general and wants to
manipulate a particular situation. The acting is often of a very high
standard, hence the wisdom of actually documenting presumed hypoglycaemia by blood glucose estimation.

Hypoglycaemia is probably the most disturbing complication of diabetes
for the adolescent who is developing the skills of social behaviour. Discussion about their fears as well as advice on reduction in insulin dose and
increase in carbohydrate where appropriate is necessary. Although undesirable, blood glucose 'running high' for a few months may have to be
accepted by the physician to help the teenager through a difficult period.

Ketoacidosis (DKA)

The classical syndrome of severe insulin deficiency, i.e. hyperglycaemia
with coexistent metabolic acidosis, is the commonest form of serious
metabolic decompensation in diabetic teenagers (Richardson & Donaldson
1989). However, it is closely followed by the syndrome of euglycaemic
acidosis, i.e. ketoacidosis without hyperglycaemia. The distinction is important since the latter syndrome often develops over a matter of hours and
carries none of the large water and electrolyte deficits expected in the
classical form.

Infection is the most common precipitating factor for DKA and its presence should be sought by all available means, including blood culture. Normal clinical pointers to sepsis are unreliable: ketoacidotic patients have a subnormal body temperature and elevated white cell count whether or not they are infected and diffuse or aberrant abdominal pain with vomiting is also an expected finding. In many cases a cause is not identified and of course the emergency is readily induced by an unhappy or alienated teenager. Sometimes the problem is recurrent and DKA can be induced by deliberate omission of insulin. It is often unwise to probe the origins too deeply if the episode has been an isolated one.

By 13 years of age, most patients have passed the stage where complicated calculations of fluid deficit are necessary and unless the child is very small, the episode can be treated as in any young adult. Isotonic (0.154 M) saline will usually be the first solution given intravenously. Soluble insulin, 3–6 units per hour depending upon severity of acidosis, is given by infusion pump and potassium supplements (20 mmol $KCl/\frac{1}{2}$ litre of infusate) commenced shortly thereafter. Treatment should not wait upon diagnosis of the underlying cause, which may never be found, and delays in the A & E Department, arranging unnecessary X-rays, are inadvisable.

Intravenous carbohydrate—usually 5% dextrose solution—will replace saline when blood glucose has declined to around 15 mmol/l and is continued until acid-base balance is normal or near normal. The use of hypotonic solutions, i.e. 0.77 M saline or 2.5% dextrose, carries the risk of inducing or aggravating cerebral oedema in children and is hardly ever necessary, except in severely dehydrated patients with an initial serum sodium > 155 mmol/l. Metabolic acidosis will usually be corrected steadily with glucose, insulin and potassium but in patients with an arterial pH $\leqslant 7$, the risk of malignant ventricular arrhythmias or cardiorespiratory arrest is enhanced and air hunger is a source of great physical distress. In such circumstances, the judicious use of sodium bicarbonate (50 ml 8.4% solution, i.e. 50 mmol bicarbonate) is appropriate and can be given over 30 minutes and repeated if necessary to restore arterial pH to 7.1–7.2. The rapid hypokalaemic effect of bicarbonate should be appreciated and serum potassium kept under continuous review.

In euglycaemic ketoacidosis, there is no fluid or electrolyte deficit to replace since osmotic diuresis has not occurred. Severely acidotic patients may walk into hospital and their air hunger is occasionally mistaken for hysterical hyperventilation by inexperienced staff. If they secure admission, they may then run the risk of partial drowning by enthusiastic and inappropriate saline infusion. Their need is for carbohydrate in concentrated form, together with potassium supplements and sufficient insulin to allow the resumption of normal aerobic metabolism. Almost all will be vomiting or have temporary gastroparesis: the treatment of choice is a hypertonic (10%) dextrose infusion, with potassium supplements and insulin infusion of 4–6 units per hour until the acidosis is fully corrected or the patient can eat once more. Recovery is usually rapid, provided that the syndrome is recognized and properly treated.

Regrettably, children still die from DKA. A few die from fulminating sepsis, either because the infection is particularly virulent (e.g. bacterial meningitis) or because hospital admission has been too long delayed. Others die from a complication of the emergency and its treatment; cerebral oedema being the prime example. The cause of cerebral oedema is unknown but modern imaging techniques, i.e. CT scan and NMR, reveal significant swelling of the brain in approximately 9% of mostly asympto-matic patients with childhood diabetes (Krane et al 1985). In this fertile ground, the risk of cerebral oedema is significantly enhanced by inap-propriate use of hypotonic replacement fluids. As noted above, these should be given with great caution only to patients who are both severely de-hydrated and hypernatraemic. The sad clinical picture is usually of the child who is not terminally ill on admission, appears to be improving biochemically but then lapses into drowsiness and deepening coma. There-after progression to coning and cardiorespiratory arrest is inexorable. The diagnosis will always be first suspected by clinical observations and if considered, should be treated as promptly and vigorously as possible. Mannitol (150–200 ml 20% solution) given over 20 minutes, dexa-methasone in high dose and inspired oxygen (100% by face mask) are the mainstays of treatment but the outcome is often disappointing. The iatro-genic nature of some cases of fatal cerebral oedema should remind clinicians that treatment of DKA is best conducted at a measured rather than breakneck pace. The longer the condition has taken to evolve—the more severe the fluid and electrolyte deficits—the greater the time we should take to replace them. DKA is always an emergency but dramatic infusion of fluids aiming for 'biochemical normality within 6 hours', is inadvisable and may contribute to the death of a child.

Unstable diabetes

Frequent, life-disrupting episodes of DKA interspersed with episodes of hypoglycaemia are rare in the adolescent period, with only the occasional patient having recurrent problems. Recurring infections are rare, with ill-health mostly related to accidents at this age. Repeated DKA, therefore, probably has its basis in insufficient insulin administration or over-indulgence of carbohydrate. These acts may be deliberate or part of a haphazard existence; all should be considered in cases of recurrent DKA.

Following the immediate therapy for DKA or hypoglycaemia or at times of difficulties with the diabetes, time should be given in the follow-up clinics or at home, to discuss with the teenager why the episode occurred.

By contrast, persistently poor control reflected by a rise in average glycated haemoglobin concentration is seen quite commonly in adolesence. Many underlying causes are likely. Changes in hormone concentration associated with the pubertal growth spurt affect insulin and glucose homoeostasis. Undoubtedly the introduction of a more flexible style of living (erratic meal times, late nights, sleeping in) stretches conventional diabetes management. At the same time, emotional and social pressures increase stress which in its turn affects blood glucose control. In the severely unstable diabetic adolescent these social factors appear to play the major part; some will come from disrupted homes (divorce, separation) or homes with little stabilizing routine (both parents working) or have difficult emotional relationships with parents, siblings, teachers or friends. Discussion around these problems are usually successful at stabilizing 'blood glucose control', although for some, suboptimal control as defined by the physician, is necessary to prevent repeated episodes of DKA and hypoglycaemia. Meticulous alteration of the diet and insulin is usually unproductive in these circumstances, frequently adding to the problems of the teenager.

Family disharmony

Most teenagers and their families cope well with the practical aspects and emotional reactions of a chronic illness, integrating into society and developing through adolescence normally. For some, however, the problems are too difficult to overcome, and emotions may dominate; fear, anger, denial, depression and guilt are common reactions. Attention to these problems is an essential part of the management of diabetes, particularly when they come to dominate the adolescent's life.

Parents frequently find this age difficult, particularly if diabetes has been present from early childhood. Handing over responsibility for control to the teenage patient is sometimes hard for the parent and in itself creates tensions. In discussion of problems of the adolescent, the parents should not be ignored, as many have a positive role to play.

MANAGEMENT: SCREENING FOR COMPLICATIONS

With the exception of neuropathy, the major complications of diabetes are due to microangiography and closely related to the duration of overt disease. Therefore it might seem inappropriate to conduct formal screening exercises within the first few years of childhood diabetes. There are grounds to take the opposite view. It is now firmly established that after a remarkably short period, sometimes under 5 years, such complications may appear and with care can be detected. Neurophysiological studies may reveal peripheral nerve dysfunction, even if asymptomatic; fundoscopy can show the few red dots that presage background retinopathy; most importantly, the earliest onset of neuropathy may be confirmed, even at the stage of renal hyperfiltration, by the finding of microalbuminuria. Adolescent diabetics with microalbuminuria are precisely the subgroup most

Table 12.5   Annual screen for complications

Biochemical	Microalbumin assay screening test (If positive → formal immunoassay of overnight urine specimen) Glycated protein assay (fructosamine or HbA1) Cholesterol (non-fasting, total plus HDL)
Retinal	Direct ophthalmoscopy (dark room, prior mydriasis)
CNS	Clinical examination (if positive or patient symptomatic → neurophysiological studies)
CVS	Blood pressure
Anthropometry	Height and weight Injection sites

likely to have coexistent elevation of blood pressure, even although this falls far short of what would be accepted as hypertension, and are prime candidates for eventual development of renal failure before middle age.

The ability to detect those early complications is matched by the knowledge that subsequent action, whether in attempts to improve ambient blood glucose levels or check a progressive rise in blood pressure, is thought to be of prime importance in preventing their progression or even reversing the pathology (Johnston 1989). The basics of a simple annual screening scheme are summarized in Table 12.5. It is not suggested that the neurological examination need proceed beyond simple clinical tests, unless that examination is abnormal or the patient is symptomatic. Other facets of screening, especially assessment of the large blood vessels, are unnecessary at this time and can be added after age 20 years. Of course the judgement of overall glycaemic control rests upon the child's records of home blood glucose monitoring and glycated protein assay at every clinic visit, not just annually. But however short the duration of disease, any defined abnormality in a teenager should lead to the most serious reappraisal of the quality of that patient's diabetic control. A trivial and ostensibly harmless complication in the teens may presage visual loss and renal failure in the thirties. No doctor should passively accept the progression as inevitable.

CONCLUSION

IDDM is an uncommon but immensely important chronic disease in childhood and adolescence. It carries the threats of short-term metabolic crises and long-term disablement with a reduced lifespan. Its proper management requires the unswerving help and support of a skilled and dedicated clinical team, underpinned by the facilities of a general hospital. The time and effort expended by staff, child and family can be immense but offers the patient the prospect that adult life will not be marred by disease or prematurely shortened. These stakes are too high to be willingly jeopardized.

REFERENCES

American Diabetes Association 1990 Prevention of type 1 diabetes mellitus. Diabetes Care 13: 1026–1027
British Paediatric Association Working Party 1990 The organisation of services for children with diabetes in the United Kingdom. Diabetic Medicine 7: 457–464
Deckert T, Poulsen J E, Larsen M 1978 Prognosis of diabetics with diabetes onset before the age of 31. Diabetologia 14: 363–370
Green A, Borch-Johnsen K, Kragh Anderson P et al 1985 Relative mortality of type 1 (insulin dependent) diabetes in Denmark: 1933–81. Diabetologia 28: 339–342
Johnston D I 1989 Personal practice: management of diabetes mellitus. Archives of Disease in Childhood 64: 622–628
Kinmonth A L, Magrath G, Reckless J P D et al 1989 Dietary recommendations for children and adolescents with diabetes. Journal of Human Nutrition and Dietetics 2, 6: 437–454
Krane E J, Rockoff M A, Wallman J K, Wolfsdorf J I 1985 Subclinical brain swelling during treatment of diabetic ketoacidosis. New England Journal of Medicine 312: 1147–1151
MacPherson J N, Feely J 1990 New drugs: insulin. British Medical Journal 300: 731–736
Richardson J E, Donaldson M D C 1989 Diabetic emergencies. Prescribers' Journal 29: 174–183

FURTHER READING

Baum J D, Kinmonth A L (eds) 1985 Care of the child with diabetes. Churchill Livingstone, Edinburgh
Craig J O 1981 Childhood diabetes and its management. Butterworths, London
Greene S A 1990 Diabetes in childhood and adolescence. In: Tattersall R B, Gale E A M (eds) Clinical diabetes management. Churchill Livingstone, Edinburgh

13. A 38-year-old crofter's wife with progressive renal impairment

J. A. Burton

End-stage renal failure has an incidence of up to 80/million population per year. Acceptance rates for dialysis vary widely in different countries. In the UK the average rate in 1988 was 55/million. The incidence in Highland Scotland is approximately 60/million. Glomerulonephritis is still the most common cause of renal failure (25%), followed by pyelonephritis (16%), multisystem disease including diabetes (16%), renal vascular disease (10%), polycystic kidney (8%) and analgesic nephropathy (3%). In the remaining patients presenting with established renal failure, the aetiology is uncertain. I shall assume that the crofter's wife probably has end-stage glomerulonephritis but that there is no histological confirmation of the diagnosis. There is now a vast literature on the treatment of end-stage renal disease. In this article, I shall try to reflect everyday practice rather than the academic state of the art.

FACILITIES AVAILABLE

My unit serves an area of 9707 square miles with a population of 201 000 and patients are also referred from the Western Isles, population 31 000. The region is therefore sparsely populated and some patients reside at considerable distances from the centre. Public transport facilities are not good. Housing standards are generally good, but the quality and source of water supplies are variable.

The original three-bedded dialysis unit soon proved inadequate and it was replaced by an eight-station, purpose-built unit. There is a large area containing four stations, and four individual rooms which can be used for either haemodialysis or continuous ambulatory peritoneal dialysis (CAPD). Also included is adequate space for storage, machine servicing and minor procedures (e.g. insertion of subclavian lines, renal biopsies) together with a small outpatient clinic and secretarial services. Staffing consists of one consultant, two sisters and five staff nurses. A full-time technician services and repairs the equipment.

End-stage renal disease causes problems in many systems and management of these patients in isolation is impossible. The base hospital has excellent facilities for investigation, including a full laboratory service, ultrasound, CT scanning, angiography and isotope scanning techniques. Easy access to such facilities is essential for the management of the crofter's wife and help may be required frequently and rapidly from colleagues, particularly surgeons, radiologists and bacteriologists. Transplantation on site is impractical with small patient numbers thus a strong link was established at an early stage with the nearest transplant unit, which is 100 miles away in Aberdeen.

PRESENTATION

The progress of renal disease is often insidious. When glomerular filtration rate (GFR) is below 20 ml/min the patient often complains of tiredness, anorexia, nausea and dyspnoea. Thirst and nocturia may be elicited by direct questioning. Symptoms may affect any system of the body, and are well known. The commonest signs are the typical muddy skin pigmentation, anaemia, dry skin with pruritus and brown lines where the nail separates from the nail bed. Hypertension and a degree of cardiac failure are often found. Earlier intervention by dialysis has made severe peripheral neuropathy and muscle wasting much less common than heretofore. Pericarditis, uraemic frost and impaired consciousness are signs of advanced renal failure and indicate the need for urgent treatment to preserve life.

ASSESSMENT

It hardly needs stating that a full history and examination are essential. Particular attention should be given to cardiovascular status, previous illnesses including abdominal surgery, family history and social and personal circumstances. These may all influence the type of dialysis preferred for the patient. Consideration of potentially reversible or treatable causes of renal failure is always worthwhile, even if the possibility seems remote. Urinary tract obstruction may be insidious particularly with uterine carcinoma, prostatic hypertrophy and sometimes calculi. Analgesic ingestion leading to nephropathy is often overlooked and requires direct questioning. Systemic lupus erythematosus, polyarteritis and Wegener's granulomatosis do not always present with florid symptoms. Treatment of these disorders can slow down or even halt decline in renal failure. Many drugs have a nephrotoxic potential and a detailed history of medication intake is essential. Acute interstitial nephritis, I suspect, is underdiagnosed and may at first masquerade as chronic renal failure. Tuberculosis still causes surprises and it is important to consider this possibility.

LABORATORY INVESTIGATIONS

The value of basic tests should not be underestimated. An ESR in excess of 100 mm is often the pointer to myeloma, systemic lupus erythematosus or polyarteritis. Granular casts in the urine are always significant and occasionally necrotic papillae may be found indicating unsuspected analgesic nephropathy. An ASO titre, anti-nuclear factor assay and DNA binding assay are routine, and more recently the test for anti-neutrophil cytoplasm antibody (ANCA) has aided the diagnosis of Wegener's granulomatosis and some cases of polyarteritis.

Creatinine clearance is a useful clinical measurement of GFR but is not essential. Serial measurements of serum creatinine are the most readily available guide to change in GFR, but certain facts about creatinine levels should be remembered. Creatinine is produced in proportion to muscle mass and in a frail lady an apparently low creatinine may accompany advanced renal failure. In a few patients tubular secretion increases with advancing failure, again underestimating the degree of glomerular failure. Conversely, unidentified compounds excreted in renal failure may interfere with the assay and overestimate the severity of failure. Plotting the reciprocal of serum creatinine against time will produce a straight line. Extrapolation of this line allows estimation of the time by which dialysis will be required. However, a serum creatinine and good clinical judgement are perfectly adequate.

All patients should be tested for HbsAg. HIV testing is not routine but the need for this must be considered by individual clinicians in the light of local circumstances.

Renal ultrasound should be performed to establish renal size. Our patient would have bilateral reduction in renal size with smooth outlines. The absence of hydronephrosis usually excludes urinary tract obstruction. Where renal size is normal, full investigation to establish the cause of renal failure is indicated. This would include percutaneous renal biopsy with ultrasound guidance. Biopsy of small end-stage kidneys is, however, inadvisable since it does not usually yield diagnostic material and a single kidney is a contraindication to biopsy.

Having reached the conclusion that the disease is irreversible and progressive, the situation is discussed fully and frankly with the patient. Her permission is requested to involve a close relative, in this case the husband. This principle is practised throughout the care of these patients over many years, and its importance is paramount—far exceeding the space allotted in this article.

TREATMENT

Prior to dialysis

Hypertension

Control of hypertension is crucial. The combination of a β-blocker, preferably one not excreted by the kidney (such as metoprolol) and a loop diuretic (such as frusemide) is commonly used. The addition of a calcium channel blocking agent is useful, and the more old fashioned methyldopa should not be forgotten. Captopril may be used in problem cases starting with low doses, following the customary test dose. If deterioration in renal function occurs with captopril it may indicate undiagnosed bilateral renal artery stenosis, and isotope renography and/or renal arteriography should be considered.

Fluid balance

Dehydration should be avoided. When diuretics are required to control oedema or left ventricular failure, frusemide is the drug of choice and progressively increasing doses occasionally up to 2–3 g/day can be used. Combination with metolazone is useful in cases of resistant oedema. Distally-acting diuretics should be avoided because of the danger of inducing hyperkalaemia.

Sodium

Reduced sodium diets are rather unpalatable and not usually necessary. If necessary sodium intake can be reduced to around 60 mmol/day by instructing that no salt should be added to food at the table.

Potassium

Hyperkalaemia is not usually a problem until the late stages of renal failure, and is usually an indication for commencing dialysis.

Dietary protein restriction

Dietary management has not retained the importance previously attached to it when dialysis facilities were restricted. Reduction of intake to 40 g protein/day produces improvement in many patients suffering from anorexia, nausea and vomiting. I regard severe symptoms as an indication for dialysis but the well-known Giandano–Giovanetti diet is useful where dialysis facilities are not readily accessible.

Anaemia

Blood transfusion should be kept to a minimum. When required on symptomatic grounds the haemoglobin should not be raised above 10 g/100 ml. Five units of blood are transfused to all patients however, since this appears to improve subsequent allograft survival. The mechanism for this is not understood. Erythropoietin is under evaluation in the pre-dialysis patient and may become routine management when the drug becomes less costly.

The treatment of bone disease and lipid abnormalities remains difficult and controversial. I do not prescribe therapy for the lipid abnormality associated with chronic renal failure. Much of the literature on bone disease deals with patients already on dialysis. If the expected time to dialysis is short, treatment with a phosphate binder and 1-α-hydroxycholecalciferol is usually postponed until dialysis has begun. Large doses of aluminium hydroxide promote aluminium retention and control of phosphate is usually poor even with the addition of calcium or magnesium carbonate until dialysis is started. Allopurinol is not given to control high serum uric acid levels unless there is clinical gout.

All staff and patients must assist in protecting the arm veins, particularly in the non-dominant arm which is the preferred site for an arteriovenous fistula.

Selection criteria

Most of the relative contraindications to dialysis have been discarded with growth in experience and facilities. Hepatitis B carrier status is my one absolute contraindication—but this is an ethical problem yet to be encountered. One major relative contraindication is poor cardiovascular status, with severe chronic left ventricular decompensation. The decision about fitness for dialysis is usually based on clinical appraisal, although echocardiography for example may help in assessing left ventricular function. Social and family circumstances are important, but living alone in an isolated area is not, per se, a barrier to successful treatment. Intellectual ability or psychiatric abnormality do not exclude dialysis within limits. Our present 38-year-old crofter's wife, presumably with a relatively fit husband, living in an isolated area, presents no real difficulties.

Time to commence dialysis

Time to start is judged by serum creatinine and clinical status. The previous starting level of 1400 μmol/l serum creatinine has been reduced to 800–1000 μmol/l on average, with the exception of diabetic patients who commence at a creatinine of not more than 800 μmol/l. This avoids the development of unwanted problems, such as pericarditis, and reduces initial morbidity and duration of hospital stay.

Plan for dialysis treatment

The strategy has changed with the advent of CAPD. Arteriovenous fistulae are not now planned 2–3 months prior to dialysis, unless haemodialysis is the only option. Quinton–Scribner shunts are rarely used but remain useful for some acute renal problems. Planned fistulae have in some patients remained unused and have thrombosed (usually after transplantation) wasting a precious site for future access. While an arteriovenous fistula can be very convenient it is now less justified if CAPD is the preferred option.

For our patient the choices are:

1. Insertion of a CAPD catheter when creatinine rises to approximately 600–800 μmol/l. Catheters will remain patent even if not used for 2–3 months.
2. Insertion of a subclavian or internal jugular dialysis catheter. This allows initial stabilization by haemodialysis. The technique is easily learned and has a low morbidity. Single-lumen catheters are much easier to insert than the double-lumen type, but the former require a machine with a double pump. After stabilization a CAPD catheter is inserted.
3. For very ill patients initial stabilization is achieved by temporary peritoneal dialysis. Although it is preferable not to breach the peritoneal cavity prior to CAPD, minor modifications to our intermittent peritoneal dialysis technique have reduced the infection risk substantially. The crofter's wife would be treated by temporary haemodialysis followed by early insertion of a CAPD catheter.

Choice of initial dialysis method

CAPD is our preferred method and growth in numbers on CAPD has paralleled that in other units. To my surprise patient acceptance is high and when the technique fails, most opt to try again.

Advantages

1. Better and smoother control of biochemistry.
2. Higher haemoglobin level and better sense of wellbeing.
3. Virtually no requirement for dietary or fluid restriction.
4. Technique easily learned—average training time 3 weeks.
5. No restriction on mobility.
6. No requirement for expensive house conversion.

Disadvantages

1. Need for surgery.
2. Peritonitis.
3. Catheter tunnel infection.
4. Herniae.
5. Extrusion of superficial cuff.
6. Subacute sclerosing peritonitis.

Technique

The standard Tenckhoff catheter with double cuffs is used, and we have found no good reason to change. Insertion is performed by an experienced surgeon at mini laparotomy and omentectomy is routine. Dialysis exchanges commence on the fifth day. Fluid exchanges earlier than this led to an unacceptable rate of fluid leak. Early heparinization of fluid was also abandoned. It led to wound haematomas and is not necessary to maintain catheter patency. Fluid exchange volumes are gradually increased to 2 litres, usually four times daily. Standard glucose fluids are used, either isotonic (347 mosm/kg, glucose 13.6 g/l) or hypertonic (486 mosm/kg, glucose 38.6 g/l). We aim to use not more than two hypertonic bags daily if required to control fluid balance.

Teaching patients the method of fluid exchange must be patient and meticulous. Dedicated enthusiastic nursing staff are the key to success. Each unit has evolved its own variations in method in the light of experience.

Once the patient is judged by the nursing staff to have mastered the technique, preparations are made for transfer home. The spouse is always invited to become involved during the training period but is not usually expected to help with CAPD unless the patient is disabled—for example in the case of one patient with spina bifida. Supplies are delivered at intervals of 2–4 weeks. Stores are bulky and provision of a garden shed has proved an economical way of providing additional space where necessary. Patients are supervized bimonthly, alternating a home visit by a dialysis sister with a hospital review by the consultant. The home visit system has proved valuable. A 24-hour on-call rota is staffed by the nurses to provide immediate advice on problems, and patients are encouraged to use this facility. A telephone is provided where required and the rental paid by the Health Service.

PROBLEMS

Peritonitis

This is the main problem. The symptoms are abdominal pain, cloudy dialysate and a positive dialysate culture. Infection usually results from contamination at the time of bag change or infection in the catheter tunnel. Gram-positive cocci are found in over 50% of episodes, particularly *Staphylococcus epidermidis* which may be difficult to treat. Fungal peritonitis can only be treated by catheter removal. All patients are taught the symptoms and signs and to start treatment immediately after telephone consultation.

Antibiotics are given intraperitoneally, and individual units have their own regimes. We usually start with cefotaxime, with a rapid change after 48 hours to vancomycin/netilmicin if no improvement occurs, and an organism has not been isolated. Urokinase 5000 units flushed through the catheter has proved useful in resistent peritonitis, presumably by removing infected debris from the catheter lumen. The unit target is to average no more than one episode of peritonitis per patient per year, however, patient susceptibility varies markedly. Some patients seem almost immune to infection and others have to abandon the technique because of recurring or resistant peritoneal infection.

Hernias

Hernias of all types may occur due to the increased intra-abdominal pressure from the CAPD fluid. They require surgical repair during a temporary period on haemodialysis.

Subacute sclerosing peritonitis

In this condition the peritoneum becomes thickened and fibrotic. The cause is unknown and the disease usually fatal. I have no personal experience of this.

Other therapeutic considerations

Hypertension

If fluid balance is properly maintained by judicious use of hypertonic 'strong' bags, antihypertensive drugs are required in very few patients. Persisting uncontrolled severe hypertension may require consideration of bilateral nephrectomy.

Anaemia

The situation is being revolutionized by the advent of erythropoietin. The manufacturers' instructions seem adequate for initiation of therapy. We are still gaining experience in the use of erythropoietin. Treatment, although effective, is expensive and for some physicians the mainstay will still be blood transfusion. Multiple transfusions may lead to iron overload and antibody production may cause problems later with organ matching. Supplements of iron and folic acid are not given routinely and do not appear to be necessary in most patients, unless there is a demonstrable deficiency. The same applies to routine vitamin supplements.

Osteodystrophy

Bone disease is difficult to control in the long term. Phosphate levels should be kept $\leqslant 2$ mmol/l. If necessary phosphate binders are prescribed. Alucaps 1 or 2 t.i.d. are most effective, but lead to aluminium accumulation. Calcium carbonate 2 g/day or magnesium carbonate 1500 µg/day are less satisfactory.

Alphacalcidol 0.25–2.0 µg/day is then added to raise serum calcium to the normal range. This aids healing of hyperparathyroid bone changes. In the longer term it may be necessary to resort to parathyroidectomy.

Transplant

All patients possible are entered on the UK Transplant Recipient List. Tissue typing is unavailable locally, but can be arranged at the Transplant Centre. Transport of patients for transplant, even in bad weather during darkness, has not been a problem due to the excellent helicopter service provided by the RAF. Transport is arranged by road or rail wherever possible.

Haemodialysis

Smaller numbers are now treated by machine. Some are transferred from peritoneal dialysis. A few are judged unsuitable for CAPD at the start, and some patients opt for haemodialysis as the preferred method. Vascular access is the key to success. A Cimino–Brescia fistula is the method of choice and Goretex grafts have proved serviceable in difficult cases. We have not had to resort to permanent internal jugular or subclavian lines.

Machines and dialysers

There are many good machines and dialysers. Choice is dictated partly by personal preference and partly by cost. A facility for bicarbonate dialysis and ultrafiltration is useful. Dialyser choice is dictated mainly by patient requirements and less by cost. Dialyser re-use is not recommended.

There are many publications on dialysis management. Our regime is 3×4-hourly haemodialyses weekly: initial twice-weekly dialysis proving unsatisfactory. Heparin dosage is established individually.

Home dialysis

All patients considered suitable are trained for home dialysis. Again there is much literature available about the practical, economical and psychosocial aspects of home treatment. We commenced with standard machines and home adaptations. This, however, is costly particularly if the patient is transplanted or dies soon after going home. If the crofter's wife requires haemodialysis in the future we would use a REDY machine. Minimal adaptation is required in most homes beyond checking the electricity supply, supplying a warning buzzer, ensuring adequate heating and lighting in the dialysis room and installing a standard washbasin with elbow operated taps. A telephone and/or extension is also fitted. We have not experienced problems with aluminium toxicity which is a theoretical hazard with the REDY machine. Because of this and the general unsuitability of water supplies in our area, water treated by reverse osmosis (RO) is supplied by the unit. Alternatively an RO plant can be placed in the house if there is adequate water pressure. All water supplies must be analysed to check contents of Al, Cu, Pb etc. Since assay results show wide fluctuations, for example in Al we always recommend using filtered and RO treated water, with a regular check to ensure that the RO plant is functioning properly. Aluminium accumulation worsens anaemia and osteodystrophy of dialysis patients. When severe it causes a specific type of dementia. When signs of cerebral damage appear the disorder is irreversible and may be rapidly fatal. A pure water supply is therefore essential.

Hopefully our crofter's wife will be transplanted after a not too lengthy period on CAPD.

CONCLUSIONS

I have tried to outline our standard plan of management but many factors may lead to change along the way. Although the approach to management reflects my personal experience it does not differ substantially, I believe, from treatment in other units. We have adhered to basic well-tried techniques partly because it is easier if all staff know the basic approach to each patient. The therapy is effective although far from perfect, but I am not convinced that newer techniques are essentially any better or any more cost-effective. The setting up of a renal service in what appeared initially to be a difficult area has not proved as difficult as expected, and has certainly been very rewarding.

My outline of the management of end-stage renal disease is of necessity very superficial in an article of this size. Although there are several excellent textbooks which form a good starting point for the uninitiated, for those wishing to progress further there is no substitute for practical 'hands on' experience which can only be gained in a large established dialysis unit.

FURTHER READING

Black D, Jones N F 1979 (eds) Renal disease, 4th edn. Blackwell Scientific Publications, Oxford
Catto G R D, Power, D A 1988 Nephrology in clinical practice, 1st edn. Edward Arnold, London
Drukker W, Parsons F M, Maher J F 1983 Replacement of renal function by dialysis. Martinus Nijhoff, Boston

14. A 65-year-old with severe psoriasis

J. Thomson

INTRODUCTION

Many forms of treatment are available for a 65-year-old with severe psoriasis. To select the most appropriate therapy for that individual involves an initial accurate clinical assessment. Psoriasis is a capricious disease which may have natural remissions or exacerbations for no known reason. Moreover, no form of treatment currently available can be deemed to 'cure' psoriasis.

PSORIASIS

Clinical assessment: history

In a condition such as psoriasis which may be easily diagnosable both by the patient and the doctor there is a tendency to abbreviate the history and move directly to clinical examination. This must be avoided, otherwise inappropriate choices of therapy may be made. Some factors which are important are as undernoted.

The patient's place of residence and transport facilities should be known as there is little point in organizing frequent attendances at hospital if the person comes from an island with a once-weekly ferry. More aggressive treatment may be indicated in someone with symptomatic, longstanding or publicly visible psoriasis. Most patients have little or no idea as to what flares their psoriasis but it is worth asking, as some can be related to factors such as stress. Most find that sunshine improves their psoriasis but occasionally it can be a precipitating factor.

A past history of previous skin conditions or general medical conditions is important. Previous sun-induced tumours would preclude treatment with ultraviolet light and gross hyperlipidaemia would rule out treatment with retinoids. Musculoskeletal disease might lead to difficulties in applying topical agents. Some drugs, such as lithium, might aggravate psoriasis, some may cause a psoriasiform eruption, e.g. beta-blockers, and some might be incompatible with proposed treatment, e.g. systemic steroids and methotrexate. Apparent over-concern might be explained by the knowledge of severe incapacitating psoriasis in the family history. It is essential to spend time on the social history. Psoriasis can be an expensive disease. Some can afford relaxing sunny holidays and others cannot. Some find the damaging of clothes and bedlinen by messy topical treatments unacceptable. Others have an excessive alcohol intake, which may be related to the depression engendered by the disease, but it may make the physician wish to avoid potentially hepatotoxic treatments. The attitude of the patient's partner or household members is important for morale and for help in the application of treatment and dealing with soiled bed linen and clothing. A 65-year-old man might have paternity desires and it would be important to know this to avoid potentially spermatotoxic drugs.

If the patient's occupation is one where psoriasis can be seen by other employees or members of the public, vigorous treatment may be important to minimize problems and to allow the person to retire on maximum pension. Similarly, psoriasis may affect the choice of new activities such as swimming at a time when this could be an important preparation for retirement.

Finally a knowledge of previous treatment is important as there is little point in suggesting one which has previously failed.

Clinical examination

A full clinical examination is essential. It may seem heretical to say that the clinician should be satisfied that the patient is indeed suffering from psoriasis. Many a doctor (senior dermatologist amongst them) have been fooled by other red, scaly rashes masquerading as psoriasis and vice versa.

The examination of the skin should initially determine the distribution patterns which are vitally important in the diagnosis. It should include looking for nail changes, which may or may not be present and for mucous membrane changes which should be absent. The type of psoriasis should be noted. In the common plaque form, some attempt should be made to assess extent. This can be done visually using the rule of nines system as for assessing burns, but is notoriously variable both between and even within observers. The Psoriasis Area and Severity Index (PASI) score (Fredriksson & Pettersson 1978) is too cumbersome for routine clinics and in any case may also be subject to assessor error (Marks et al 1989).

Having an objective measurement is a help in assessing progress particularly if different doctors review progress. An absolute number is not the 'be all and end all', e.g. 1% psoriasis on the face may demand more treatment than 40% psoriasis on covered areas. Simple diagrammatic records are often easier to assess progress than numerical calculations. The type of psoriasis found on examination will have a very great influence on the selection of subsequent treatment.

Guttate psoriasis

Guttate psoriasis with its scattered small 'raindrop' lesions is much less common in the elderly. It may be a sequel to minor infections such as a streptococcal sore throat. It usually clears spontaneously in approximately 6 weeks and thus little treatment may be necessary.

Plaque psoriasis

Plaque psoriasis has a predilection for the elbows, knees, scalp and sacral region but it may affect all skin or any area. Individual plaques have a clear demarcation with normal skin. They are covered by silvery scales, the colour being enhanced by light scraping. Removal of the scales can lead to bleeding (Auspitz's sign). Treatment is proportional to the extent and degree of visibility.

Pustular psoriasis

A localized form may affect palms and/or soles which may be socially or professionally devastating. Generalized pustular psoriasis renders the patient very unwell, pyrexial and toxic, and urgent hospital admission is required.

Erythrodermatous and/or exfoliative psoriasis

There is widespread redness and scaling. The patient is very unwell, pyrexial and toxic requiring urgent hospital admission.

Nail psoriasis

There may be sporadic and variable involvement. The pathognomonic type is with linear sharp pits (pepper pot pitting). Variants, not unique to psoriasis, include detachment of the nail plate (onycholysis) or thickened crumbly nails. The treatment is proportional to the extent and the patient's social and working circumstances.

Intertriginous/genital psoriasis

Raw painful areas may cause profound disabilities disproportionate to the area extent.

Psoriatic arthropathy

A minority of patients have the coexisting, occasionally disabling, arthritis. Sometimes clearing the psoriasis may help the arthritis.

Patient education

In Biblical times, psoriasis was often mistaken for leprosy and to a certain extent the 'leper complex' remains today. There are many misconceptions in the public mind about psoriasis. Until patients are aware of the behaviour of their disease, it can be a very frightening condition with, at times, its rapid spread. Often its manifestations are visually extensive and can result in other people avoiding direct or indirect body contact. It is thus essential that the disease and possible therapies are explained to the patient. Comments such as 'it's only a skin disease and won't do your general health any harm' are unhelpful and incorrect. Even if the lesions can be covered, the accompanying aroma, scale shedding and bleeding soiling clothes and bed linen are all embarrassments.

In such a potentially long-term disease, sympathy and understanding from the physician are paramount. Rapport with the patient is all important. Some, though not all, find attending self-help groups beneficial.

Some common questions and possible replies are undernoted.

Question: Why have I developed psoriasis?

Reply: It may run in your family. It is a very common disease, approximately 2% of the population being affected. The cause is not known.

Q: Why do I scale?

R: The outer layers of your skin are turning over in 3–4 days (the normal is 28 days). Thus the outermost layer is incompletely formed and more easily detached.

Q: Is it infectious?

R: No.

Q: But if I cut my skin I sometimes get psoriasis in the healing cut.

R: This occurs in a number of skin conditions including psoriasis. It is called the Koebner phenomenon and is not due to infection.

Q: Does this mean I will not heal easily after surgery?

R: No. It has little or no effect on wound healing and strength.

Q: Can you cure psoriasis?

R: No. It may clear spontaneously but we cannot predict the course. We can help considerably and most people can lead a normal life.

Q: Will I give it to my children?

R: Not necessarily, but they will have an increased chance of developing it, especially if the other parent is also affected.

Q: Does diet affect it?

R: Probably not. Many diets have been tried but there is no proof of help. Trials of fish oil are not concluded.

Q: Should I avoid sun?

R: Not in moderation. Most psoriatics are helped by sun and thus ultraviolet light is used in some forms of treatment. If you are one of the few patients whose psoriasis is aggravated by sunlight obviously you should avoid it.

Q: Can patches of psoriasis turn into cancer?
R: This is almost unheard of in psoriasis and tar has been used for many years.
Q: But if I use coal tar on my psoriasis, is that not a cancer producing substance?
R: Again, almost unheard of in psoriasis, and tar has been used for very many years.
Q: I have scalp psoriasis. Will I lose my hair?
R: No. It may thin a little if your scalp is very red but will revert to normal.

Treatment

By this stage, the clinician has a considerable knowledge about the patient, as a person, with his/her modus vivendi and the type and extent of the disease. The first decision is whether to use topical or systemic (second-line) treatment. Commoner topical agents would include the undernoted.

Emollients such as yellow soft paraffin or aqueous cream

These are the only feasible topical treatment in erythrodermatous and exfoliative psoriasis. They may be useful also, with or without polythene occlusion, in removing scale from crusted plaque psoriasis. The disadvantages are that they are non-specific and will rarely control the condition on their own.

Tars

Coal tars made up in 5–30% in yellow soft paraffin are a long established treatment, particularly in plaque psoriasis. They may act synergistically with ultraviolet light therapy. They are very messy and malodorous and they may cause tar folliculitis especially in closed areas such as axillae. Cleaner extracted tars and proprietaries are less messy but generally less effective. Wood tars such as oil of cade 6–12% emulsion have long been used in the treatment of scalp psoriasis but suffer from the same cosmetic problems.

Dithranol (Anthralin in USA)

This is useful in plaque psoriasis and was traditionally held in place by mixing 0.1% up to about 5% in stiff Lassar's paste. The disadvantages are a marked surrounding pigmentation, burning in sensitive areas and discoloration of hair, clothes and baths. Some of these disadvantages are lessened by the use of proprietary dithranol in a cream base which is washed off after about half an hour. This is called short contact therapy.

Salicylic acid

10–20% is mixed in yellow soft paraffin. It is cleaner than Dithranol and tar but often less effective and occasionally absorption may lead to salicylism. For the scalp it can be mixed with aqueous cream but this has a very short shelf life.

Topical steroids

Topical steroids work in psoriasis and are liked by patients because they are clean and produce a rapid response. The problem is that the more potent ones are more effective and there is therefore a likelihood of side effects such as skin atrophy. Their efficacy tends to be time-limited requiring escalation to more potent ones. There is often a rapid rebound on cessation, thus their use should be minimal. They may be used with discretion in exposed sites or axillae and groins.

Ultraviolet light

UVB (280–320 nm) can be listed under topicals because it is usually used alone. It helps many patients suffering from guttate or plaque psoriasis. Its effect can be potentiated by topical tar or enhanced by applying an emollient such as coconut oil to the scaly plaques.

Other topicals

Topical vitamin D analogues, cyclosporin A, etc. are at present not fully assessed.

In all topicals with messy agents, light bandaging such as Tubegauze helps to stop the preparation being rubbed off and reduces the soiling of clothes.

Systemic treatment

The decision to use systemic therapy is usually based on:

Failure of topical treatment
Severe forms of psoriasis, e.g. erythrodermatous or widespread pustular psoriasis
A marked reduction in individual patient's quality of life

Treatments available are:

PUVA
Methotrexate
Retinoids

Hydroxyurea
Systemic steroids
Others

PUVA

PUVA is an acronym for *P*soralen (the photosensitivity agent) and ultra violet radiation of the *A* range (320–400 nm). It harnesses the fact that most psoriatics are improved by sunshine. Some may go to the sunny shores of the Dead Sea Centre where there is a spectral shift to longer wave lengths. Some are treated with UVB (280–320 nm) with no systemic medication though the effect is enhanced by topical tar. Psoriatics generally seem to respond best to the wave lengths of approximately 300–315 nm. Lower wave lengths have little or no effect. The therapeutic cut-off in longer wave lengths is less clear, tailing off sharply at about 320 nm and then more gradually to approximately 360 nm. UVA given alone may be effective but is impractical due to the large doses requiring an inordinate time exposure to achieve this. UVA is thought to be less damaging to the skin in general.

The psoralen is activated by UVA (but not UVB). Thus PUVA therapy seems to offer the most beneficial effects with the least number of adverse factors.

The psoralen may be applied locally but due to practical difficulties, oral administration is commonest except where small areas of, say, pustular psoriasis occurs on the palms and soles. Currently 8-methoxy psoralen (8MOP) is the usual drug though others are available and may supersede it. It inhibits cell replication by combining with DNA (Walter et al 1973).

PUVA is a clean form of treatment, highly effective (90%) in plaque psoriasis, but usually avoided in severe exfoliative erythrodermatous or generalized pustular psoriasis. It does, however, require well-maintained suitable equipment, usually hospital based. The physician must be familiar with the apparatus used. It is time-consuming and very wasteful of medical time unless some of the supervision can be done by trained ancillary staff, usually nurses.

Treatment regimes vary considerably in different centres. The orthodox dose of 8MOP would be 0.6 mg/kg body weight taken 2 hours before treatment. If taken with a small meal there is better absorption and less nausea. The minimal phototoxicity dose (MPD) is determined by exposing areas of untanned (usually buttock) skin to increasing dose of UVA after giving 8MOP. The dose of UVA is measured in joules per square centimetre (J/cm^2). The MPD is the dose required to produce a just visible erythema which should ideally be assessed at 72 hours after testing, the time of the maximum phototoxicity (Wolff et al 1977). The therapy is commenced at the MPD with three sessions per week. The psoralen dose is then held and the UVA exposure increased in steps of 0.5 to 1.5 J/cm^2 according to the response, ensuring at least a 72-hour gap between alterations. Once satisfactory clearance has been achieved exposures can be reduced to say one or two per week.

PUVA therapy is well established but there is still concern about the long-term effect on the skin. It thus seems prudent to be cautious about inaugurating it in the young, especially those who burn easily in the natural sun. The same caveat would apply to its use in persons with evidence of past sun damage such as solar-induced skin tumours. Previous arsenic intake may be cumulative with UVA in producing cutaneous malignancies.

It should not be used in those where light may be a trigger in aggravating their disease such as lupus erythematosus or porphyria cutanea tarda. Prior to treatment it is worth ensuring that there is not a high anti-nuclear antibody titre. Photosensitivity may be unexpectedly enhanced if the patient is receiving, or subsequently commences on, a potentially photo-sensitizing drug such as tetracycline or antihistamine etc. The drug list should be checked before and during treatment.

Psoralen excretion may be grossly impaired in severe renal or hepatic disease. High blood levels of the drug would therefore ensue. The pre-treatment checks should include liver and renal function tests and should be followed during treatment at intervals of about 3–4 months.

There is dispute as to whether PUVA treatment leads to cataract for-mation in humans. Nevertheless it is wise to organize a pretreatment ophthalmic assessment and at 6–12 month intervals thereafter. Existing cataracts should preclude PUVA. UVA opaque glasses should be worn during the entire period of increased photosensitivity.

The commonest side effects are nausea, erythema, hyperpigmentation, which may be of a blotchy nature, and occasionally severe pruritus. Less commonly, dizziness, headaches, burns or blisters may occur. Rarely photosensitive dermatoses may be induced.

Methotrexate

Methotrexate (MTX) is a cytotoxic antimetabolite acting in the 'S' phase of cell division by competitively inhibiting dihydrofolate reductase. This stops cellular replication by blocking the reduction of dihydrofolate to tetrahydrofolate. MTX has been used in the treatment of some forms of psoriasis for about 30 years. It is readily available worldwide.

It can be used for the treatment of severe erythrodermic or pustular psoriasis but may have a place in some localized forms and in psoriatic arthropathy. It can be given orally or parenterally and has the advantage of rapid action. Changes in the lesion start within 24 hours of commencing intravenous MTX. While 100% clearing is the optimum, this is rarely achieved. MTX needs to be given by experienced clinicians and requires careful supervision and monitoring. It is essential to explain about the drug to the patient. Many of the problems reported have arisen because of poor supervision or a lack of awareness of side effects and drug interactions. The full blood count must be checked pretreatment. Leucopenia or thrombo-cytopenia would be contraindications. Because abrupt falls may occur unexpectedly, regular checks are essential every 2 weeks or so.

High serum levels, with increased chance of toxicity, may occur in patients with renal impairment and lower doses should thus be employed. MTX itself may be nephrotoxic and its concurrent administration with other such drugs should be avoided. It may also cause a distressing mucositis of the renal tract or other mucous membranes which is reversible with leucovorin.

Unexpectedly high levels of MTX may occur when it is administered along with other drugs which displace it from its protein binding. These drugs include salicylates, acid anti-inflammatories, diuretics, hypoglycae-mics, sulphonamides, tetracyclines, chloramphenicals, β-aminobenzoic acid and diphenylhydantoins. Cumulative immunosuppressive effects may occur if it is given along with other cytostatic drugs or systemic corti-costeroids.

The main hazard in the use of MTX in dermatology is its potential hepatotoxicity with the development of changes very similar to that seen in alcoholic liver disease. Careful pretreatment assessment and subsequent monitoring is mandatory. Ideally there should be normal liver function tests and a normal liver biopsy prior to treatment. If the overlying skin is too inflamed occasionally the biopsy may require to be delayed. It should be repeated every 1500 mg MTX. Liver ultrasound examinations and other non-invasive tests cannot at present substitute for liver biopsy, though there is hope that analyses of serum aminoterminal propeptide of type III procollagen (P111NP) might (Zachariae 1990).

Potentiating risk factors to liver damage include heavy alcohol intake, obesity, other hepatotoxic drugs, and previous arsenic administration. In all such patients MTX, if used at all, should be used with caution.

MTX is spermatotoxic and if our 65-year-old was a male with paternity desires, it should not be given.

The commonest side effects are nausea or abdominal discomfort and occasionally vomiting. Less commonly fatigue and headache occur. Some patients complain of mucous membrane lesions or a burning sensation in the plaques. Rarely there may be fever, depression or hair loss. To counter the acute side effects leucovorin (folinic acid) should be readily available. This is a metabolite of folic acid and an essential co-enzyme for nucleic acid synthesis. If given within 12–24 hours in a dose of up to 120 mg/day it may counter some of the toxic effects.

There are health hazards and legal requirements for personnel handling the drugs, especially females in the childbearing years. Appropriate protec-tive measures and emergency equipment should be provided.

Many regimes have been described. It is probably best for each depart-ment to adhere to one regime although it may require alteration in indi-vidual patients. A fairly standard regime would be as follows:

Pretreatment checks
Low test dose, e.g. 2.5–5 mg to exclude idiosyncratic reactions
10–25 mg orally, intravenously or intramuscularly ONCE weekly.
Some centres use an intermittent weekly oral schedule in divided doses.

MTX is an effective, well-tried, generally safe drug but careful monitoring, especially in the early stages, is necessary. A flow chart with cumulative doses and appropriate headings for concomitant drugs is highly recommended.

Retinoids

Vitamin A (Retinol) has a number of essential functions in man including the maintenance and differentiation of epithelial tissues. Various natural derivatives plus synthetic ones are called retinoids and some have been found to have useful therapeutic effects. Different diseases seem to respond better to different retinoids. As far as psoriasis is concerned, the most useful at present is etretinate (Tigason®; Tegison® USA).

Used in adequate doses, it is a useful drug particularly in generalized pustular psoriasis where some therapeutic effect is apparent in 1–2 weeks with full benefit in approximately 5 weeks. It also has a place in the treatment of disabling localized psoriasis, a lesser place in exfoliative psoriasis, and a lesser place in plaque psoriasis.

As far as the UK is concerned, it is available only on a hospital prescription due to the fear of its inadvertently being taken by pregnant women with potentially disastrous tetratogenic effects. Patients taking retinoids must not be blood donors in case the blood were used in pregnant females. Etretinate has a long half-life and this embargo must remain for at least 2 years after it is stopped.

The drug is bound to a specific transport protein. Higher than expected blood levels may occur in severe renal impairment leading to diminished excretion. Although etretinate is much less hepatotoxic than MTX, severe dysfunction would be a contraindication and the liver function tests require to be monitored. Great care is necessary if other potentially hepatotoxic drugs are administered along with it.

All retinoids may increase blood lipid levels and etretinate for psoriasis — being fairly long-term treatment — may do this. Risk factors are a strong family history of hyperlipidaemia, obesity, alcohol abuse, heavy smoking or diabetes mellitus. Lipid levels must be monitored. Fasting levels are more easily compared and are carried out pretreatment and then monthly, reducing to 3 monthly. Significant rises may require dose reduction or treatment cessation but may respond to tackling the risk factors or to diet. It is still not clear if adequate reductions occur with Fish Oil Capsules or bezafibrate.

The patient's drug history must be ascertained before and during treatment. A high intake of vitamin A will be additive and may precipitate hypervitaminosis A. Some drugs may interfere with the action leading to a diminished clinical effect. These include anti-epileptics, salicylates, indomethacin and tetracycline. Hepatotoxic drugs have been mentioned previously.

Common side effects are hacking of the lips and dry nasal, oral or eye mucosae. Usually simple remedies will alleviate these. Less commonly hair thinning and alopecia may occur, usually reversible. Myalgia and arthralgia can be associated with reduced tolerance to exercise. Calcification of ligamentous structures may occur. In the para-vertebral arc this may be one cause of the DISH syndrome (diffuse idiopathic skeletal hyperostosis). With the desire to reduce radiation to a minimum a reasonable compromise might be pretreatment X-rays of the spine, tendon Achillis and wrist with repeat examination as indicated.

Very occasionally nausea, headache, malaise, drowsiness and sweating have been noted. Persistent headaches should alert the physician to the possibility of benign intracranial hypertension.

Once again, there are many individual variations, but the standard therapy is to start with an oral daily dosage of 1 mg/kg body weight per day up to a maximum of 75–100 mg/day. Once control is achieved, the dose can be reduced to 0.5 mg/kg body weight per day. If etretinate is given as the only treatment modality, a rebound is common on cessation of treatment.

Hydroxyurea

Hydroxyurea is an orally active drug which causes a marked reduction in the rate of DNA synthesis.

It is a potent mutagen. Though slower acting than MTX it has a useful place in treating patients with plaque psoriasis and to a lesser extent pustular psoriasis. It is useful in patients who cannot be given MTX.

Hydroxyurea is myelosuppressive being most toxic to the leucocytes, then the platelets and then the red blood cells. Haematological assessment pretreatment and weekly during therapy is required. Severe anaemia before therapy should be corrected by transfusion. Hydroxyurea may lead to early and usually transient megaloblastic appearances.

Both renal and liver function require to be assessed and monitored. The drug should be used with caution in severe renal impairment. Whilst less hepatotoxic than MTX it can occasionally lead to elevation of the liver enzymes. Hydroxyurea can lead to an increased level of urate in the blood provoking gout or even uric acid nephropathy. Appropriate estimates should be performed before and during treatment and the patient encouraged to maintain a high fluid intake. It may damage spermatozoa.

Side effects are relatively rare. There may be anorexia, nausea or diarrhoea and a variety of skin rashes have been described. The usual dose regime is 20–30 mg/kg body weight or 0.5–2 g/day in a single dose. Lower doses should be given to the elderly. Dosage regimes based on intermittent administration every third day may be less toxic to the white blood cells.

Systemic corticosteroids

Systemic corticosteroids have a very limited place in the treatment of psoriasis. They act quickly, but the price to pay is that the pendulum will almost inevitably swing to produce a more severe form of the disease, e.g. plaque psoriasis being converted to pustular psoriasis which is more recalcitrant to treatment. Perhaps their only place is to 'buy time' in life-threatening psoriasis when the chosen treatment will take a little time to act, but they should not be given without great thought. Systemic steroids administered for other reasons to psoriatic patients will cause the same problems.

Cyclosporin

Cyclosporin A (CyA) is a fungal metabolite and potent immunosuppressant. It has been in limited use for the treatment of psoriasis for about 7 years, but its exact role will require more time and study. Because of its immunosuppression, it should not be given to patients with current or previous malignancies (British Journal of Dermatology, Editorial 1990). Patients should not over-expose themselves to the sun. Other concurrent drugs may alter bioavailability. Possible reduction in blood levels occurs with rifampicin, anti-epileptics (phenobarbitone; phenytoin, primidone) and barbiturates. By contrast, the blood levels may increase with erythromycin, ketoconazole, calcium channel blockers (diltiazam; nicardipine; verapamil), danazol and progestogens. Hyperkalaemia can be a problem aggravated by ACE inhibitors, potassium-sparing diuretics and potassium salts themselves. Far and away cyclosporin's greatest side effect is nephrotoxicity with a rise in serum creatinine and blood pressure. This risk is increased if there is simultaneous administration of aminoglycosides, co-trimoxazole or amphotericin.

The kidney damage may be reversible on drug withdrawal or dose reduction. Unlike many other anti-psoriatic drugs, it is considered to have virtually no toxic effects on the marrow.

The current thoughts are to keep the dose below 5 mg/kg body weight. Baseline values of blood pressure, serum creatinine, liver function tests, electrolytes and urea, serum magnesium, uric acid and urinary protein levels are needed. Preferably renal function tests should be done. For the first 3 months, fortnightly follow-ups with particular emphasis on blood pressure and serum creatinine are required. It is considered that a rise of 30% of the serum creatinine above the patient's own individual baseline is important even if this level is still within the normal range.

Side effects which may be troublesome include hypertrichosis, gastro-intestinal disturbances, tremor, gum hyperplasia.

Razoxane

This drug should *not* now be used to treat psoriasis in view of its association with the development of leukaemias.

Combination treatments

The commonest combination is a systemic drug with some topical therapy as an adjunct. However, the physician is usually endeavouring to withdraw topical therapy to obviate the need for frequent local applications of messy preparations.

Mixing systemic treatments may be helpful, e.g. retinoids plus PUVA. Such regimes lie in the realms of the expert and are not without added risk, for example, methotrexate and etretinate may lead to life-threatening hepatitis (Zachariae 1990).

Choice of treatment

It is impossible to give a 'best buy' suitable for all patients. Suggested starting treatments and progressions are discussed below, but must be modified in accordance with individual circumstances.

Guttate psoriasis

Bland topicals, clean tars or salicylic acid preparations are usually all that are required till spontaneous settling occurs.

Plaque psoriasis

In all forms of stable plaque psoriasis topicals should be tried first of all, with PUVA as the second-line choice. The decision to move on to this depends on the patient's individual circumstances and the degree of skin involvement. Methotrexate or etretinate are further choices which may be employed, with hydroxyurea and cyclosporin to be considered thereafter. If plaque psoriasis is red and unstable bland topical treatments may be worth a trial, but the likelihood is that second-line treatment in the form of methotrexate or perhaps etretinate will be necessary sooner rather than later. Cyclosporin would be a third-line choice.

Pustular psoriasis

In a localized variety topical treatment should be tried. Topical steroids may be useful in this particular type of psoriasis, failing which PUVA to the localized area may be tried or methotrexate, failing which cyclosporin. In generalized pustular psoriasis the only topicals used should be bland and it is likely that early intervention with etretinate or methotrexate may be necessary. Less evaluated treatment would be with hydroxyurea of cyclosporin.

Erythrodermatous or exfoliative psoriasis

Topical bland preparations may be soothing but are unlikely to be very effective and it is usually necessary to move to methotrexate. If this fails hydroxyurea may be considered. The retinoids do not usually work so well but a trial may be indicated.

Psoriatic arthropathy

It may be appropriate to treat the psoriasis and arthritis separately. Methotrexate or etretinate for the psoriasis may occasionally help the joints as well, failing which a trial of PUVA may be indicated, although this does not often help the joints.

Nail psoriasis

Topical strong steroids around the nail bed may help, failing which the steroid can be injected into the nail bed. In some patients who have severe problems a trial of methotrexate or etretinate would be indicated.

Scalp psoriasis

This will usually respond to intensive topical therapy but occasionally etretinate requires to be employed.

CONCLUSION

The management of disabling psoriasis remains a therapeutic challenge. In general, the psoriatic of the present day is less willing than previous generations to tolerate disfiguring, disabling psoriasis or to treat with messy topicals. The search is on for a safe oral therapy. Some of those discussed in this article are still being assessed.

REFERENCES

Anonymous 1990 A consensus report: Cyclosporin A therapy for psoriasis. British Journal of Dermatology 122: Suppl. 36 1–3
British Journal of Dermatology 1990 Editorial 122(36): 1–3

Fredriksson T, Pettersson U 1978 Severe psoriasis—oral therapy with a new retinoid. Dermatologica 157: 238–244

Marks R, Barton S P, Shuttleworth D 1989 Assessment of disease progress in psoriasis. Archives of Dermatology 125: 235–240

Walter J F, Voorhees J J, Kelsey W H, Duell E A, Arbor A 1973 Psoralen plus black light inhibits epidermal DNA synthesis. Archives of Dermatology 107: 861–865

Wolff K, Gschnait F, Honigsmann H, Konrad K, Parrish J A, Fitzpatrick T B 1977 Phototesting and dosimetry for photochemotherapy. British Journal of Dermatology 96: 1–10

FURTHER READING

Fitzpatrick T B, Eisen A Z, Wolff K, Freedberg I M, Austen K F 1987 Dermatology in general medicine, 3rd edn. McGraw–Hill, New York, pp 461–491; 1441–1451; 1522–1529

Rook A, Wilkinson D S, Ebling F J G, Champion R H, Burton J L 1986 Textbook of dermatology, 4th edn. Blackwell Scientific Publications, Oxford, pp 1469–1532

Van de Kerhof P C M, Mier P D 1986 Textbooks of psoriasis. Churchill Livingstone, Edinburgh

Zachariae H 1990 Management of difficult psoriasis. In: Champion R H, Pye R J (eds) Recent advances in dermatology, Chapter 1, No. 8. Churchill Livingstone, Edinburgh, pp 1–20

15. A 50-year-old with non-Hodgkin's lymphoma

A. C. Parker

In this age group non-Hodgkin's lymphoma (NHL) is heterogeneous in terms of clinical presentation, extent of disease at diagnosis and in pathological classification. These factors have an important bearing on management and will be outlined before therapeutic strategies are delineated for specific but common clinical presentations.

INCIDENCE

In most developed countries the incidence of NHL has a wide range which may reflect true differences due to environmental and genetic causes or may be artefactual. In various series the incidence ranges from 10 to 20 per 100 000 of the population. In many countries there has been an increase over the last four decades which may be partially explained by improvement in diagnosis. In addition, as this disorder has an increased incidence with age, the shift to a more elderly population may help to explain the rise. There has been a slower increase in mortality probably because of the improvement in survival with modern therapy.

PRESENTATION

In practical terms a useful classification is into patients with nodal and extranodal lymphoma.

In an unpublished review of cases from the East of Scotland registry, 16% of a total of 845 patients analysed had extranodal disease only. The three tissues most commonly involved were GI tract (5.3%), bone (2.8%) and skin (2.7%). The other organs involved (1% or less) were thyroid, genitourinary tract, CNS, liver, muscle, lung, salivary glands and breast. This type of extranodal involvement in NHL contrasts markedly with the situation in Hodgkin's disease where amongst 384 patients there were only 4 with extranodal disease (1%). This demonstrates a major biological difference between the two disorders of profound importance therapeutically and prognostically. Examples of skin involvement are shown in Fig. 15.1.

In the same survey 250 patients with NHL had 'pure' nodal disease

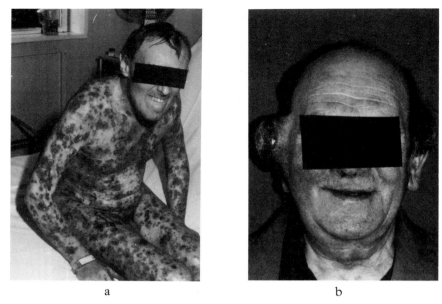

a   b

Fig. 15.1   (a) Patient with generalized skin lymphoma. (b) Patient with large 'localized' skin lymphoma.

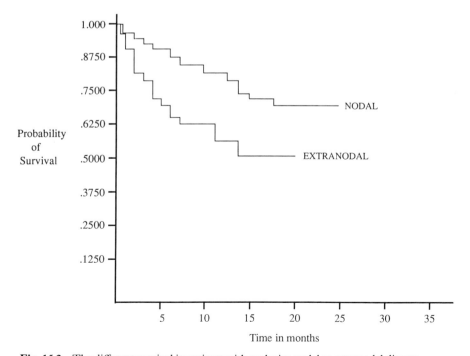

Fig. 15.2   The different survival in patients with exclusive nodal or extranodal disease.

(29%). Although there was a tendency for supraclavicular nodes to be most commonly involved, in general, nodal involvement was almost equally represented in axillary and inguinal regions.

In the remaining 55% of patients there was a combination of nodal and extranodal involvement. In these the most commonly involved extranodal organ was bone followed by gut, liver, lung and skin. This analysis showed a difference in survival between patients with nodal as against patients with extranodal disease (Fig. 15.2).

Definition of involvement in terms of tissue affected is thus of prognostic importance as is the assessment of 'bulk' of disease.

STAGING

Measuring the 'bulk' of disease in NHL is dependent on a combination of clinical and laboratory assessment, called staging. In adult lymphoma the most commonly used system is the Ann Arbor classification (Table 15.1).

Although it has proven to be of major use in establishing a logical approach to lymphoma patients the Ann Arbor criteria do not cope adequately with other individual prognostic factors which have either independent or interdependent effects on survival. These factors include tumour volume, which as it increases, adversely affects prognosis, patient performance status, serum lactic dehydrogenase level at presentation and the proliferative potential of the tumour. Other adverse prognostic factors are increasing age and cytogenetic abnormality, the latter perhaps indicating clonal evolution (Yunis et al 1987). Histology is helpful in defining prognostic subgroups. Staging is of importance in terms of management. The procedures utilized are dependent upon available resources but much information can be gained from relatively simple tests.

Clinical examination and history are essential to define the extent of the disease, the performance status of the patient and the presence or absence of 'B' symptoms (Table 15.1). The latter are relatively strong adverse prog-

Table 15.1   The Ann Arbor staging classification for malignant lymphoma

Stage	Definition
I	Involvement of a single lymph node site or of a single extranodal organ or site (I_E).
II	Involvement of two or more lymph node regions on the same side of the diaphragm, or localized involvement of an extranodal site or organ (II_E) and one or more lymph node regions on the same side of the diaphragm.
III	Involvement of lymph node regions on both sides of the diaphragm, which may also be accompanied by localized involvement of an extranodal organ or site (III_E) or spleen (III_S) or both (III_{SE}).
IV	Diffuse or disseminated involvement of one or more distant extranodal organs with or without associated lymph node involvement.
	Fever $> 38°C$, night sweats and/or weight loss $> 10\%$ of body weight in the 6 months preceding admission are defined as systemic symptoms and denoted by the suffix B. Other patients are denoted by the suffix A.

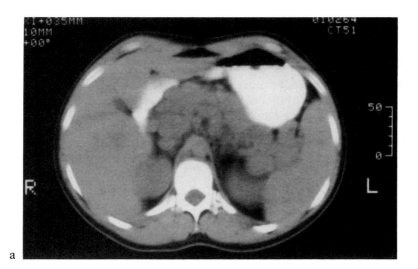

a

nostic indicators. In many cases the clinical assessment will indicate, without any ancillary help, an impending, potentially disastrous complication such as extradural spinal cord compression. In all cases, if only as a baseline, measurement of biochemical tests and liver, renal and bone marrow function together with serum LDH and uric acid are particularly useful. Any abnormalities in these measurements require appropriate further investigation.

In terms of radiological investigations all patients should have routine PA and lateral chest X-rays and thoracic, abdominal and pelvic CT scan. A typical scan showing intra-abdominal involvement in a patient with NHL is shown in Fig. 15.3a. The sensitivity of CT scanning is improved, particularly in defining liver and splenic involvement, using ethiodized oil emulsion (Fig. 15.3b, c). This technique is not widely available.

The use of ultrasound can be complementary to, or can, in a particularly thin patient, replace CT scanning. It is highly operator dependent and interpretation can be difficult, however in reliable hands, it is repeatable and thus can assess tumour responsiveness rapidly.

Lymphography is used for the assessment of lymphoma in a few centres. It is time consuming, relatively invasive and does not define extranodal disease or nodal involvement in the upper abdomen. It is, however, sensitive and as the dye remains in the nodes for some months, follow-up assessment of progress by plain abdominal X-rays is feasible.

For logistical and economic reasons radio-isotope scans should be selected carefully. In some centres such scans are considered an essential part of the basic work up in NHL.

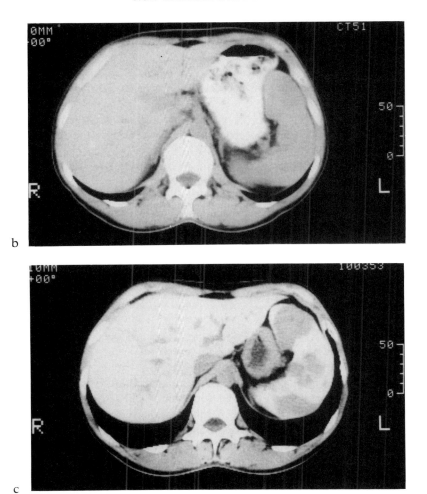

b

c

Fig. 15.3   (a) Abdominal CT scan showing extensive nodal enlargement due to lymphoma. CT scan before (b) and after (c) ethiodized oil emulsion demonstrating clearly intrasplenic deposits after the procedure.

HISTOLOGICAL INVESTIGATIONS

As the incidence of bone marrow involvement in NHL is much higher than in Hodgkin's disease, bone marrow aspiration and biopsy should be carried out. It is sometimes recommended that multiple sites should be biopsied but this should only be done if it is likely to change management. In most cases patients who have bone marrow involvement have an abnormal peripheral blood count.

It is useful to examine any other accessible abnormal tissue for example, pleural fluid. Cerebrospinal fluid does not require to be examined routinely although there is controversy about the population of patients who should undergo the procedure. Central nervous system (CNS) involvement in low grade NHL is uncommon and usually of the extradural type. CNS involvement is commoner in high or intermediate grade NHL and more commonly shows a diffuse leptomeningeal pattern. In one series 7/213 with high or intermediate grade disease had CNS involvement; of these, 6 had stage IV disease (Sheehan et al 1989). Thus consideration of CSF examination should be given in advanced intermediate/high grade lymphoma particularly in the younger patient.

The examination of blood and marrow by means of molecular biological techniques is new, developing and potentially of major importance. Detection rates of tumour cells using the polymerase chain reaction can be 1 in 10^6 cells with technology presently available in certain defined types of lymphoma (Lee et al 1987). The significance of positive results by such sensitive techniques is at present unclear in terms of initial staging, for deciding on therapeutic options, for follow-up in defining remission and in deciding on intensive therapeutic manoeuvres such as autologous bone marrow transplantation.

Histology

Histology has an important part to play in helping management decisions. Although there is a tendency for lymph node aspiration to be increasingly used for diagnostic purposes, such an approach has little or no part to play in the diagnosis and classification of malignant lymphoma. It would be foolhardy to accept the implications of the diagnosis of malignant lymphoma based on such a technique in other than exceptional circumstances.

Node or appropriate tissue biopsy is at present essential for proper and reliable diagnosis of this clinical condition. Once removed such tissue can yield a large amount of information, much of immediate clinical importance. The most widely used and clinically helpful classification is the working formulation, shown in a simplified version in Table 15.2. For accuracy, according to this scheme it is vital to have adequate, atraumatized material. In most hospital pathology departments where significant numbers of patients with malignant lymphoma are seen, fresh tissue is usually sent by the surgeon for examination. This allows immunological methods to be performed, cytogenetics to be defined and molecular, viral and other studies to be carried out in addition to standard histology.

It is a moot point at present whether the extensive application of monoclonal (monospecific) antibodies has been a major advance in terms of steering clinical decisions. They are extensively used. Predominantly these antibodies are used on frozen sections but some very useful antibodies react with formalin-fixed tissue namely leucocyte common antigen (CD 45) and leu M1 (CD 15). The leucocyte common antigen is very useful in differen-

Table 15.2 An abbreviated form of one of the most commonly used classifications in non-Hodgkin's lymphoma—the working formulation

---

LOW GRADE
A. Small lymphocytic (CLL)
B. Follicular/small cleaved cells
C. Follicular/small cleaved/large cells

INTERMEDIATE GRADE
D. Follicular—large cell
E. Diffuse—small cleaved
F. Diffuse—mixed small/large
G. Diffuse—large cleaved

HIGH GRADE
H. Large cell/immunoblastic
I. Lymphoblastic
J. Small non-cleaved cell

---

tial diagnosis of lymphoma from undifferentiated carcinoma. Leu M1 is found on neoplastic cells in Hodgkin's disease and can be used to differentiate Hodgkin's disease from high grade NHL. The precise significance of the immunophenotype in terms of clinical prognosis is by no means clear. Many T cell tumours within the same subgroups have not been shown to be worse prognostically than their B cell counterparts, which is in contrast to opinions previously held and based on preliminary evidence.

For practical and clinical purposes the important division is between low and intermediate/high grade lymphomas according to the working formulation. Low grade lymphomas usually follow an indolent course and are often disseminated at diagnosis. They form a 'bridge' between easily recognized chronic lymphatic leukaemia and intermediate grade lymphomas. However, intermediate and more especially high grade lymphomas are aggressive neoplasms which more commonly involve extranodal sites. It is important to emphasize that many of these patients can be cured by appropriate treatment despite unfavourable histology.

It is important to define the extent of disease in an individual. Often patients are being entered into prescribed ethical studies with standard investigational protocols, if not, staging investigation should be tailored to clinical findings and other simple investigations. This minimizes discomfort, inconvenience and expense.

It is extremely important to have excellent histological advice. In the case of malignant lymphoma, which is a difficult field, adequate tissue is required and the opinion of a pathologist experienced in this field is of utmost importance. The role of the many additional investigations which can be performed on such tissue has been discussed briefly but at present plays a subsidiary role in guiding therapy.

THERAPEUTIC OPTIONS IN A PATIENT WITH NHL

As the variation in this disorder is so great the most logical way of illustration is to list types of treatment available and indicate their role in a few clinical vignettes.

Radiotherapy

Although radiation oncologists may disagree the role of this modality in the treatment of NHL is not well defined in terms of providing curative therapy in any stage or histological subtype. Its most important use at present, which may well change with the publication of prospective randomized trials, is in dealing with symptomatic local problems that do not respond to multi-agent therapy. Radiotherapy is also important when considering combined modality therapy and has a role in conditioning for certain cases undergoing bone marrow transplantation.

Chemotherapy

When treatment is required, this approach is the one most commonly used in NHL. The use of single agents is now infrequent and multi-agent chemotherapy, of which there are numerous combinations, is the most effective.

Chemotherapy and radiotherapy

Combined modality therapy can be used with curative intent or with palliative objectives. If the results of an increase of secondary tumours in patients receiving combined treatment in Hodgkin's disease can be transcribed to NHL then caution will have to be the byword (Kaldor et al 1990). The fact that local control with radiotherapy is excellent, i.e. relapse in treated areas is rare, is however important to bear in mind when considering treatment of relatively localized bulk disease particularly after treatment with chemotherapy. Nodal recurrence in sites of previous disease is quite common following chemotherapy.

Bone marrow transplantation

This mode of treatment is being increasingly utilized in younger patients with high risk disease. At present it is predominantly utilized for patients who have relapsed but who continue to be sensitive to chemotherapy (Philip et al 1987). Two types of transplantation can be performed: allogeneic—using bone marrow from an HLA identical sibling and autologous—using the patient's own bone marrow. The results to-date are relatively disappointing and for improvement it seems likely that better definition of poor prognosis patients from the start, allowing earlier utilization of this treatment, is going to be the most fruitful approach.

Miscellaneous

Various other approaches are possible but their use is limited by uncertainty, logistics, expense and toxicity. They include the use of interferons, cytokines such as interleukin-2, anti-idio type antibodies and 'targeted' drug delivery. There are anecdotal reports about such therapies in the literature. There is most information about interferon which certainly appears to be an important member of the family of biological response modifiers (Foon et al 1984). These methods of treatment will not be covered further in this article, but it is possible they will be important in certain clinical scenarios in the future.

Clinical vignettes

(a)   50-year-old with low grade lymphoma—bulky abdominal/thoracic disease with marrow involvement (Stage IVA).

There is much controversy about the approach in such patients. There is no controversy about the principle mode of treatment, which is chemotherapy, but there is much dubiety about the intensity of therapy to use and when to treat.

At present an acceptable approach is to monitor for disease progression. It is certainly still acceptable to adopt a 'wait and see' policy in this clinical situation. Median survived overall in these patients is 10–12 years. If there is obvious progression of disease demonstrated by either clinical or radiological means, then therapy is indicated. There is at present no good evidence for the use of non-aggressive therapy such as a single alkylating agent, with or without steroids, as against a more intensive approach with cyclophosphamide, hydroxydaunorubicin, vincristine, prednisolone (CHOP)-based regimens.

There is some preliminary evidence on a closely related disorder, chronic lymphocytic leukaemia (French Cooperative Group 1 1989) This shows no difference in survival between patients receiving chlorambucil and those receiving cyclophosphamide, vincristine and prednisolone (COP). More recent experience of the same authors (French Cooperative Group 2 1990) and others, however, indicates that CHOP gives superior results to both chlorambucil and COP.

It follows that in low grade NHL there are ongoing trials with many combinations, chlorambucil ± prednisolone, chlorambucil ± interferon and intensive CHOP-based regimes. Final answers from these trials will not be avilable for a number of years and until that time the approach to these difficult patients unless they are participating in such trials has to be individualized.

In a 50-year-old with static disease, a 'wait and see' policy is presently acceptable. If the disorder shows evidence of progression then present preliminary evidence from closely related disorders indicate that an intensive approach results in higher remission rates. This is achieved with limited toxicity but there is as yet no truly convincing evidence that survival is prolonged by such treatment.

(b) 50-year-old with 'localized' intermediate/high grade lymphoma affecting the left supraclavicular region—but bulky disease (>5 cm in diameter) with no systemic symptoms (Stage IA).

This vignette assumes the fact that the disorder is localized after the most extensive investigative work-up. The use of staging laparotomy has not been discussed in this review but it does not have a role in NHL as an investigational procedure. In NHL because intra-abdominal disease is a presenting feature in up to 20% of patients they often undergo laparotomy because of an emergency presentation such as obstruction or perforation, or the investigation of an intra-abdominal mass. Even in this clinical situation, often because of the patient's condition, extensive exploration is not performed at laparotomy. In a few cases of true localized gastrointestinal lymphoma resection can be a curative procedure.

As there is this limitation on staging and most investigators believe that diffuse intermediate/high grade lymphomas are systemic disorders at diagnosis, chemotherapy is the primary approach required in the majority of patients. CHOP-based regimens are most effective. At the present time, there is no definite evidence that second or third generation derivatives of this regime are superior to the basic combination. Most studies which have looked at the use of additional localized radiotherapy to the site of initial bulk disease have been non-randomized or retrospective (Miller and Jones 1987). In such trials there has been a trend to an increase in disease-free and overall survival but the differences could have arisen by chance. Thus the approach to these patients is somewhat flexible. The use of adriamycin-containing combinations such as CHOP, together with limited but involved field radiation therapy, is recommended and can result in 80% long term, disease-free survival.

(c)   50-year-old patient with bulky, diffuse high grade NHL (Stage IV B).

The only approach in this clinical situation when curative therapy is contemplated is chemotherapy. There is only suggestive evidence that the use of CHOP alone is inferior to second or third generation derivatives with added drugs given in non-cross resistant schedules. CHOP and two examples of more intensive schedules are shown in Table 15.3. A general assumption, tending to become accepted dogma, is that these schedules are superior to CHOP. As there has not been a prospective randomized trial using CHOP in one arm this is not yet proven. This supposition reflects the tendency to push chemotherapy towards the limits of patient tolerance.

Table 15.3 The regimen 'CHOP' contrasted with its more intensive derivatives MACOP-B and ProMace-MOPP

Acronym		Day(s)	
CHOP			
—cyclophosphamide	750 mg/m² i.v.	1	
—adriamycin	50 mg/m² i.v.	1	
—vincristine	1.4 mg (max 2 mg)/m² i.v.	1	
—prednisolone	100 mg p.o.	1–5	
Cycle repeats every 21 days			
MACOP-B			
M—methotrexate*	400 mg/m² i.v. then (100 mg/m² i.v. then 300 mg/m² i.v. over 4 hours	8, 36, 64	Repeat every 84 days
A—doxorubicin (Adriamycin)	50 mg/m² i.v.	1, 15, 29, 43, 57, 71	
C—cyclophosphamide	350 mg/m² i.v.	1, 15, 29, 43, 57, 71	
O—vincristine (Oncovin)	1.4 mg (max 2 mg) m² i.v.	8, 22, 36, 50, 64, 78	
P—prednisone	75 mg/m² p.o.	1–84	
B—bleomycin	10 u/m² i.v.	22, 50, 78	
ProMACE-MOPP			
Pro—prednisone	60 mg/m² p.o.	1–14	Repeat every 28 days
M—methotrexate*	1500 mg/m² i.v. (over 12 hrs)	15	
A—doxorubicin (Adriamycin)	25 mg/m² i.v.	1, 8	
C—cyclophosphamide	650 mg/m² i.v.	1, 8	
E—etoposide	120 mg/m² i.v.	1, 8	
Followed by MOPP after maximal response			
M—mechlorethamine	6 mg/m² i.v.	1, 8	Repeat every 28 days
O—vincristine (Oncovin)	1.4 mg/m² i.v.	1, 8	
P—procarbazine	100 mg/m² p.o.	1–14	
P—prednisone	40 mg/m² p.o.	1–14	

* Leucovorin rescue is given 24 hours after each methotrexate dose.
i.v. intravenously; p.o. by mouth.

With second generation regimens there is undoubtedly a price to pay both in terms of toxicity and expense. Perhaps the result of a trial presently being conducted comparing CHOP, M-BACOD, ProMACE-CYTABOM and MACOP-B (to name a few!) will allow us to advise patients objectively, rather than assuming that 'more' is better.

It is important that if the more intensive regimes are used on an ad hoc or individual basis, that the medical and nursing teams involved are experienced in caring for patients with myelosuppression and that there are appropriate support facilities available to deal with complications, both physical and psychological. Such regimens have significant morbidity and a mortality rate due to toxicity of 4–5%. In good hands the complete remission rates using such regimens is 60–70% and 10-year survival somewhat less in patients fitting into this vignette.

PRINCIPLES IN FIRST-LINE THERAPY

The foregoing vignettes have outlined the therapy of newly presenting patients with NHL—most of them commonly encountered. As can be seen there is much variability in approach both to differing clinical situations and within individual scenarios. In general once a patient relapses following properly given and appropriate chemotherapy the outlook for long-term survival is bleak. In some relapsed patients marrow transplantation can be considered.

Because the prognosis after relapse is poor it is important that initial chemotherapy is given as effectively as possible. There is good evidence that precise scheduling and drug dosage are vital in certain types of lymphoma (DeVita 1987). Reducing dosage of drugs below 70% of that planned and excessive delays in therapy can result in significantly inferior results. As treatment can have major unpleasant side effects, support, counselling and effective anti-emetic treatment are all very important. Patients benefit from a clear explanation of 'their' disease and the objectives and potential results of therapy.

In general terms the rule of thumb is to use 6 complete cycles of chemotherapy. Although the rapidity of response can be quite gratifying in some cases, there is no hard data in NHL to indicate that rapidity of response correlates with long term remission.

RELAPSED PATIENTS

In the clinical context of low grade lymphoma, clinical remissions are as yet not frequently seen, as potentially remission-inducing therapy is not commonly used. Thus 'relapse' in this type of NHL is not the problem which it is in intermediate and high grade lymphomas. In the latter group patients who are refractory to therapy from the start, that is patients who achieve less than a partial response to first-line therapy are relatively uncommon, but are very difficult to manage and their prognosis is poor.

A different clinical problem is that of recurrence of lymphoma in a patient who has achieved remission. Patients who relapse early, within 6–12 months of stopping therapy are less likely than patients relapsing later to respond satisfactorily to reinduction. Other adverse prognostic factors are high lactic dehydrogenase level, numerous previous relapses and bulky disease with many separate anatomical sites involved.

In the context of relapsed disease patients have to be considered in terms of the presence or absence of these prognostic indicators. It may be appropriate to re-utilize standard chemotherapy in a late relapse with few adverse prognostic signs and inappropriate to use such an approach in a patient who has relapsed early.

In the latter situation one possible approach which is being evaluated is bone marrow transplantation. The last clinical vignette outlines the objectives and possible results of such an approach in a 50-year-old with relapsed NHL.

Clinical vignette

(d)   50-year-old with relapsed high grade lymphoma—relapse occurring 9 months following cessation of therapy—bulky intra-abdominal disease.

This is a clinical situation in which bone marrow transplantation can be considered. As procedure-related morbidity and death increase considerably in allogeneic transplantation with age above 20 an autologous procedure is most appropriate.

One of the most important factors related to success is whether the lymphoma is responsive or non-responsive to standard chemotherapy. Patients with responsive disease are most likely to benefit, particularly if they can be brought into clinical remission prior to transplantation. This result is not unexpected if one draws a parallel with the results in leukaemia, where patients in remission, with good performance status, have much improved outcomes compared to patients transplanted in relapse and in poor clinical condition.

If the patient is responsive to chemotherapy then bone marrow transplantation should be seriously considered. Bone marrow transplantation is technically simple but complex in terms of aftercare and support required.

For an autologous transplant bone marrow has to be removed from the patient, usually electively, when in remission. In some cases it is possible to identify high risk patients early and bone marrow can be removed in first remission as an insurance. Otherwise if there is no obvious marrow contamination, harvesting can be performed at a convenient time prior to transplant. In most centres performing this procedure, marrow can be harvested and preserved for future use by cryopreservation.

Bone marrow transplantation allows high doses of drugs and/or radiotherapy to be given. The dosage chosen is sufficient to 'ablate' the bone marrow but to have reversible toxic effects on other tissues. Theoretically because of the steep dose-response curve to therapy in lymphoma, 'eradication' of residual lymphoma is more likely than with conventional treatment.

Numerous schedules are used for such ablation, but as yet in NHL the classic regime developed by Professor Thomas and his team in Seattle of cyclophosphamide, 60 mg/kg on 2 successive days followed by total body irradiation has been the most frequently used approach.

Following ablation, the harvested bone marrow is reinfused intravenously and within 3 weeks engraftment normally takes place. During this period major support with blood products and antibiotics is required. Increasingly, cytokines are used to accelerate recovery of the bone marrow, thus reducing morbidity and length of inpatient stay.

The results of such an approach are preliminary and are of course undergoing constant re-evaluation. There is a tendency for transplantation to be moved 'up front' in the therapeutic armamentarium, particularly in patients identified as high risk. In fact autotransplantation is showing a dramatic increase in usage for NHL but as stated the interpretation of results from various centres is difficult.

In a series reported by the European Bone Marrow Transplant Group the following points were highlighted (Goldstone et al 1988). From a total of 393 adults with intermediate and high grade lymphoma a complete remission was obtained in 53% of patients. Of these patients the projected 5-year survival was 56%. In essence approximately one-quarter of all patients treated had a good long term response. For patients in first remission the death rate from toxicity was 9% and for patients transplanted in relapse this rose to 20%. Thus transplantation is a procedure with considerable mortality and even more morbidity. Recommendations as to its use must depend on careful evaluation and the patient must be made fully aware of the risks involved.

CONCLUSIONS

This article is a personal review of the present approach to management of NHL in a middle-aged patient. There are perhaps some contentious points. One of the major ones is the role of radiotherapy and undoubtedly if this article were written by a radiation oncologist it would have had a different emphasis. Patients with NHL are often very dependent on radiotherapy for various reasons but I strongly believe that chemotherapy should be a major part of the initial treatment in all patients with diffuse, intermediate or high grade lymphoma. It is perhaps premature to consider early transplantation in this disease situation. It is, however, likely that with improvements in diagnostic classification, identification of minimal disease and the potential use of cytokines, autologous transplantation will be used earlier and more frequently.

There are many developing approaches including immunological techniques and others based on the use of interleukins which might improve the lot of patients with NHL. Results of trials involving these techniques will not be available for a number of years and our continuing effort should be to maximize the results obtainable by conventional treatment. This can be done by improving scheduling and providing adequate support if and when complications arise.

It is important to recognize that the diagnosis of lymphoma and consequences of that diagnosis are major life events (Devlen et al 1987). They have profound consequences for the patient and immediate relatives. Most centres are aware of the need for a 'holistic supportive' approach to patients. In many cases however the resources are not available to provide the level of support required. At present some of the inadequacies of conventional medicine due to financial restraints are being corrected by outside and charitable sources It is questionable whether this is a wholly satisfactory solution. Continuity of care for such patients is of the utmost importance and should be fully supported and encouraged.

REFERENCES

Devlen J, Maguire P, Phillips P, Crowther D, Chambers H 1987 Psychological problems associated with diagnosis and treatment of lymphomas. British Medical Journal 295: 953–957
DeVita V T 1987 The evolution of lymphomas in adult leukaemia. Leukaemia 1(6): 467–485
Foon K A, Sherwin S A, Abrams P G et al 1984 Treatment of advanced non-Hodgkin's lymphoma with recombinant leukocyte A interferon. New England Journal of Medicine 311: 148–152
French Cooperative Group on Chronic Lymphocytic Leukaemia 1989 Long term results of the CHOP regimen in stage C chronic lymphocytic leukaemia. British Journal of Haematology 73: 334–340
French Cooperative Group on Chronic Lymphocytic Leukaemia 1990 A randomised clinical trial of chlorambucil versus COP in stage B chronic lymphocytic leukaemia. Blood 75: 1422–1425
Goldstone A H, Singer C R J, Gribben J G, Jarrett M 1988 Fifth report of EBMTG experience of ABMT in malignant lymphoma. Bone Marrow Transplantation 3: 33–36
Kaldor J M, Day N E, Clarke A et al 1990 Leukaemia following Hodgkin's disease. New England Journal of Medicine 322: 7–13
Lee M S, Chang K S, Cabanillas F et al 1987 Detection of minimal residual cells carrying the t(14; 18) by DNA sequence and amplification. Science 237: 175–178
Miller T P, Jones S E 1987 Initial therapy for clinically localised lymphomas of unfavourable histology. Blood 62: 413–418
Philip T, Armitage J O, Spitzer G et al 1987 High dose therapy and autologous bone marrow transplantation after failure of conventional chemotherapy in adults with intermediate grade or high grade non-Hodgkin's lymphoma. New England Journal of Medicine 316: 1493–1498
Sheehan T, Cuthbert R J G, Ludlam C A, Parker A C 1989 Central nervous system involvement in haematological malignancies. Clinical and Laboratory Haematology 11: 331–338
Yunis J J, Frizzera G, Oken M M et al 1987 Multiple recurrent genomic defects in follicular lymphoma. New England Journal of Medicine 316: 79–84

FURTHER READING

Magrath I T (ed) 1990 The non-Hodgkin's lymphomas. Edward Arnold, London

History of medicine

16. Gallstones in the 20th century

I. A. D. Bouchier, A. Cuschieri

AETIOLOGY OF GALLSTONES (*I. A. D. Bouchier*)

HISTORICAL

Gallstone disease is as old as man himself and gallstones have been identified in mummies unearthed in Egypt and China. Furthermore, gallstones are essentially a human disease. They are rarely encountered in any other animal species and although the prairie dog is a popular and useful animal model of gallstone disease demonstrating most of the clinical antecedents of the human disorder, their cholesterol gallstones are only produced by feeding a highly artificial diet (Brenneman et al 1972).

Although it is claimed that Alexander the Great died from the complications of gallstone disease, the first recording of gallstones is by the Greek physician Trallianus (525–605) who described gallstones in the bile ducts. Gentile da Foligno who was Professor of Medicine in Padua demonstrated gallstones while conducting a public dissection in 1341. In 1556, Realdo Colombo of Cremona (1510–1559) found gallstones when performing an autopsy on St Ignatius, Founder of the Jesuit Order. The English physician Thomas Sydenham (1624–1659) confused biliary colic with hysteria. It was some 200 years later that Bernard Naunym who had succeeded Kussmaul in the Chair of Medicine in Strasburg laid the scientific foundations for the study of cholelithiasis in a treatise on cholelithiasis published in 1896. He clearly enunciated the role of the gallbladder in the genesis of gallstones, the importance of stasis, the place of infection and the potential for sloughed epithelial cells to act as a nidus for stone formation. He also noted the association of gallstones with diabetes mellitus (Beal 1984). However, recognition should also be given to Thudichum who first proposed the nidus theory of gallstones in 1862 (Drabkin 1958).

MODERN CONCEPTS

In more recent times, important monographs relating to gallstone disease have come from Tera (1960) who developed further the concept of bile stasis, and Bogren (1964) whose studies defined the crystalline composition of gallstones emphasizing the presence of bile pigment in the centre of not only pigment but also cholesterol gallstones.

This review deals only with the formation of cholesterol stones, the most common type of gallstone found in Western countries.

Our understanding of gallstone disease has expanded greatly over the past 30 years beginning in the 1960s with the publications of Danielsson, Sjovall, and Hofmann which defined the chemistry and biology of bile salts. At this time too Small, working in Paris at the laboratories of Dervichian, clarified the biophysics of lipidic associations and this led directly to the seminal paper of Admirand & Small (1968) which defined the physico-chemical basis for cholesterol gallstone formation. This most influential paper used micellar theory and triangular plots to show a complete separation of normal from cholesterol stone-forming bile on the basis of biliary cholesterol saturation. It appeared as if the micellar relationship of cholesterol, bile salts and phospholipids was all that determined whether or not gallstones would form. Unfortunately, neither the observation nor the claim has stood the test of time but the paper stimulated a spate of studies on biliary lipids in cholelithiasis and undoubtedly formed the basis for the modern approach to gallstone disease.

METABOLIC CHANGES

Three major fields of interest occupied workers in the 1970s, attempts to understand why there is a relative excess of cholesterol in the bile of gallstone formers, the importance of nucleation and cholesterol crystals, and the definition of forms of cholesterol transport in bile other than in mixed micelles. The essential feature of cholesterol gallstone disease is the relative excess of cholesterol in bile. This may come about from an excess of cholesterol or a lack of bile salts or alterations in the phospholipids in bile. Many gallstone subjects have a diminished total bile acid pool size (Vlahcevic et al 1970) for reasons which have never been adequately explained but may be related to alterations in the metabolism of the secondary bile acid deoxycholic, which is excreted in excess amounts in gallstone patients (Pomare & Heaton 1973). Recent thinking, however, gives primacy to the concept that hypersecretion of cholesterol by the liver is the most important event in producing bile saturated with cholesterol and this can arise for many reasons of which race, increasing age, and obesity are the most important.

NUCLEATION

In 1973, Holzbach and his colleagues demonstrated that supersaturated bile was frequent in individuals who did not have gallstones and they subsequently developed the concept that the nucleation of cholesterol crystals from supersaturated bile was a critical factor in gallstone formation

(Holan et al 1979). This observation led to a further appraisal of the complex interaction of cholesterol, bile salts and phospholipids in the aqueous medium comprising bile, and an appreciation that the excess cholesterol in supersaturated bile is carried in the form of phospholipid-cholesterol vesicles (size $\sim 630\,\text{Å}$) which, parenthetically, had been observed before but their significance had not been fully appreciated (Howell et al 1970). It is from these vesicles that cholesterol nucleation and continued crystal growth occur (Somjen & Gilat 1985). The difference between those who form single stones and those with multiple stones is that the former have a more modest tendency to nucleation while the latter have much shorter nucleation times.

THE ROLE OF THE GALLBLADDER

The 1980s have seen the gallbladder emerge from the shadow of the liver as being of prime importance in the pathogenesis of gallstone disease. The gallbladder can influence stone formation in many ways: disturbed motility, absorption, secretion, alteration of normal metabolites in bile and the provision of nucleating agents for crystal formation. The development of isotopic and ultrasonographic techniques to study gallbladder muscle function in vivo has shown with reasonable certainty that patients with gallstones have defective gallbladder motility which persists after the gallstones have been removed by non-surgical techniques which leave the gallbladder intact (Spengler et al 1989). It is also of interest that this defective motility is related to the degree of cholesterol saturation. Studies on prairie dogs suggest that the abnormality is primarily one of muscle activity and not a receptor defect (Doty et al 1983). Another factor of major significance is mucus secretion by the gallbladder (Bouchier et al 1965). Human and animal studies indicate that gallbladder mucin is produced in excess prior to the development of gallstones (Lee 1981). A possible link between these two events lies in disturbances of biliary phospholipid metabolism which occurs in stone-forming gallbladders and, again, appears to be a primary event preceding crystal deposition and stone growth. Patients with gallstones have a change in the type of biliary phospholipids with increased amounts of arachidonyl lecithin and it is believed that continued absorption of arachidonic acid by the gallbladder mucosa initiates prostanoid synthesis by the mucosa. Prostanoids are potent mucin secretogogues and also influence muscle contractility (Carey 1988, Kalminski 1989).

Another factor of importance is the relationship between the pH of bile and calcium. The human gallbladder actively secretes hydrogen ions (Plevris et al 1988), and by acidifying bile (the mean pH of hepatic bile is 7.7 while that of gallbladder bile is 7.25) reduces the possibility that calcium carbonate will precipitate. Actively concentrating gallbladders will absorb calcium and indeed cholesterol to some extent as well (Jacyna et al 1987) thereby reducing the risk of gallstone formation. On the other hand, as bile becomes more concentrated the phospholipid-cholesterol vesicles become larger which makes them more prone to precipitate out cholesterol in crystalline form, and in concentrated bile with a low pH, the solubility of calcium bilirubinate may be exceeded. This may be a reason for the presence of bilirubinate in the centre of most gallstones. The gallbladder mucosa, during periods of digestion, secretes electrolytes and water and this will serve to dilute biliary contents and wash out particulate matter (Jacyna et al 1989). Finally, there is the important phenomenon of the inhibition of crystal formation. Bile contains factors preventing nucleation; they are probably proteins. Their precise nature remains to be determined as well as whether they are secreted by the liver or the gallbladder or arise from both sources.

Thus, the formation of cholesterol gallstones is almost fully understood. It is the end process of a series of checks and balances existing mainly in the gallbladder, on a system which is inherently precarious—that is the tendency for most adults in developed countries to produce bile that is supersaturated with cholesterol.

REFERENCES

Admirand W H, Small D M 1968 The physiochemical basis of cholesterol gallstone formation in man. Journal of Clinical Investigation 47: 1043–1052
Beal J M 1984 Historical perspective of gallstone disease. Surgery, Gynaecology and Obstetrics 158: 181–189
Bogren H 1964 The composition and structure of human gallstones. Acta Radiologica Suppl. 226 pp 1–75
Bouchier I A D, Cooperbrand S R, El Kodsi B M 1965 Mucus substances and viscosity of normal and pathologic bile. Gastroenterology 49: 343–345
Brenneman D E, Conner W E, Forker E L, Den Besten L 1972 The formation of abnormal bile and cholesterol gallstones from dietary cholesterol in the prairie dog. Journal of Clinical Investigation 51: 1495–1503
Carey M C 1988 Formation of cholesterol gallstones: the new paradigms. In: Paumgartner G, Stiehl A, Gerok W (eds) Trends in bile acid research. Kluwer, Dordrecht, pp 259–281
Doty J E, Pitt H A, Kuckenbecker S L, Den Besten L 1983 Impaired gallbladder emptying before gallstone formation in the prairie dog. Gastroenterology 85: 168–172
Drabkin D L 1958 Thudichum. Chemist of the Brain. University of Pennsylvania Press, Philadelphia
Holan K R, Holzbach R T, Hermann R E, Cooperman A M, Claffey W J 1979 Nucleation time: a key factor in the pathogenesis of cholesterol gallstone disease. Gastroenterology 77: 611–617
Holzbach R T, Marsh M, Olszewski M, Holan K 1973 Cholesterol solubility in bile: evidence that supersaturated bile is frequent in healthy man. Journal of Clinical Investigation 52: 1467–1479
Howell J I, Lucy J I, Pircla R C, Bouchier I A D 1970 Macromolecular assemblies of lipid in bile. Biochimica Biophysica Acta 210: 1–6
Jacyna M R, Ross P E, Bakar M, Hopwood D, Bouchier I A D 1987 Characteristics of cholesterol absorption by human gallbladder: relevance to cholesterolosis. Journal of Clinical Pathology 40: 524–529
Jacyna M R, Ross P E, Hopwood D H, Bouchier I A D 1989 Effects of secretin on sodium ion transport in the human gallbladder. Alimentary Pharmacology and Therapeutics 3: 293–297
Kalminski D L 1989 Arachidonic acid metabolites in hepatobiliary physiology and disease. Gastroenterology 97: 781–792

Lee S P 1981 Hypersecretion of mucus glycoprotein by the gallbladder epithelium in experimental cholelithiasis. Journal of Pathology 134: 199–207

Naunym B 1896 A treatise on cholelithiasis. The New Sydenham Society, London

Plevris J N, Hayes P C, Bouchier I A D 1988 Evidence of acid secretion by the human gallbladder in vitro. Gut 29: A1455

Pomare E W, Heaton K W 1973 Bile salt metabolism in patients with gallstones in functioning gallbladders. Gut 14: 885–890

Somjen G J, Gilat T 1985 Contribution of vesicular and micelle carriers to cholesterol transport in human bile. Journal of Lipid Research 26: 699–704

Spengler U, Sackmann M, Sauerbruch T, Holl J, Paumgartner G 1989 Gallbladder motility before and after extracorporeal shock-wave lithotripsy. Gastroenterology 96: 860–863

Tera M 1960 Stratification of human bile in vivo. Acta Chirugica Scandinavica Suppl. 256

Vlahcevic Z R, Bell C C Jr, Buhac I, Farrar J T, Sell L 1970 Diminished bile acid pool size in patients with gallstones. Gastroenterology 59: 165–173

SURGICAL MANAGEMENT OF DUCTAL STONES
(*A. Cuschieri*)

The first successful endoscopic extraction of a stone impacted in the ampulla was reported by Anazawa et al in 1972 and endoscopic papillotomy was introduced in Japan in 1973 and Germany in 1974. Since then this technique has become firmly established in clinical practice as it permits ductal clearance without the need for operative intervention. Endoscopic stone extraction is now the procedure of choice in the emergency treatment of patients with cholangitis (Carr-Locke 1986), acute pancreatitis and ampullary stone impaction (Neoptolemos et al 1986). It is also employed routinely for retained ductal stones after cholecystectomy and in elderly or poor risk patients with symptomatic ductal calculi even in the presence of a functioning gallbladder.

In addition, there are some surgeons who consider endoscopic ductal stone extraction (in the postoperative period) to be a safer option than operative exploration of the common bile duct in patients with narrow common duct and small ductal calculi encountered during cholecystectomy. By contrast, duct exploration during cholecystectomy is advisable in patients with a dilated common bile duct, in the presence of large calculi or a big stone load within the ductal system. In these patients endoscopic ductal clearance often poses technical problems and is accompanied by a definite failure rate (5–10%) and a higher morbidity.

A standard diagnostic endoscopic retrograde choledochopancreatography (ERCP) followed by endoscopic papillotomy and stone extraction is the established initial approach in all patients with ductal calculi. Ductal clearance immediately or within a few weeks is achieved in 80% of cases. Problems are however encountered in some 15–20% of cases. These arise either where a conventional papillotomy is not technically feasible, or with large stones (< 2.0 cm) where some form of fragmentation is necessary.

THE DIFFICULT PAPILLA

Despite experience and the use of the appropriate equipment, standard papillotomy is difficult and carries a higher risk in the presence of certain anatomical configurations:

Papillary variants, e.g. polypoid papilla
Abnormal location of the papilla within duodenum
Presence of duodenal diverticulum
Location of papilla on the margin or within diverticulum
Previous gastric surgery/reconstruction

The presence of a duodenal diverticulum often changes the orientation of the lower part of the common bile duct and thus renders deep cannulation difficult. The problem is exacerbated if the papilla is situated on the margin or within the diverticulum itself. Some patients with previous gastric surgery and Billroth II (Polya) reconstruction may be impossible to approach endoscopically.

In all these situations ancillary or alternative techniques are necessary which require special expertise. There is a case for referral of such complex patients to major centres where procedures such as transpapillary wire-guided papillotomy, transhepatic guided endoscopic papillotomy and, more rarely, descending percutaneous papillotomy can be initiated.

CLEARANCE OF LARGE DUCTAL CALCULI

Ductal calculi in excess of 2.0 cm or impacted/occluding ones are often difficult to remove with the standard extraction technique despite an adequate papillotomy. The methods available for the management of this situation are:

Nasobiliary drainage and dissolution with methyl tert-butyl ether
Mechanical lithotripsy
Extracorporeal shock wave lithotripsy
Intracorporal electro-hydraulic lithotripsy
Pulsed laser lithotripsy

RETAINED DUCTAL STONES AFTER CHOLECYSTECTOMY

Although the incidence of missed stones in a prospective study conducted by members of the International Biliary Association was 4.5% (Denbesten & Berci 1986), a higher incidence (approximating to 10%) is encountered in routine clinical practice since many surgeons do not employ operative cholangiography routinely and fewer still undertake completion choledochoscopy after common bile duct exploration. The management of these patients is no longer surgical in the first instance and depends on the presence or absence of an indwelling T-tube. Endoscopic papillotomy and stone extraction is the treatment of choice in patients without a T-tube in situ.

The first option for patients with an indwelling T-tube in whom the calculi are small (< 1.0 cm) consists of flushing with heparinized saline and concomitant relaxation of the sphincter by ceruletide or secretin. This simple technique is effective in 30% of patients. Alternative approaches when this measure fails are percutaneous stone extraction via the T-tube tract or endoscopic stone extraction.

Percutaneous stone extraction via the T-tube tract can be performed using a steerable radio-opaque catheter introduced under fluoroscopic control (Burhenne 1973). The main disadvantage of this method is the radiation exposure required to direct manipulations. An alternative technique involves insertion of a flexible choledochoscope over a guide wire. This is safer, permits visually controlled extraction and is successful in 90–95% of cases (Oliver 1976).

MINIMAL ACCESS SURGICAL MANAGEMENT OF GALLSTONES

The newer minimal access alternative procedures to conventional open cholecystectomy for the treatment of symptomatic gallstone disease are:

Percutaneous stone extraction
Percutaneous cholecystostomy for severe acute cholecystitis
Laparoscopic cholecystectomy

Percutaneous stone extraction

The advantage of percutaneous stone clearance over extracorporeal shock wave lithotripsy is that the method is applicable to all stones irrespective of composition, calcification, size and load. The essential prerequisite for this form of treatment is a functioning gallbladder with an adequate lumen. In the majority of reported cases, the procedure has been performed under fluoroscopic/ultrasound control (Kellet et al 1988) but the laparoscopic approach is preferred in some centres including our own because of its greater safety margin.

Various techniques can be used according to the surgeon's preference and experience; however, irrespective of the technique used, stones larger than 1 cm require fragmentation. The methods available for gallstone lithotripsy include mechanical crushers, ultrasonic fragmentation, electrohydraulic splitting and laser fragmentation. The simplest and most effective is ultrasonic fragmentation which powders the stone and permits simultaneous suction of the debris. This technique requires a continuous irrigation system. The vibrating ultrasound probe transmits energy to the stone causing the formation of cavities at the interface of media with different acoustic impedance (fluid-stone). This results in a crumbling disintegration of the stone with the formation of tiny pieces which are sucked through the hollow ultrasound probe.

It is difficult to define the precise role of percutaneous cholecystolitho-tomy since the procedure has been superseded by laparoscopic cholecystec-tomy. However, in the author's view it is a viable option in poor risk patients after percutaneous drainage of an empyema of the gallbladder. In addition, some surgeons perform gallstone lithotripsy at the time of laparo-scopic cholecystectomy.

Percutaneous cholecystostomy for severe acute cholecystitis

In essence this is a percutaneous cholecystostomy, performed either under visual control through a laparoscope or with radiological/ultrasound guid-ance. The other alternative to formal open surgery for poor risk patients is the minicholecystostomy technique of Burhenne & Stoller (1985).

Although routine elective cholecystectomy in the fit adult is safe and carries a low mortality, emergency surgery for acute cholecystitis in the elderly carries a reported mortality of 10–12%, usually from postoperative cardiorespiratory complications (Glen 1981, Sullivan et al 1982). Further-more these patients are at a greater risk from developing empyema which doubles these mortality figures (Fry et al 1981). In addition to being immunocompromised, elderly patients often have intercurrent cardio-respiratory disease which enhances the anaesthetic risk and contributes significantly to the postoperative mortality. Cholecystectomy is also a high risk procedure in cirrhotic patients (Aranha et al 1982). Ultrasound-guided percutaneous transhepatic cholecystostomy has been employed success-fully and without complications in 6 patients suffering from acute acalcu-lous cholecystitis (Eggermont et al 1985). In 4 of these patients the tube cholecystogram was normal and subsequent follow-up investigation at 4–30 months showed no evidence of gallbladder disease. Percutaneous cholecystostomy may well turn out to be the treatment of choice in these critically ill patients.

In all these high risk patient groups a relatively minor percutaneous intervention which can effectively and safely drain the acutely inflamed gallbladder can tide the patient over the critical period. The indications for percutaneous gallbladder drainage are as follows:

> Progressive acute obstructive cholecystitis in poor-risk/
> elderly patients
> Empyema of the gallbladder
> Acute acalculous cholecystitis

If local expertise in laparoscopy is available, this is best achieved by laparoscopic drainage of the gallbladder. The approach is safer since the risk of damage to the hepatic flexure of the colon is obviated. In this respect, a CT study of the relevant anatomy in 100 patients demonstrated that the fundus of the gallbladder was positioned posterior to the liver in 70% and the right colon was interposed between the gallbladder and the abdominal wall in 13% (Warren et al 1983). Laparoscopic cholecystostomy can be performed under local anaesthesia (right lower intercostal block) and intravenous sedation. Under visual guidance the gallbladder is evacuated and a balloon catheter inserted. Alternatively (but in the author's opinion less satisfactorily) this treatment can be carried out by an interventional radiologist under fluoroscopic/ultrasound control. Drainage is usually followed by marked improvement of the patient's condition within 24 hours and should be maintained for at least 7 days. With experience and the necessary precautions, percutaneous drainage of the gallbladder, whether performed radiologically or through the laparoscopic approach, is safe. The reported complications include catheter dislodgement, bile leakage into the peritoneal cavity, bleeding and damage to the hepatic flexure of the colon. These complications underline the importance of a tube cholecystocholangiogram 24 hours after insertion of the gallbladder catheter.

A different combined surgical-radiological approach 'the minicholecystostomy' is practised by Burhenne & Stoller (1985). The gallbladder and liver edge are located by ultrasound scanning and their position marked on the skin. Under local anaesthesia, a small oblique incision (approximately 5.0 cm) is made over the gallbladder fundus in which a purse string suture is inserted. A Foley catheter is then introduced and the purse string tightened and used to anchor the catheter. These authors report no deaths or significant wound infections in 21 patients (Gibney et al 1987). This minimally invasive procedure is a safe and viable alternative to percutaneous drainage in poor risk patients. Prospective trials comparing it with radiological and laparoscopic catheter drainage are needed.

A cholecystocholangiogram is essential 24 hours after the execution of a percutaneous cholecystostomy to check on the position of the catheter, the extent of the stone load, the patency of the cystic duct and the presence of ductal calculi.

The subsequent management of these patients varies depending on the extent of improvement and the severity of the co-morbid cardiorespiratory disease. In some an interval cholecystectomy can be performed. Others remain at risk from this operation. In these, the options include percutaneous stone extraction or dissolution with methyl tert-butyl ether.

Laparoscopic cholecystectomy

There is little doubt that the advent of laparoscopic cholecystectomy will be regarded in the future as a milestone not only in the treatment of gallstone disease but in the evolution of surgical treatment. It became possible with the technological advances in optics (the Hopkins rod-lens system) and the introduction of the miniature electronic chip endotelevision camera. Although the technique had been established experimentally in the pig in Dundee, the first human case was performed successfully by Phillipe Mouret in Lyon in 1987 (personal communication). Early centres to establish the programme in clinical practice included those in Paris, Bordeaux, Nashville and Dundee (Cuschieri 1990).

The advantages of laparoscopic cholecystectomy are several. In the first place it provides a definitive treatment for gallstone disease equivalent in all respects to open cholecystectomy and obviating the problems of stone recurrence common to all the other 'non-surgical' options. By abolishing the trauma of access, handling/exposure and retraction of abdominal viscera, it is followed by a remarkably rapid recovery with early hospital discharge and return to full activity within 10–14 days of the operation. The most extreme examples which the author has encountered include a 25-year-old female who got married 6 days after a laparoscopic cholecystectomy and a businessman who travelled to the West coast of America from Dundee 5 days after his operation!

There are other perceived benefits of the new approach. Early ambulation is likely to be accompanied by a reduced incidence of postoperative deep vein thrombosis and chest infection. There is virtual abolition of all wound related complications, early and late.

The author has recently reviewed over 12 000 cases of laparoscopic cholecystectomy from seven European centres where there were no deaths, the total morbidity was 1.5%, and only 7 postoperative complications required laparotomy. The conversion rate (to open operation) due either to technical difficulties precluding the laparoscopic approach or because of the onset of a complication during the procedure was 3.5%. Patients spent a median of 3 days in hospital and returned to full activity 11 days after discharge (Cuschieri et al in press).

There are undoubtedly some unresolved problems. Perhaps the most pertinent concerns the management of ductal calculi encountered during laparoscopic cholecystectomy. In some of these patients, if the anatomy of the extrahepatic biliary tract permits and the stones are small (< 4.0 mm), it is possible to dilate the cystic duct, introduce a flexible choledochoscope (3.5 mm) and undertake guided extraction of the stones. Otherwise the cholecystectomy is completed and endoscopic stone extraction performed postoperatively. The presence of large and multiple calculi is, however, an indication for conversion to open surgery and bile duct exploration. It seems likely that techniques to perform this procedure laparoscopically will be introduced shortly.

CONCLUSIONS

Within the foreseeable future the standard treatment for symptomatic gallstone disease will be laparoscopic cholecystectomy. This is likely to be applicable in over 95% of patients with non-complicated disease. Percutaneous drainage of the inflamed gallbladder is a sensible option in the poor risk patient with acute obstructive cholecystitis/empyema since it tides the patient over a critical episode. Subsequent management will vary depending on improvement and fitness for surgery and anaesthesia. Percutaneous stone extraction or dissolution with methyl tert-butyl ether are indicated for those who remain at risk because of co-morbid disease. Otherwise interval cholecystectomy is performed.

It is difficult to envisage a substantial role for either oral dissolution or ESWL in the primary management of gallstones. ESWL will remain a viable option for ductal calculi when endoscopic extraction is not feasible for technical reasons.

REFERENCES

Anazawa W, Takagi K, Kuno K (1972) Endoscopic removal of gallstone impacted at the major papilla: a case report. Stomach and Intestine 7: 64
Aranha G V, Sontag S J, Greenlee H B 1982 Cholecystectomy in cirrhotic patients. American Journal of Surgery 143: 55–60
Burhenne J J 1973 Nonoperative retained biliary tract stone extraction. American Journal of Roentgenology 117: 388–399
Burhenne H J, Stoller J L 1985 Minicholecystostomy and radiologic stone extraction in high risk cholelithiasis patients. American Journal of Surgery 149: 632–635
Carr-Locke D L 1986 Endoscopic management. In: Bateson M (ed) Gallstone disease and its management. MTP Press, Lancaster, pp 173–202
Cuschieri A 1990 The laparoscopic revolution. Journal of the Royal College of Surgeons of Edinburgh 34: 295
Cuschieri A, Dubois F, Mouret F et al 1991 Laparoscopic cholecystectomy: the European experience. American Journal of Surgery 161(3): 385–387
Den Besten L, Berci G 1986 The current status of biliary tract surgery: an international study of 1072 consecutive patients. World Journal of Surgery 10: 116–122
Eggermont A M, Lameris J S, Jeekel J 1985 Ultrasound guided percutaneous transhepatic cholecystostomy for acute acalculous cholecystitis. Archives of Surgery 120: 1354–1357
Fry D E, Cox R A, Harbrecht P J 198 . Empyema of the gallbladder: a complication in the natural history of acute cholecystitis. American Journal of Surgery 141: 366–369
Gibney R G, Fache J S, Becker C D et al 1987 Combined surgical and radiologic intervention for complicated cholelithiasis in high risk patients. Radiology 165: 715–719
Glen F 1981 Surgical management of acute cholecystitis in patients 65 years of age and older. Annals of Surgery 193: 56–59
Kellet M J, Wickham J E A, Russell R C G 1988 Percutaneous cholecystolithotomy. British Medical Journal 296: 453–455
Oliver W J 1976 Postoperative choledochoscopy via the T-tube tract. Journal of the American Medical Association 236 2781–2782
Neoptolemos J P, London N, Slater N D, Carr-Locke D L, Fossard D P and Moosa A R 1986 A prospective study of ERCP and endoscopic sphincterotomy in the diagnosis and treatment of gallstone acute pancreatitis. Archives of Surgery 121(6): 697–702
Sullivan D M, Hood T R, Griffin W O 1982 Biliary tract surgery in the aged. American Journal of Surgery 143: 218–220
Warren L P, Kadir S, Dunnick N R 1988 Percutaneous cholecystostomy: anatomic considerations. Radiology 168: 615–616

NON-SURGICAL TREATMENT OF GALLSTONES
(*I. A. D. Bouchier*)

Before 1972 there was no rational therapy for gallstones other than cholecystectomy, or in some circumstances a cholecystostomy. No other effective treatment existed although it had long been the dream of physicians that

Table 16.1   Historical events of importance in the treatment of gallstones

1867	First cholecystostomy	Bobbs
1881	First cholecystectomy	Langenbuch
1895	Discovery of X-rays	Roentgen
1898	Gallstones first described on X-ray	Buxbaum
1924	First cholecystogram	Grahan & Cole
1952	Cholescintigraphy introduced	
1970	Ultrasonography introduced	
1972	First oral dissolution of gallstones: chenodeoxycholic acid	Danziger
1975	Use of ursodeoxycholic acid	Makino
1985	Use of methyl tert-butyl ether	Thistle
1986	Introduction of extracorporeal shock-wave lithotripsy	Sauerbruch

oral therapy might be used to dissolve gallstones. Gallstones do not disappear spontaneously or if this does happen it is an exceedingly rare event. Spa therapy, laxatives, diets, often low-fat or weight-reducing and bile salt mixtures have been tried for generations without success. The important milestones in the non-surgical treatment of gallstones are summarized in Table 16.1. Of prime importance was the development of X-rays which paved the way for the oral cholecystogram thereby permitting for the first time an accurate diagnosis of gallstones. Later studies on the physiology and metabolism of bile salts led to the introduction of oral chenodeoxycholic acid therapy as a means of dissolving gallstones (Hofmann 1989, Bouchier 1990).

The non-surgical treatment of gallstones includes both dissolution therapy and stone fragmentation therapy. This is a somewhat arbitrary classification because some types of dissolution therapy require invasive radiological techniques and both dissolution and fragmentation therapy may be combined with an endoscopic papillotomy, an account of which has been given in the previous section. Whereas chemical dissolution therapy of stones is restricted entirely to cholesterol stones, shock-wave fragmentation may have a place in the management of lightly calcified stones. Consequently it is important to identify before treatment whether gallstones are predominantly formed of cholesterol. Stones which are radiolucent on plain X-ray and which 'float' or layer in the presence of radiolucent contrast material are usually predominantly cholesterol. While the ultrasonic scan is not a good guide to stone type, computed tomography is an extremely accurate technique for determining the presence of calcium. There is at present no method of distinguishing pigment stones prior to therapy.

Unless specifically indicated, all forms of therapy mentioned in this review will apply to cholesterol gallstones.

DISSOLUTION THERAPY

Gallbladder gallstones can be dissolved by the oral administration of bile acids or by direct contact dissolution using methyl tert-butyl ether.

Oral dissolution therapy

Only three bile acid preparations are in general use to dissolve cholesterol gallstones: chenodeoxycholic acid, ursodeoxycholic acid and a combination of the two. Neither cholic acid nor deoxycholic acid are effective and there is very limited experience with ursocholic acid and 7-ketolithocholic acid. Rowachol, an inexpensive preparation of six cyclic monoterpines, has some success in dissolving cholesterol gallstones (Bell & Doran 1979) and the efficacy can be improved when used in combination with bile salts but its use has not become popular and in the UK. Rowachol is licensed only for the treatment of common bile duct stones in combination with chenodeoxycholic acid. It will not be discussed further.

Chenodeoxycholic acid (CDCA)

It was the demonstration by Danziger and his colleagues in 1972 that CDCA could dissolve cholesterol gallstones which initiated the modern era of oral dissolution of cholesterol gallstones. Their results have been confirmed in countless studies during the last two decades. CDCA is a naturally occurring dihydroxy bile acid with hydroxyl groups in the 3- and 7-alpha positions. Absorption occurs to some extent in the jejunum by passive non-ionic diffusion but mainly via an active transport system situated in the distal ileum. CDCA enters the enterohepatic circulation, returning via portal blood to the liver where it is excreted in bile having been conjugated to glyine or taurine. The majority of the conjugated CDCA is reabsorbed in the distal ileum but some is deconjugated by intestinal bacteria. Part is then reabsorbed to mix with the pool of endogenous CDCA while the remainder is dehydroxylated in the 7-alpha position by colonic bacteria to form the monohydroxy lithocholic acid. Four-fifths of this is lost in the stool. One-fifth is reabsorbed, conjugated and sulphated by the liver, secreted into bile and lost from the body in the passage of the stool.

Ingestion of CDCA in therapeutic doses enriches the total bile acid pool by 80%. CDCA reduces the cholesterol saturation of bile by a number of mechanisms: suppression of endogenous bile acid synthesis and also hepatic cholesterogenesis. Cholesterol secretion is reduced but biliary bile acid output is relatively unchanged. The dose which is necessary to unsaturate bile is 12–15 mg/kg/day (Bouchier 1990, Lanzini & Northfield 1990).

Ursodeoxycholic acid (UDCA)

UDCA is also a naturally occurring bile acid but is found in only very small amounts in human bile. The name is derived from the fact that this bile acid was first isolated from polar bear bile. It is the 7-beta-epimer of CDCA and undergoes a similar intrahepatic circulation, but absorption is less complete and in therapeutic doses it comprises only 50% of the total bile acid pool. UDCA reduces cholesterol saturation in bile because it acts primarily to reduce cholesterol absorption. It suppresses neither cholesterol nor bile acid biosynthesis; indeed it may increase hepatic conversion of cholesterol to bile acid. The therapeutic dose is 8–10 mg/kg/day.

CDCA and UDCA differ in the way in which they remove cholesterol from gallstones. CDCA solubilizes cholesterol into a micellar phase, whereas UDCA enhances the transport of cholesterol in the liquid crystalline phase as well as mixed micelles. UDCA has the additional benefit of retarding crystal nucleation time (Tazum et al 1989). Because they differ both in the way in which they reduce biliary cholesterol saturation, and remove cholesterol from gallstones it is now common practice to administer both bile acids together in dose of 6–8 mg/kg/day of each. This is taken as a single bed-time dose for greater clinical efficiency because night-time administration prevents the reduction of hepatic bile acid secretion and consequent supersaturation of bile with cholesterol that normally accompanies overnight interruption of the enterohepatic circulation (Lanzini et al 1988). The combination treatment reduces the daily cost by 25% because UDCA is about twice as expensive as CDCA. A low cholesterol diet may enhance the effect of oral bile acid therapy.

Side effects

UDCA is free from any unwanted side effects during the normal course of therapy which is maximally for 2–3 years. CDCA does have side effects, the most important being dose-dependent diarrhoea which occurs in 30–60% of patients but mild elevations in liver enzymes occur in 30% of patients and a modest increase in low density lipoprotein cholesterol is also observed. Mixed UDCA and CDCA is free from toxic effects.

Patient selection

Experience over two decades has identified with certainty those patients who are likely to respond to oral bile acid dissolution therapy. The gallbladder must be functioning on cholecystography indicating the presence of a patent cystic duct. The stones must be radiolucent indicating that they are formed mainly of cholesterol; the stones should be less than 15 mm in diameter; and the patient must not be suffering from acute symptoms. Most gastroenterologists believe that patients must be symptomatic to receive therapy. Fertile women should be using adequate contraceptive methods.

Stones with calcium or pigment will not dissolve and the recent use of computed tomography to identify calcium in radiolucent stones is cost-effective because it prevents a period of ineffective and consequently unnecessary therapy. The more rapid dissolution rate for small stones is because they have a greater surface:volume ratio—this is important in relation to extracorporeal shock-wave lithotripsy.

Efficacy

It is difficult to identify overall efficacy of oral dissolution because of different points of entry into studies and various ways of expressing outcome: partial dissolution, complete dissolution, intention to treat, ideal conditions for dissolution and achievement of unsaturated bile. A reasonable estimate is that complete dissolution is achieved in 30–40% of patients using CDCA and 20–30% on UDCA (Gleeson et al 1990). Dissolution with UDCA or CDCA averages a change of 1–2 mm per month in stone size. While dissolution may be faster initially with combined therapy there is no evidence at present that it is more effective than the single bile acid.

There are many reasons why bile acid therapy has not been as effective as hoped and consequently why it has not become a popular form of therapy although as discussed below, bile acid therapy has undergone a renaissance since the introduction of extracorporeal shock-wave lithotripsy. It has become apparent using careful selection procedures, that only 30% of all patients with gallstones and gallbladder disease are suitable for oral bile salt therapy. Another problem is the inevitable and inappropriate treatment of those radiolucent stones which are formed by bilirubin. About one-third of all radiolucent stones are of the pigment type and at present cannot be clearly differentiated from cholesterol stones. Gallstones tend to calcify with calcium bilirubinate during therapy, particularly with UDCA (Bateson et al 1981). This reduces their chance of dissolving and the most recent experience suggests that calcification occurs in up to 22% after 4 years, the material being calcium carbonate (Gleeson et al 1990). Therapy is usually required for 2 years, seldom less than 1 and is unnecessary if stones have not dissolved within 2 years. A 6-month cholecystogram which fails to show any reduction in stone size indicates a very low probability of success. Other difficulties include non-compliance and 'drop-out' is frequent. Obese patients, who form a large number of gallstone subjects, are relatively resistant to therapy because their bile fails to become desaturated on conventional doses of bile acid. The development of a blocked cystic duct during therapy as evidenced by pain and non-functioning of the gallbladder radiologically is another reason for failed therapy. Finally, as discussed below, there is the problem of gallstone recurrence once bile therapy has been discontinued.

HMG-CoA reductase inhibition

The recent introduction of agents such as lovastatin and simvastatin, which competitively inhibit 3-hydroxy-3-methyl-glutaryl coenzyme A (HMG-

CoA) reductase thereby reducing serum, low-density-lipoprotein cholesterol levels has relevance to the therapy of gallstones. Limited experience
with these drugs suggests that the inhibitors do not affect other enzymes
involved in cholesterol metabolism such as cholesterol 7-alpha-hydroxylase
and acyl-coenzyme A; cholesterol O-acyltransferase and should not have a
lithogenic potential (Reihner et al 1990). Indeed, it is possible that the
combination of these agents and UDCA might be a more powerful combination to dissolve gallstones that UDCA alone (Logan & Duane 1990).
Time will tell whether these agents are safe and have a role in gallstone
therapy.

Direct contact dissolution

Two agents are available: methyl tert-butyl ether (MTBE) which is used to
dissolve cholesterol gallbladder stones and mono-octanoin which has a role
in the dissolution of common bile duct stones.

MTBE, and ether which is liquid at body temperature, is a highly
effective dissolving agent for cholesterol gallstones; a 4 cm stone can be
dissolved within 2–3 hours. Small amounts of calcium in cholesterol stones
do not prevent dissolution. The solvent does not damage the gallbladder
mucosa. MTBE is instilled directly into the gallbladder via a radiologically
placed percutaneous transhepatic catheter, a technique which should be
familiar to most experienced interventional radiologists. Using small
volumes, 3–7 ml, which are continually infused and aspirated, any number
of cholesterol gallstones can be dissolved within a matter of hours (Allen et
al 1985). The material from the gallbladder, essentially sludge of dissolved
cholesterol is aspirated until the gallbladder is free of stones. Small fragments of non-cholesterol material which remain may require transcatheter
or extracorporeal fragmentation prior to aspiration or extraction.

The hazards of the procedure are few in experienced hands. MTBE is
both a general anaesthetic and potentially explosive. Precautions must be
taken to avoid spilling or using excessive volumes. The agent should not be
allowed to spill into the duodenum to any extent because it will induce a
duodenitis and if absorbed causes narcosis. Most experience with MTBE
has been acquired by J L Thistle and his colleagues in the Mayo Clinic and
they have developed an automatic infusion-aspiration pump which rapidly
mixes MTBE and bile in the gallbladder, doubling the rate of dissolution
and adding to the safety of the procedure (McCullough et al 1989).

The advantage of MTBE is the rapidity with which it dissolves cholesterol gallstones, the fact that gallstone size or number is not a limiting
factor, and its relative safety. General anaesthesia is not required for the
procedure and the patient may only be hospitalized for a couple of days.
The problems are the requirement of skilled interventional radiologists and
the retention of stone fragments which would favour recurrence. It remains

to be seen whether MTBE contact dissolution of gallstones will be widely adopted in competition with the other technologies that are emerging.

STONE FRAGMENTATION METHODS

The publication by Sauerbuch and colleagues describing the fragmentation of gallstones by extracorporeal shock waves was another milestone in gallstone management and set in motion a remarkable rapid evolution in lithotripsy technology (Sauerbuch et al 1986). In concept the methodology is simple; because small stones have a greater surface: volume ratio the fragmentation of gallstones will speed up dissolution. Extracorporeal shock-wave lithotripsy (ESWL), therefore, is not by itself, sufficient to eradicate gallstones. The treatment must be combined with dissolving agents. Oral bile acid therapy has emerged from a period of neglect as having an important place in gallstone treatment and indeed it is in combination with ESWL that bile acids are most frequently used to treat gallstones.

The original Dornier HM3 machine, developed in Germany, required that the anaesthetized patient be immersed in a water bath. However, second generation lithotripters do not require a water immersion tank for they have a compressible mobile water bath and the patients require either no analgesia or only mild sedation. The principle of ESWL is simple. Shock waves are single pressure impulses of high amplitude which are focused by reflectors to form a small volume of high-intensity waves on or close to the gallstone. Cavitation forces—the collapse of small bubbles around the gallstones—produce tearing and shearing forces that lead to stone fragmentation. The analogy with depth-charge destruction of a submarine can be made. Three different methods may be used to generate shock waves in water: the original spark gap electrode, electromagnetic forces and the piezoelectric system which induces shock waves by the rapid expansion of electrically stimulate ceramic tiles (Katz 1990).

ESWL can only be used to fragment cholesterol stones. Brown or black pigment stones which are soft, putty-like, pit but do not fracture and this may also be a reason why some pure cholesterol stones will not respond to ESWL therapy. The criteria for stone selection are similar to those for oral dissolution therapy—symptomatic radiolucent gallstones in a functioning gallbladder. Best results are obtained when the gallbladder has no more than three stones which are less than 30 mm diameter. This accounts for only 30% of all gallstone patients and indeed this is the same group who are suitable for oral bile acid therapy. The majority of stones may be fragmented at one sitting but occasionally two or more sessions are necessary. The gallbladder with its folds and dysmotility is usually unable to expel all the stone fragments and oral bile acid therapy, usually the combination of CDCA and UDCA in the dose indicated above, is essential in order that retained fragments can be dissolved. This is another reason why pigment or heavily calcified stones are not able to be treated with ESWL. Dissolution agents are commenced 12 days before lithotripsy and continued for 3 months after the stones have dissolved.

Adverse effects with ESWL are claimed to be few but 30–60% of patients experience biliary pain, skin petechiae (20%), haematuria (8%) and pancreatitis (2%). Further studies are required on the renal effects of gallstone lithotripsy.

ESWL has rapidly become a very popular form of treatment without having undergone controlled evaluation in comparison with other methods for treating gallstones. Does it have advantages over other non-surgical technologies? Is it preferable to cholecystectomy or the newer minimally invasive surgical procedures? Is it cost-effective? What is the recurrence rate of gallstones? Before we are seduced into accepting this new and expensive technology, it is essential that these questions are answered satisfactorily.

DIET

Little requires to be said about diet for there is no dietary therapy that has proved to be effective in the treatment of gallstones. A low fat, low calorie, high fibre diet is traditionally prescribed but the efficacy of this has yet to be demonstrated. It is not always appreciated that strict low calorie diets in obese individuals can induce cholesterol excretion into bile which becomes markedly supersaturated and such diets are therefore potentially lithogenic. There is no evidence that high fibre diets are of therapeutic benefit.

RECURRENCE

Extensive experience with oral bile acid therapy and the more recent experience with ESWL demonstrates clearly that as long as the gallbladder remains in situ after gallstones have been eradicated the stone may recur, and the recurrence rate is similar regardless of how the stones have been treated. Bile returns to the supersaturated state within 4 weeks of discontinuing bile salt therapy. The recurrence rate is about 10% per year for the first 3–5 years after which stones do not develop. The overall recurrence rate is 50%; of course, the other way of looking at the data is to infer that 50% of patients have been cured of their gallstones. Gallstones recur three times more frequently in those patients who had multiple stones prior to stone dissolution compared to those with single stones. Stones that recur are usually asymptomatic (O'Donnell & Heaton 1988, Villanova et al 1989, Sackmann et al 1990).

Once stones have dissolved it is not considered safe nor is it economic to continue on full dose therapy with bile acids. Experience gained by the British-Belgian Gallstone Group suggests that neither a high fibre diet nor low dose UDCA prevents recurrent stone growth although UDCA may delay recurrence. The problem of gallstone recurrence needs to be resolved; it will need to be considered when comparing different methods of treating gallstones some of which leave the gallbladder in situ.

OTHER METHODS OF STONE REMOVAL

Stones in the gallbladder can be fragmented using a percutaneous transhepatic or subhepatic cholecystostomy approach. Skilled radiological support is essential.

BILE DUCT STONES

The same principles for treating gallstones in the gallbladder apply to stones in the bile ducts and these can be dissolved or fragmented. There is a great variety of technologies which may be used to fragment bile duct stones including ESWL, removal of stones via oral endoscopic procedures, the use of mechanical lithotripsy, electrohydraulic lithotripsy, tunable dye lasers or ultrasound techniques. All of these require an ERCP and sphincterotomy which is described in the preceding section. Such mechanical approaches have almost entirely replaced chemical means of dissolving bile duct stones, for example the use of mono-octanoin (Neoptolemos et al 1986, Johnson & Hosking 1987).

CONCLUSION

As we approach the 21st century we can take considerable satisfaction from the progress that has been made in the past 20 years in the management of cholelithiasis. The options for treating gallstones are now considerable and the patient who is unable or unwilling to face either a general anaesthetic or major surgery can be offered an effective alternative to cholecystectomy. But there are many problems yet to be solved. We need an accurate method of identifying the precise composition of gallstones in vivo; there are as yet no effective agents to dissolve either calcified or pigment stones; if the non-invasive methods of treating gallstones are to become established, a means of preventing recurrence in the retained gallbladder must be found; and the different therapeutic modalities need to be properly compared and costed. Perhaps in the process of sorting out these issues, we may achieve the ultimate goal which is the primary prevention of gallstone formation.

REFERENCES

Allen M J, Borody T J, Bugliosi T F, May G R, la Russo N F, Thistle J L 1985 Rapid dissolution of gallstones in humans using methyl tert-butyl ether. New England Journal of Medicine 312: 217–220
Bateson M C, Bouchier I A D, Trash D B, Maugdal D P, Northfield T C 1981 Calcification of radiolucent gallstones during treatment with ursodeoxycholic acid. British Medical Journal 283: 645–646

Bell G D, Doran J 1979 Gallstone dissolution in man using an essential oil preparation. British Medical Journal 279: 24

Bouchier I A D 1990 Gallstones. British Medical Journal 300: 592–597

Danziger R G, Hofmann A F, Schoenfield L J, Thistle J L 1972 Dissolution of cholesterol gallstones by chenodeoxycholic acid. New England Journal of Medicine 286: 1–8

Gleeson D, Luppin D C, Saunders A, Murphy G M, Dowling R H 1990 Final outcome of ursodeoxycholic acid treatment in 126 patients with radiolucent stones. Quarterly Journal of Medicine 76: 711–729

Hofmann A F 1989 Medical dissolution of gallstones by oral bile acid therapy. American Journal of Surgery 158: 198–204

Johnson A G, Hosking S W 1987 Appraisal of the management of bile duct stones. British Journal of Surgery 74: 555–560

Katz S 1990 Biliary lithotripsy: more questions than answers. American Journal of Gastroenterology 85: 497–509

Lanzini A, Facchinetti D, Northfield T C 1988 Maintenance of hepatic bile acid secretion rate during overnight fasting by bedtime bile acid administration. Gastroenterology 95: 1029–1035

Lanzini A, Northfield T C 1990 Review Article: bile acid therapy. Alimentary Pharmacology and Therapeutics 4: 1–24

Logan G M, Duane W C 1990 Lovastatin added to ursodeoxycholic acid further reduces biliary cholesterol saturation. Gastroenterology 98: 1572–1576

McCullough J E, Lesma A, Thistle J L 1989 A rapid stirring automatic pump system for dissolving gallstones using methyl tert-butyl ether (MTBE): in vitro comparison with the manual syringe method. Gastroenterology 96: A629

Neoptolemos J P, Hofmann A F, Moosa A R 1986 Chemical treatment of stones in the biliary tree. British Journal of Surgery 73: 515–524

O'Donnell L D J, Heaton K W 1988 Recurrence and re-recurrence of gallstones after medical dissolution: a longterm follow up. Gut 29: 655–658

Reihner E, Rudling M, Stahlberg D et al 1990 Influence of provastatin, a specific inhibitor of HMG-CoA reductase, on hepatic metabolism of cholesterol. New England Journal of Medicine 323: 224–228

Sackmann M, Ippisch E, Sauerbruch T, Holl J, Brendel W, Paumgartner G 1990 Early gallstone recurrence rate after successful shock-wave therapy. Gastroenterology 98: 392–396

Sauerbruch T, Delius M, Paumgartner G et al 1986 Fragmentation of gallstones by extracorporeal shock waves. New England Journal of Medicine 314: 818–822

Tazuma S, Sasaki H, Mizuno S et al 1989 Effect of ursodeoxycholic acid administration on nucleation time in human gallbladder bile. Gastroenterology 97: 173–178

Villanova N, Bazzoni F, Taroni F et al 1989 Gallstone recurrence after successful oral bile acid treatment. Gastroenterology 97: 726–731

20th century Scottish physicians

17. Dr A. Rae Gilchrist, CBE

M. F. Oliver

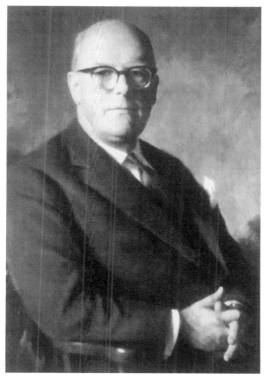

Dr A Rae Gilchrist

Rae Gilchrist's life spans this century, having been born in 1899. His imprint on the practice and teaching of clinical medicine and cardiology in Edinburgh was profound at the time, and has continued since he retired nearly 30 years ago. His rigorous training of numerous cardiologists and physicians who now occupy senior posts (or are even retired themselves) in many parts of the world, reflect credit on the Edinburgh medical scene.

Dr Rae Gilchrist was one of the 'greats' in Edinburgh medicine during the war and post-war period. His influence dominated some 25 years of medical students and young graduates. There was a trio, perhaps better called a triumvirate because they really were the adjudicators for the careers of so many, during these years: Sir Stanley Davidson, Sir Derrick Dunlop and Rae Gilchrist. They were the mentors of many, perhaps most, medical graduates of those days. During and immediately after the war medical students in their last term of second year were exposed to a weekly lecture from one of the 'chiefs'. We paraded for the first time into the great (as we regarded it) Royal Infirmary with our stethoscopes sticking out of our jacket pockets to hear these men. Each had their own inimitable style and Rae Gilchrist's was the one that attracted most of the medical students. The lists for enrolment in his clinic were usually the biggest—it was the students not a computer, who made the selection. He was a superb demonstrator of clinical signs. There are so many lectures to recall—for example, 'Red, white and blue'. This was a demonstration of polycythaemia, anaemia and cyanosis in the most simple and clear way.

Rae Gilchrist was one who would brook no equivocation. An ambiguous answer, even if it concealed real doubt, to one of his commanding questions by the bedside would be met by scorn. This bred a discipline and orderliness of mind that few other teachers achieved. Thus, on being asked to examine the crooked and misshapen hand of some poor lady with advanced rheumatoid arthritis to say that the hands 'are a little stiff, Sir' would provoke suffusion of the face, tension of the lips and the reply 'Look out of the window, is it raining or isn't it raining? It is not a little raining'. This is but one example of numerous forceful exchanges which introduced precision into the minds of many woolly-headed students and doctors—although not all were able to stay the course! Of course, he bullied us but it taught us not to vacillate and when you had learned to stand up to him, which was difficult for some since he stood 6 foot in height and well over 16 stones in weight, he responded with his high intelligence to encourage the young doctor to explore the subject from a different point of view and in greater depth. There is little better in a teacher than one who is seen by the enquirer or learner as showing respect for the questioning. Mutual respect between the teacher and the student is an inspiring investment for both.

Rae Gilchrist was always excited by clinical diagnosis and treatment. He could not let it alone. He would make a round of some 50 patients almost every day. He would examine them in great detail, possibly spending as much as 30 minutes at one patient's bedside. Sometimes he infuriated his young staff for making a diagnosis for which there would seem very little basis. When pushed, he might say 'But I have seen this before. Sister, do you remember the woman about the third bed on the left at the top some 5 or 6 years ago?' and Sister and Rae Gilchrist would compare notes and recognize the similarity of the clinical features. This was, of course, quite beyond the young doctors he had in training but the essence of an experienced physician. An individualist and not a clubbable man, he could be overawing but always kind. Except perhaps for occasions when in thick snow and low temperatures, his house physician had to stand in the Royal Infirmary car park outside his Rolls Royce in order to get further instruction about some of the patients he had just seen. The Rolls, incidentally, seemed to be as large as its owner. Stories used to abound concerning Rae Gilchrist, Stanley Davidson and Derrick Dunlop—the three prima donnas of the post-war years—and they all had a huge influence in moulding those generations of doctors. It is as well that all three lived and taught in the time they did because all would be infuriated and totally intolerant of the pettiness, narrowness and lack of vision of some of today's managers. None of the three 'greats' suffered fools gladly.

Gilchrist, a son of the manse, qualified in 1921. After a house surgeon appointment in Addenbrocke's Hospital, Cambridge, a year of paediatrics in The East London Hospital for Children, a neurological training in Queen's Square, a year at the hospital of the Rockefeller University in New York, he returned to Edinburgh. He was appointed to the Staff of the Royal Infirmary at the age of 31. 'I was very lucky. It was my greatest achievement because I could now practise real medicine and really help sick people'. This early promotion was not only due to his talent but also the premature death from lobar pneumonia of four senior physicians. 'The pneumococcus was not yet controlled.'

Rae Gilchrist established cardiology in Edinburgh with the opening of a new department, dedicated to the subject, in 1953. This was the culmination of the increasing incidence of heart disease and sophistication in its diagnosis and treatment. The interest in cardiology in Edinburgh goes back to 1898 when George Alexander Gibson, in whose honour the Gibson Lecture at the Royal College of Physicians is named, became a national and international authority. He is particularly remembered for his description of the continuous murmur of patent ductus arteriosus (the Gibson murmur) and his account of the natural history of heart diseases. He was followed by Ritchie, who applied physiology to heart disease and was the first to recognize and describe the condition of atrial flutter; and by Jonathan Meakins, a Canadian graduate trained in cardiology by Thomas Lewis in London and in respiratory function by Haldane in Oxford. Meakins was appointed to the first Chair of Therapeutics in Edinburgh: an inspired teacher who introduced biochemical analyses and respiratory function tests to the Royal Infirmary. He passed on his excitement of enquiry to many students and not least won the lasting loyalty and admiration of his house physician in 1924, Rae Gilchrist. Gilchrist's earlier work on oxygen therapy in paroxysmal ventricular tachycardia, digitalis, the treatment of complete heart block and experimental work on atrial fibrillation all followed from this stimulus. He took a particular interest in cardiac problems in pregnancy and established the Antenatal Cardiac Clinic in the Simpson Memorial Maternity Pavilion. This provided an unique experience to many young physicians and obstetricians, as well as many publications on the subject.

Early in his career, Gilchrist became particularly interested in electro-cardiograms and there is a story that in 1928 a very well groomed clinical young tutor arrived in the Doctors Room carrying the long glass plates then used for recording the ECG. The young man—Rae Gilchrist—had recognized the pattern of anterior myocardial infarction in the three limb leads used at that time and explained to the physician in charge of one of the wards in the Royal Infirmary (Dr Edwin Matthew) that his patient had suffered a coronary thrombosis. Dr Matthew had never heard of this condition nor had any of the other physicians in the Royal. Gilchrist had read about the condition, although he had not previously seen a case and did not see any during the year in New York when he visited several hospitals, in addition to the Rockefeller. By 1930 he was able to report 7 cases of myocardial infarction in the Edinburgh Medical Journal. He is convinced that the experienced physicians and cardiologists of those early days were not failing to diagnose the condition, although some patients may have been missed, but that the disease itself either changed dramatically from Heberden's days or emerged in the late 1920s and 1930s towards the proportions that we now know. When I was Gilchrist's resident in 1947, there was no specific treatment for coronary thrombosis and many died. Anticoagulants improved the prognosis by reducing pulmonary thrombo-embolism and Gilchrist and Tulloch pioneered this therapeutic approach. But we really felt helpless. D.C. cardiac shock therapy was not introduced until 1963. Thus, Gilchrist advised me in 1952 'To find out all you can about coronary thrombosis but study it properly'. On this advice I spent nearly 3 years with George Boyd in the Department of Biochemistry—an investment which has proved invaluable throughout my professional life. Gilchrist's interest in electrocardiograms and his clinical acumen led him to be an international authority on heart block.

In the 1930s, Gilchrist was called upon to advise on heart disease in schoolchildren. This was the start of paediatric cardiology in Edinburgh and the basis of Robert Marquis' career. Bobby Marquis was his closest clinical colleague and friend for many years and carried on his tradition, teaching and practise of cardiology after Gilchrist retired. Shortly after Gilchrist's appointment in 1939 as Physician-in-Charge of Ward 25, he introduced Sir John Fraser to the idea of surgical ligation of a persistant ductus. As a result, cardiac surgery was introduced into the Royal Infirmary the next year. Dr Gilchrist was the Royal College of Physicians' Gibson Lecturer in 1944 and the subject of his lecture was 'Patency of the Ductus Arteriosus and its Surgical Treatment'. The end of the war in 1945 witnessed increasing cardiological activity centred on Ward 25 (the cardiological ward). The staff consisted of the chief (Rae Gilchrist) the sub-chief (I. G. W. Hill—later Professor Sir Ian Hill of St Andrews University and Dundee), the clinical tutor (Henry Matthew, son of Professor Edwin Matthew) and a changing collection of research fellows and unpaid clinical assistants. These included Sheila Sherlock (Professor Dame Sheila

Sherlock) who subsequently went to Hammersmith and later became a world authority on liver disease, James Lowe from Auckland and John Tulloch, a future professor of medicine in Uganda; Bobby Marquis, who succeeded Gilchrist as head of the department of cardiology, Hamish Watson, the author of several books on congenital heart disease and cardiologist at Ninewells Hospital Dundee; Bruce Paton, who turned from being physician to being Chief-in-Charge of Cardiac Surgery in Denver; two who went to New Zealand—Gavin Kellaway, an international clinical pharmacologist and Olav Simpson an authority on hypertension and professor of medicine in Dunedin. Desmond Julian was one of the stars. He initiated the Coronary Care Unit and many innovatory studies on intensive care of acute infarction, became professor of cardiology at the University of Newcastle and is now medical director of the British Heart Foundation. Part of John Richmond's formative experience was as house physician to Rae Gilchrist and, in due course, he became professor of medicine in Sheffield. Ian Hill, John Richmond and I all had the privilege of becoming Presidents of the Royal College of Physicians of Edinburgh thus, with Gilchrist himself, four presidents came through the same unit in the Royal Infirmary!

Rae Gilchrist is the longest serving Fellow of the Royal College of Physicians of Edinburgh, having been elected in 1929; he was President during the years 1957–1960 and in 1990 was made an Honorary Fellow. When President, he would come to the wards on the morning of the Quarterly Meeting dressed in a black swallow coat and striped trousers. He says that 'The College was really a light relief' from the very heavy load of clinical work in the Royal and in private practice. Today's Presidents might envy him! The portrait of Rae Gilchrist which hangs in the Great Hall is superb and he admits that he quite likes it himself. It is of a formidable man whom you approach if you dare but who might just roar with laughter or, alternatively, dismiss your enquiry with a scoff. But laughter was the usual response and once he had started to laugh, his laughter became so infectious that he made everyone the better for the encounter.

Another quality was his perspective in recognizing new advances. This led to free use of his green-inked pen in correcting and criticizing the emerging works of his young staff. To be prolix was fatal. To be confused was nearly as bad. Of clinical medicine, he says, there is nothing more fascinating. He would not have chosen another career and looks back with satisfaction and fulfilment. His greatest interest in its practice was to give confidence to his patients and 'to try to understand their fears and needs'.

Rae Gilchrist decided to retire just before his 65th birthday after a major heart attack, from which he really had no right to survive. But he is a great survivor and is clearly indestructible—having illnesses which would have sent lesser men to their grave. At ninety-one, he writes with an entirely steady and totally legible hand. His memory—and more important his judgement—is unimpaired. Anecdotes of the past are plentiful. While he has had to give up his pleasure of fly-fishing and is no longer very active perhaps he will be the first President of the Royal College of Physicians to receive a telegram from the Queen.

Cardiology flourishes today in the Royal Infirmary through men such as Hugh Miller, Michael Godman and Keith Fox, all trained by those whom Gilchrist trained. We salute this great clinician and teacher, recognizing his immense influence on Edinburgh medicine and cardiology over this century. Those of us privileged to have worked with the 'big red man' have much to thank him for and not the least is his generous and magnanimous company.

18. Dr Joseph H. Wright, CBE

R. Fife

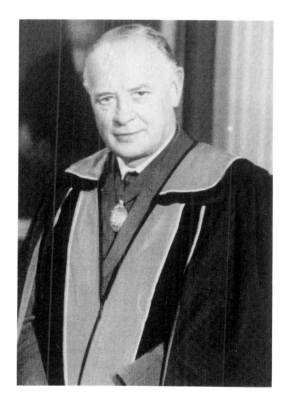

Dr Joseph Wright

Joseph Houston Wright was born in the Townhead District of Glasgow on the 27th November, 1899 and lived to enjoy his 90th birthday with his family. Physically he had of late lost some of his former robustness, but his phenomenal memory remained intact. He died after a short acute illness on the 21st December, 1989.

He went to the University of Glasgow during the First World War, intending to take a degree in Mathematics and Physics. However, after a few months he enlisted in the Army and the next year was spent in the Tank Corps. In later life he did not drive a car, alleging with tongue in cheek that this was a result of his experience in driving tanks!

By the time he returned to his classes, his thinking had changed, and he applied for a transfer to medicine. He graduated MB then ChB in 1922, and he became house physician to Dr W. K. Hunter in the Royal Infirmary.

After a spell as an assistant in general practice in Maryhill, he set up on his own in Bath Street. From the outset, he had felt that he would return eventually to the Royal Infirmary. In those days, clinical appointments to the teaching hospitals were part-time and were paid only a small honorarium. A general practice post, near to the hospital and not too onerous, was the usual means in Glasgow of maintaining a livelihood during the earlier years.

An unexpected opportunity arose in 1927. It was the custom at the time for the 'Chief' of a unit to employ a personal assistant of his own to help with the teaching. Dr A. W. Harrington had just been appointed in 1926 as a visiting physician to the Royal Infirmary, and he was looking for the customary assistant. The young Dr Wright was the successful applicant, and this was the beginning of a lasting friendship and collaboration.

His appointment involved assisting with the teaching of a large clinic of students, with the bonus of access to the wards to examine and study the patients. The only official ward staff at that time were the Chief, the first assistant and the house physician. The physicians to outpatients and their assistants had a role in the wards only if invited by the Chief. Most of them had their main source of income from general practice, which, however, had to be given up if and when they were appointed to the position of first assistant. For many this was an impecunious phase in their lives while they were building up a private consulting practice. One Chief, for example, quoted three guineas as the total of his first year's fees!

At this stage in his career, Dr Wright was attracted by what he perceived as the mathematical logic of clinical neurology. However, by chance he saw a notice in the hospital entrance hall indicating that the Infirmary required the services of a 'cardiographer', and offering the salary of £25 per year. This turned out to be his humble point of entry to the specialty of cardiology. A paper with Harrington in 1931 on aspects of the clinical presentation of coronary thrombosis confirmed the direction of his future career. He proceeded to FRFPS (Glas) and to MD in 1933.

His teaching duties were on the basis of an honorary clinical teacher appointment at the Royal Infirmary. He later became the first assistant to Professor Harrington, until the latter's retiral in 1945. At that time, the University opted for a major change in direction to a full-time post, and Professor L. J. Davis was appointed as the first full-time professor of medicine. Dr Wright and his immediate colleagues, including the late Dr Anne Aitkenhead, moved out of the unit to give the new Professor freedom of choice of staff. Dr Aitkenhead later became a Consultant Physician at Law Hospital.

Until the appointment of L. J. Davis, all clinical posts in the main teaching hospitals, including these of the professors, had been part-time. If the individual had the aptitude, it was usual for him or her to engage in private consulting practice also. Dr Wright had by this time built up a large consulting practice widely over the West of Scotland. He undoubtedly enjoyed this pattern of life and was very successful in it.

He was well aware of the significance for the future of the change in the type of appointment to the Chair of Medicine in the Royal Infirmary, and in later years it was clear that he came to agree with the new thinking. His relationship with Professor Davis was seen by the junior staff as being one of somewhat guarded mutual respect. By the time of the latter's retirement, however, it had developed into close personal friendship, and they were on visiting terms from that time onwards.

It is salutary to recall that prior to 1948 the total hospital budget was quite small by present standards. The Chiefs received an honorarium of £50 per year, and the first assistants £25 per year. New thinking on staffing was on the way however.

During the next 2 or 3 years, Dr Wright shared the charge of a small investigative ward with the biochemist, the endocrinologist, and the neuro-surgeon. He used his share of the beds for the investigation of patients with hypertension, looking particularly for possible unilateral renal disease and other potentially remediable primary causes. This work later formed the basis of his Honeyman–Gillespie Lecture to the Royal College of Physicians of Edinburgh.

Moving on to 1948, we find that the start of the National Health Service was almost synchronous with the appointment of Dr Wright as Physician-in-Charge of Wards 6 and 7, a general medical unit in the Royal Infirmary. This was a decisive moment in his career. It gave him a secure base with sufficient staff and 'clout' to start moving towards his hitherto undisclosed ambition, namely the creation of a thoroughly modern cardiology department, incorporating all the emerging new technology. He was aware of a sense of urgency, feeling that he was already 48 years of age, and that there was so much to be accomplished in a limited time.

Young men had returned from the Services after World War II or after post-war military service; they were looking for opportunities and for career ideas. Postgraduate grants were available, and the National Health Service was just getting into gear. There were new thoughts on specialist training, and many were studying for higher qualifications. Memberships had become essential for even fairly junior posts.

Dr Wright found the role of 'provider of opportunities and ideas' both satisfying and productive. It was accompanied, however, by a ceaseless driving thrust for results, which was received at times with mixed feelings. He was in the hospital every morning including Saturday, and very often on

Sunday mornings also. As all of the staff were expected to be in attendance, this single-minded enthusiasm made a lasting impression on the younger married doctors and their spouses!

Cardiac catheterization was just in its infancy at the time, and the late Dr George Aitken was given the task of 'getting on with it'. There were trips to London to see John McMichael and Sharpey Shafer, pioneers in the procedure. There were no non-medical scientists around at the time, and the sparse technical staff was without experience in the new technology. Equipment had to be acquired, mastered and brought into used from scratch. Pressure measurements and blood gas measurements were done by the medical staff, usually after normal working hours. Cooperation with radiologists had to be built up, and a start made in the training of technical staff.

The rapid expansion of cardiac surgery for congenital and rheumatic heart disease, even with only 'closed' cardiac surgery available at first, provided a powerful stimulus to the production of reliable data on large numbers of cardiac patients. In the early days in the Royal Infirmary, these included children as well as adults, and George Aitken studied and followed up a large group of those. Interesting observations emerged, and some were reported to the British Cardiac Society, but unfortunately this work was interrupted by his early death. Over the years, successive generations of trainee cardiologists learned the arts of the catheter room in the Royal Infirmary Cardiology Department. Joint discussions with radiologists and cardiac surgeons were a new feature, educative to all, but not without their moments of tension!

Life had its amusing incidents, though these were not always seen to be so at the time by the individuals concerned. A certain registrar, being sought by the great man for some piece of information, was discovered indulging in a rather late post-prandial game of bridge instead of being in the wards. It seemed for a moment as if his career would end that week, but fortunately a more tolerant view emerged, and he survived to become a senior cardiologist elsewhere in the city.

Another junior member was identified unexpectedly on the television screen while standing by the 16th green at Turnberry during the Walker Cup. As it was a working day, the comments on the following morning were blunt! He also survived, however, to become a Professor of Paediatrics in the Midlands.

With the signs of increased activity within the unit, there came a number of requests to Dr Wright from younger physicians in other units for facilities to carry out projects, usually for MD theses in the first instance. The late Dr John Ramage, afterwards consultant physician in Greenock, in this way developed phonocardiography in the hospital. Similarly, the late Dr Alastair Cameron, later to be the senior cardiologist in the Western Infirmary, did very meticulous work on the effects of posture on the electrocardiogram. These examples are picked out to indicate that a surprisingly large number of individuals who later became consultants else-where in this country or abroad had a significant part of their formative years in cardiology under the aegis of JHW.

Not all projects arrived at a happy fruition. A proposal was floated for a large-scale 'before and after surgery' study of all the rheumatic valvular cases in the West of Scotland. Dr Wright tried to persuade all the cardio-logists in the city to accept a common plan of investigation, to include right heart and pulmonary artery pressure measurements in all cases. Standard proformas were prepared and printed, but curiously enough, the plan failed to get general agreement. Several senior cardiologists at the time were against the idea of making right heart catheterization obligatory because of 'unnecessary hazard'. Or was it simply a clash of personalities, or even fear of a take-over bid? It was certainly an opportunity lost.

Dr Wright took a personal interest in all of these projects, and he made himself readily available for discussion. His comment was always worth-while, though he was not without his prejudices. From an early date he had had a particular interest in two facets of the work. The mathematical basis of electrocardiography had always intrigued him, and he encouraged Dr Veitch Lawrie, later to be the first Walton Professor of Medical Cardiology, to pursue further his interest in the theory and practice of vectorcardiology.

It was soon found that more sophisticated mathematical participation was going to be required, and Dr Wright made an approach to Professor Sneddon, the professor of mathematics of Glasgow University. After some study, the latter agreed that a PhD project in mathematics could be defined in this area. He introduced Peter Macfarlane, a young honours graduate in mathematics, who was looking for such a project at the time. Twenty-five years later, he is a Titular Professor in Medical Cardiology.

The collaboration between Veitch Lawrie and Peter Macfarlane proved very effective, culminating in the recent production of a three volume work, 'Comprehensive Electrocardiology', by an international panel of well-known cardiologists. This is likely to be a standard work of reference for years to come, and it must have been a source of satisfaction to Dr Wright, who could be said to have sown the seed.

The other major interest within the unit was on the place of 'cholesterol' in the aetiology of atheroma. Amongst others, the late Dr Robert Pirrie worked on this aspect in the early days, and had a 'hands on' experience of the biochemical assays, again often outwith the normal working hours.

A remark made by Dr Wright that nobody had looked seriously at the atheromatous plaque since the days of the classical morbid anatomists, was the starting point of an interesting investigation by another registrar in the unit, now a consultant elsewhere in the city. He used the newly available techniques of histochemical staining to try to elucidate the function of the cells around the plaque.

There was a continuing effort in the area of clinical trials of drugs. Dr Wright was a member of the Steering Committee for the MRC Trials of

Anticoagulant Therapy in Myocardial Infarction, and the unit participated in these trials. Hypertension and Angina Clinics were a steady source of drug trials in addition to their diagnostic and therapeutic function. They added a heavy work load to the staff, however, and the justification for this was debated at times with some heat. Several small trials were done in cooperation with a group of general practitioners, invited to participate by Dr Wright, who of course knew them all. These experiments were very educative to all parties, particularly to the younger hospital staff, who, in the new era, had no experience of general practice.

With the introduction of the National Health Service, a new administrative organization was brought into being, and Dr Wright spent a good deal of time as one of the original members of the Western Regional Hospital Board. His great asset at a meeting was his ability to cut through the side issues and irrelevancies and to concentrate on the core of the problem. He was Chairman of the Committee on the Medical Staffing Structure of the Scottish Hospitals, which produced 'The Wright Report' in 1964. This secured for many years a very favourable staffing position for the Scottish hospitals.

He was President of the then Royal Faculty of Physicians and Surgeons of Glasgow in 1960–1962, steering it through the vital period of the discussions leading to the change of name to 'Royal College'. His driving force was never more needed that at that time, and it is clear that he was largely responsible for the successful outcome of these negotiations. His portrait as President, by Alberto Morrocco, is regarded by all as showing good insight into a formidable personality. His personal friendship with the Fraser family was no doubt a factor in the generous benefaction of the Fraser Library to the College.

He had been a Fellow of the Royal College of Physicians of Edinburgh from 1953, and he became a Fellow of the London College in 1964. He was awarded the CBE in 1962. He was an active member of the University Court for some years, and he was awarded the Honorary LLD of the University of Glasgow in 1966.

At the peak of his career, his large chauffeur-driven Austin Princess car with its number 'GYS 1' was well known in the West of Scotland medical scene, and it allowed him to do a great deal of travelling without undue fatigue. In himself, he was a quiet and unostentatious man. He always gave the impression of being rather proud of his humble origins and early poverty. Though he dressed quite formally, he did not have an elegant or effusive manner. His reassurance of patients was brief, but it was remarkably effective because of his aura of strength and competence. He was not, however, a man to be lightly crossed!

The younger generation of postgraduates in the years from 1948 were fascinated by his clinical acumen. His ability to pick out a case with a hidden problem which others had missed was legendary. He was at his best when teaching a small group by the bedside, or in discussion around a table.

His wide clinical experience and his extensive personal reading were noteworthy. Indeed, he is probably most remembered as an outstanding clinician. His lectures to a larger group were logical and well prepared, and his material was always worth writing down. His delivery was not outstanding, however; perhaps he lacked the histrionic talent of the natural orator.

When there was a dispute on a point of fact, his juniors were intrigued to find a Chief who would insist on sending for 'the books', that they could be consulted on the spot; and this could occur in the middle of a ward round. There was never any reluctance to admit the need to look up something, and original sources would be sought out if necessary. Similarly, it was a surprise to find a busy consulting clinician subscribing personally to a range of American journals, both cardiac and general. These were brought into the hospital from week to week, with articles marked off to be read by one or other junior. A bookcase full of recent textbooks followed from his own personal library in order to have an up-to-date collection for reference at the wards. All this was very helpful to the junior staff, and it quietly laid down a standard.

The teaching of students was high in the priorities, and both with students and at postgraduate level there was continuing emphasis on the basic clinical skills. Junior staff in specialties such as dermatology and ophthalmology, wishing to widen their experience for their own higher examinations, were welcomed to the fold, to the mutual benefit of all. A trickle of postgraduates came to registrar posts from Australia and the Far East, adding their own unique contribution. Two brothers from Australia appeared in succession and made their mark on the local scene before moving on later to achieve University Chairs, one in Neurology and the other in Epidemiology, in the United States.

The juniors were reminded periodically by JHW of their ignorance of the history of medicine in Glasgow, and in particular of the history of cardiology in the Royal Infirmary. Amongst former distinguished physicians, Sir William Gairdner had worked in the Royal from 1862 till 1874, and he had published a number of papers of cardiological interest. More recently, Dr John Cowan had worked from 1906 till 1930 in the wards currently run by JHW. He was, in fact, still remembered in 1948 by one of the senior Sisters, who had been a Student Nurse there in Dr Cowan's time. One of her tasks had been the smoking of his kymograph drums, and the subsequent 'fixing' of his tracings. To spoil a tracing was a heinous crime! She was able to produce his original MacKenzie polygraph from her cupboard, and it was still in good working order.

John Cowan was the co-author with W. T. Ritchie of Edinburgh of a well-known textbook of cardiology. He was also one of the founder members of the Cardiac Club, which later evolved into the British Cardiac Society, of which Dr Wright was Chairman and host to the meeting in Glasgow of 1951. On reflection, it is perhaps not unfair to say of the eminent early Glasgow cardiologists that they were distinguished individuals rather than the founders of a continuing cardiological tradition or school.

Dr Wright had looked after several members of the Walton family, and the desire had been expressed to establish an appropriate memorial in the family name. After discussions, the Walton Chair of Medical Cardiology was founded following a gift to the University of Glasgow from Mr Isidore Walton. The first incumbent was appointed on the retiral of Dr Wright, and it was his colleague and protege, Dr Veitch Lawrie. He also is now in retirement, having firmly established the new regime. At the end of the day, the facilities in the Queen Elizabeth Building of the Royal Infirmary, including those of the University Department there, have perhaps come up to the early aspirations of JHW. It must have been satisfying to him to have seen the full fruition of his efforts, even if the final stage came after his own retiral.

All this was not accomplished without a certain amount of trauma to those involved. Dr Wright himself was prone to migraine, and one humorous resident, now in the United States, would warn the waiting staff that 'the hat sign' was in evidence. If the Chief sat down at his desk to open his mail and hear the morning report without remembering to take off his hat, his migraine was troubling him and the weather forecast for the day was unsettled! On one occasion, when soothing words were produced in response to some irate riposte, 'I'll stick to the method of the irritant' was the reply! This was not an exaggeration, as those whose feelings were trampled on could confirm! Yet there was a sense of loyalty within the unit, and many who passed through it, both local and from abroad, remember Dr Wright and their stay in the Royal Infirmary with pleasure. Much of his own satisfaction was in the achievements of those he had guided and helped. Great kindness in a personal way was another facet of his complex personality.

Despite a very busy life, JHW still managed to fit in fairly regular games of golf, and most of his younger colleagues had the experience of playing as his guest on Douglas Park at one time or another. Many also enjoyed the friendly hospitality of his wife and himself in the relaxed domestic atmosphere at Bath Street, and later at Kirklee Road. His two daughters are both married and active in the practice of medicine, and there are six grandchildren.

All in all, those who took part in the unit in those days enjoyed a memorable experience; and JHW's continuing awareness after his retirement of current happenings in the local scene suggested that many were still in touch with their former mentor.

Dr Wright made contributions on four main fronts: firstly he was an outstanding clinician, both in general medicine and in cardiology. He could be regarded as the founder of the continuing tradition of specialist cardiology in the Royal Infirmary. Secondly, he had a keen eye for the principles and strategy of administration in the medical context; his work in relation to

'The Wright Report' is the example that comes to mind. Thirdly came his work for the Glasgow College, then the Royal Faculty of Physicians and Surgeons of Glasgow. During his Presidency, he played a leading part in the negotiations to become a 'College' rather than a 'Faculty' and in the acquisition of the Fraser Library. And fourthly, his services to the University, including his part in the University Court and his role in founding the Walton Chair of Medical Cardiology.

The writer would add to these, however, his great influence on the lives and attitudes of many younger physicians, both local and from abroad.

Index